MILITARY PSYCHOLOGY

MILITARY PSYCHOLOGY

CLINICAL AND OPERATIONAL APPLICATIONS

SECOND EDITION

edited by
Carrie H. Kennedy
Eric A. Zillmer

Foreword by Thomas C. Lynch

THE GUILFORD PRESS
New York   London

© 2012 The Guilford Press
A Division of Guilford Publications, Inc.
72 Spring Street, New York, NY 10012
www.guilford.com

Printed in the United States of America

This book is printed on acid-free paper.

Last digit is print number: 9 8 7 6 5 4 3 2

The authors have checked with sources believed to be reliable in their efforts to
provide information that is complete and generally in accord with the standards
of practice that are accepted at the time of publication. However, in view of the
possibility of human error or changes in behavioral, mental health, or medical
sciences, neither the authors, nor the editors and publisher, nor any other party
who has been involved in the preparation or publication of this work warrants
that the information contained herein is in every respect accurate or complete,
and they are not responsible for any errors or omissions or the results obtained
from the use of such information. Readers are encouraged to confirm the
information contained in this book with other sources.

Library of Congress Cataloging-in-Publication Data

Military psychology: clinical and operational applications / edited by Carrie H.
Kennedy and Eric A. Zillmer.—2nd ed.
    p. cm.
  Includes bibliographical references and index.
  ISBN 978-1-4625-0649-1 (cloth : alk. paper)
  1. Psychology, Military. 2. United States—Armed Forces—Medical
care. 3. Operational psychology—Moral and ethical aspects. 4. Psychological
warfare—United States. I. Kennedy, Carrie H. II. Zillmer, Eric.
  U22.3.M487 2012
  355.001′9—dc23

                                                    2012017933

The views presented in this book are those of the authors and do not reflect the
official policy or position of the U.S. Air Force, U.S. Army, U.S. Marine Corps,
U.S. Navy, the Department of Defense, the U.S. Government, or any other
institution with which the authors are affiliated.

To the men and women who serve
in the Pennsylvania National Guard

About the Editors

Carrie H. Kennedy, PhD, ABPP, is a Commander in the Medical Service Corps of the United States Navy and is the Group Psychologist for the Marine Corps Embassy Security Group in Quantico, Virginia. She has served at the Naval Medical Center in Portsmouth, Virginia; the National Naval Medical Center in Bethesda, Maryland; the United States Naval Hospital in Okinawa, Japan; the University of Virginia (Duty Under Instruction; Neuropsychology Fellowship); and the Naval Aerospace Medical Institute in Pensacola, Florida. Dr. Kennedy has deployed with the Detention Hospital in Guantanamo Bay and with the 1st Medical Battalion to Helmand Province, Afghanistan. She is a Fellow of the American Psychological Association (Division 19, Military Psychology) and the American Academy of Clinical Psychology. Dr. Kennedy is coeditor of the books *Military Neuropsychology, Wheels Down: Adjusting to Life after Deployment,* and *Ethical Practice in Operational Psychology: Military and National Intelligence Applications* and serves on the editorial boards of the journals *Military Psychology* and *Psychological Services.*

Eric A. Zillmer, PsyD, is the Carl R. Pacifico Professor of Neuropsychology and Director of Athletics at Drexel University in Philadelphia. He is a clinical psychologist and a Fellow of the College of Physicians of Philadelphia, the American Psychological Association, the Society for Personality Assessment, and the National Academy of Neuropsychology, for which he has also served as president. Dr. Zillmer has written extensively in the areas of sports psychology, neuropsychology, and the psychology of terrorists. He is the author of several books, including *Principles of Neuropsychology* and *The Quest for the Nazi Personality: A Psychological Investigation of Nazi War Criminals,* and the coauthor of two psychological assessment procedures: the d2 Test of Attention and the Tower of London test.

Contributors

Victoria Anderson-Barnes, BS, Department of Psychology, The Pennsylvania State University, State College, Pennsylvania

Teresa M. Au, MA, VA Boston Healthcare System, and Department of Psychology, Boston, University, Boston, Massachusetts

Colonel Bruce E. Crow, Warrior Resiliency Program, Southern Regional Medical Command, San Antonio. Texas

Benjamin D. Dickstein, MA, VA Boston Healthcare System, and Department of Psychology, Boston, University, Boston, Massachusetts

Commander (Ret) Anthony P. Doran, PsyD, United States Navy, Psychological Consulting Services, Millersville, Maryland

Louis M. French, PsyD, Defense and Veterans Brain Injury Center, Walter Reed National Military Medical Center, Bethesda, Maryland

Michael G. Gelles, PsyD, ABPP (United States Navy, 1986–1993), Deloitte Consulting LLP, Arlington, Virginia

Lieutenant Colonel Revonda Grayson, PhD, United States Air Force, Wilford Hall Ambulatory Surgical Center, Lackland Air Force Base, San Antonio, Texas

Captain Patricia J. Hammond, PsyD, United States Army, John F. Kennedy Special Warfare Center and School, Fort Bragg, North Carolina

Colonel Sally Harvey, PhD, United States Army, Intelligence and Security Command, Fort Meade, Maryland

Laurel L. Hourani, PhD, MPH, Research Triangle Institute International, Research Triangle Park, North Carolina

Captain (Sel) Gary B. Hoyt, PsyD, United States Navy, Naval Special Warfare Development Group, Virginia Beach, Virginia

Lieutenant Colonel Ann S. Hryshko-Mullen, PhD, ABPP, United States Air Force, Wilford Hall Ambulatory Surgical Center, Lackland Air Force Base, Texas

Jamie G. H. Hacker Hughes, PsychD, FBPsS, Joint Medical Command, Ministry of Defense, Visiting Professor of Military Psychological Therapies, Anglia Ruskin University, Heybridge, Essex, United Kingdom

Captain David E. Jones, PhD, ABPP, United States Navy, Navy Medicine East, Portsmouth, Virginia

Lieutenant James M. Keener, PsyD, ABPP, United States Navy, Oceanside, California

Commander Carrie H. Kennedy, PhD, ABPP, United States Navy, Quantico, Virginia

Lieutenant Commander Melissa D. Hiller Lauby, PhD, ABPP, United States Navy, Center for Security Forces/SERE West, Naval Base Coronado, San Diego, California

Brett T. Litz, PhD, VA Boston Healthcare System, Massachusetts Veterans Epidemiological Research and Information Center, Boston, Massachusetts

Teresa L. Marino-Carper, PhD, Orlando VA Medical Center, and University of Central Florida College of Medicine, Orlando, Florida

Shawn T. Mason, PhD, Wellness and Prevention, Inc., Johnson and Johnson Company, Ann Arbor, Michigan; Department of Psychiatry and Behavioral Sciences, Johns Hopkins University School of Medicine, Baltimore, Maryland

Captain (Ret) William A. McDonald, MD, United States Navy, Psychiatry Department, Navy Medicine Operational Training Center Detachment, Naval Aerospace Medical Institute, Pensacola, Florida

Donald D. McGeary, PhD, ABPP, Department of Psychiatry, University of Texas Health Science Center at San Antonio, San Antonio, Texas

Lieutenant Colonel Jeffrey A. McNeil, PhD, United States Army Special Operations Command, Fort Bragg, North Carolina

Commander (Ret) Mark C. Monahan, PhD, United States Navy, Comprehensive Combat and Complex Casualty Care, Naval Medical Center, San Diego, California

Bret A. Moore, PsyD, ABPP, (United States Army, 2003–2008), Behavioral Readiness Division, Warrior Resiliency Program, Southern Regional Medical Command, San Antonio, Texas

Charles A. Morgan III, MD, Department of Psychiatry, Yale University School of Medicine, and National Center for Posttraumatic Stress Disorder, New Haven, Connecticut

Russell E. Palarea, PhD, Operational Psychology Services, LLC, Bethesda, Maryland

Lieutenant Commander Ingrid B. Pauli, PhD, United States Public Health Service, Department of Psychology, Naval Medical Center, Portsmouth, Virginia

Lieutenant Colonel (Ret) Alan L. Peterson, PhD, ABPP, United States Air Force, Department of Psychiatry, University of Texas Health Science Center at San Antonio, San Antonio, Texas

Colonel James J. Picano, PhD, United States Army Reserve, Department of Veterans Affairs, Northern California Health Care System, Fairfield, California

Lieutenant Mathew B. Rariden, PsyD, ABPP, USS Theodore Roosevelt (CVN-71), Naval Station, Norfolk, Virginia

Greg M. Reger, PhD, (United States Army, 2003–2007), National Center for Telehealth and Technology, Joint Base Lewis-McChord, Tacoma, Washington

Colonel (Ret) Robert R. Roland, PsyD, United States Army

Lieutenant Colonel Kirk L. Rowe, PhD, ABPP, United States Air Force, Wright-Patterson Air Force Base, Ohio

Laurie M. Ryan, PhD, Neuroscience and Neuropsychology of Aging Program, National Institute on Aging, Bethesda, Maryland

Nancy A. Skopp, PhD, National Center for Telehealth and Technology, Joint Base Lewis-McChord, Tacoma, Washington

Commander Aaron D. Werbel, PhD, United States Navy, USS Dwight D. Eisenhower (CVN-71), Naval Station, Norfolk, Virginia

Colonel (Ret) Thomas J. Williams, PhD, United States Army War College, Leader Feedback Program, Carlisle, Pennsylvania

Lieutenant Colonel (Ret) Thomas M. Zazeckis, PhD, United States Air Force, Behavioral Analysis Service, Lackland Air Force Base, San Antonio, Texas

Eric A. Zillmer, PsyD, Department of Psychology and Department of Athletics, Drexel University, Philadelphia, Pennsylvania

Foreword

Less than one quarter of the 35 million Americans between the ages of 17 and 24 have the necessary qualifications for service in the U.S. armed forces. These men and women volunteers of the U.S. military meet high standards, and together they compose what I believe to be the finest military organization ever produced. And yes, this includes the "greatest generation" who won World War II and is now regrettably passing from the scene, as well as my own generation who confronted and won the Cold War. For the most part, the Cold War was just that. We trained the way we were going to fight—through all types of weather and battlefield conditions without pulling the trigger—with some exceptions. We were physically fit, motivated, and well prepared for any eventuality. With the fall of the Berlin Wall in 1989 and the subsequent demise of the Soviet Union, we rejoiced (naïvely) because we believed that our vigilance saved the next generation of Americans from experiencing the holocaust of war. How wrong we were!

Today's soldiers, sailors, airmen, and Marines realize that from the moment they take the oath to protect and defend the United States of America against all enemies foreign and domestic they become our shield as they serve on the frontlines of our current war on terror and, therefore, may expect frequent deployments, continual violence, and the daily threat of death. I marvel at their courage, determination, and resilience.

The daily news brings Americans reports of the most recent suicide bombing, improvised explosive device attacks, and other combat actions with their resultant casualty count. After a while, the news becomes numbing. Even though we know the physical toll these events take on our personnel, the unseen psychological effects are just as devastating to the individual warfighter and the military unit itself, and more difficult to detect and address.

The authors have described these effects in the following pages. I encourage every operational military commander to read this book because, much the same as a football coach roaming the sidelines, the commander must know at all times, to the best of his or her ability, the mental as well as the physical readiness of the unit. I believe that the football analogy is an apt one. Today in the National Football League and in organized sports in general we have been awakened to the debilitating effects that nerve injuries and multiple concussions may have on an individual. No longer do we consider a stinger injury or "having your bell rung" symptoms of courage or displays of toughness to be ignored. We now understand, for example, the harmful damage that successive concussions may have on the brain. Specially trained corpsmen, medics, medical officers, and psychologists are called immediately to evaluate an injured individual, much as a physician, not a coach, determines if a player is fit to resume play. So it must be with an operational commander who needs to be aware of and continually assess individual and unit mental readiness.

The men and women serving in our military today are, as were their forefathers, a reflection of our society. They are but a very small percentage of the population, but they protect our way of life, and they are being stressed as never before. This book does not provide easy solutions, but it will serve the commander, anyone in a leadership position (which includes most men and women in uniform), and our medical and mental health providers invaluable information that can be applied on the battlefield, after returning from deployment, and later in traditional clinics and hospital settings. We all must become informed about, aware of, and attentive to the stressors experienced by our men and women in the armed forces, and for that I am indebted to the authors.

THOMAS C. LYNCH
Rear Admiral (Ret), United States Navy
Commander of the Eisenhower Battle Group
during Operation Desert Shield,
Superintendent of the U.S. Naval Academy
(1991–1994), and captain of the Navy
football team (1963)

Preface

Military psychology represents the practical application of psychological science. As with any applied field, growth occurs in response to real world needs. The Global War on Terror has now lasted over a decade, and military psychologists have had to adapt to changes in service member and organizational requirements, necessitating greater numbers of military psychologists, working as researchers and clinicians, in both military facilities and the theater of operations. The amplified need for psychological science and clinical services has resulted in more formal training programs, professional opportunities and responsibilities, and increased utilization of military psychologists.

These requirements have grown largely because of terrorist tactics employed in current wars. The physical and psychological injuries incurred in battle, and even on the home front, present a serious challenge to allied forces. Clinical military psychologists have played center stage from the beginning of this war, addressing issues as diverse as combat stress, blast concussion, virtual reality treatments, telehealth, and detainee mental healthcare.

Both the clinical practice of psychology and its operational applications have grown tremendously in response to the war. Fighting terrorism requires creative nontraditional tactics, and psychologists have proven to be a powerful force in counterterrorism and counterintelligence efforts. Furthermore, military psychologists continue to hone crisis negotiation strategies, procedures for training service members at high risk of enemy capture, and assessment and selection procedures for special duty personnel. In addition to their wartime responsibilities, military psychologists continue to support peacekeeping missions and disaster response efforts (e.g., the Haiti earthquake).

With the increase in both the numbers and duties of military psychologists has come a greater acceptance of mental health professionals and behavioral scientists as integrated members of military and operational commands. Embedded psychologists are now a regular part of Marine ground units, Navy aircraft carriers, and special operational forces, and interaction with psychologists and mental health professionals of all stripes is becoming routine and less stigmatizing.

The second edition of *Military Psychology: Clinical and Operational Applications* has been revised to incorporate many of the changes in the practice of military psychology since the first edition was published in 2006. The book expands on the history of military psychology and updates the areas of assessment and selection of special duty personnel; military health psychology; military neuropsychology; substance abuse prevalence and treatment; suicide prevention; survival, evasion, resistance, and escape (SERE) psychology; and hostage negotiations. In addition, there are new chapters on the assessment and management of acute combat stress on the battlefield, addressing common mental health problems postdeployment, modern disaster response, and military psychology ethics, as well as a how-to chapter on conducting the fitness-for-duty evaluation.

The second edition is again an edited volume owing to the vast scope of the field of military psychology. We carefully selected contributors for their proven expertise in their subject and are indebted to each of them for taking the time away from their wartime duties, civilian employments, and families to cover this timely information. We present this practical manual as a road map to help meet the needs of our service members and optimize our military potential using the principles of military psychology.

Contents

MILITARY PSYCHOLOGY

CHAPTER 1

A History of Military Psychology

Carrie H. Kennedy
Jamie G. H. Hacker Hughes
Jeffrey A. McNeil

The history of military psychology is particularly rich. Although military history reaches back thousands of years, formal military psychology is only a recent development, less than a century old. The development of psychology in the United States and elsewhere has had a similar trajectory as that of military psychology in the United States and in other nations, and it is easy to conclude that their history and growth are undeniably linked. However, the growth of military psychology has occurred in spurts, each related to the demands, psychological as well as military, of the conflicts of different nations.

Whereas formal psychology has been only recently introduced to militaries, organizational, clinical, and operational psychological concepts are inextricably intertwined with the historical development of war. Despite the fact that the history of formalized military psychology is relatively short, its impact pervades the practice of psychology. Military psychology has evolved from that of limited participation in wars of the past to today's war, where it has been an indispensable asset in combat readiness and policy development. This chapter briefly describes the development of the profession of military psychology and the various roles of the military psychologist through the years. The following chapters also provide some history of specific issues, to which the reader is directed.

EARLY HISTORY OF U.S. MILITARY PSYCHOLOGY:
THE REVOLUTIONARY WAR

still see today During the American Revolutionary War, almost no attention was paid to the emotional toll of battle. In fact, adverse reactions to combat were often deemed a defect of character or cowardice. However, the war did see one of the first U.S. psychological operations campaigns: The colonials distributed enticement leaflets where they would be seen by British troops, encouraging their desertion. The leaflets advertised "seven dollars a month, fresh provisions and in plenty, health, freedom, ease, affluence and a good farm" at Prospect Hill, whereas at Bunker Hill one would receive "three pence a day, rotten salt pork, the scurvy, and slavery, beggary, and want" (Walters, 1968, p. 23). The British retaliated with a propaganda campaign of cartoons, which depicted the colonials as "a mob of cowardly, undisciplined, whiskey drinking, and mostly unkempt renegades" (Johnson, 1997, p. 9). Since then, psychological operations in the U.S. military have evolved to highly organized endeavors that have been credited for significantly influencing the outcome of war and conflict since World War II (Joint Chiefs of Staff, 2003).

THE U.S. CIVIL WAR

During the U.S. Civil War, military medicine was in its infancy, although military physicians were responsible for the medical screening of recruits. If a physician missed an illness or failed to detect a malingered malady, he was fined (Lande, 1997), apparently because soldiers received a bonus for enlisting and occasionally would then reveal a physical illness or mental health condition to avoid service. It was during the Civil War that the first steps were taken to address the effects of combat and war on servicemen. The concept of nostalgia was first described, and military doctors reported treating other such psychological concepts as phantom pain in amputees (Shorter, 1997), acute and chronic mania, alcoholism, suicidal behavior, and sunstroke (Lande, 1997). While there is no documentation of the number of nostalgia cases, one anecdote depicts the numbers of psychiatric casualties of the Civil War.

> Both the Union and Confederate Armies attempted to utilize hospital ships to evacuate their wounded situated in areas near the Atlantic coastline. It has been reported that both armies had to abandon the use of such ships because a large number of individuals suffering from what was then called "nostalgia" practically clogged the gangplanks. This precluded such ships' properly caring for the physically sick and wounded. (Allerton, 1969, p. 2)

Following the war, soldiers who presented themselves for mental health care were often diagnosed with chronic mania. Formal programs to address veterans' problems were scant. These servicemen were mostly cared for at home—although at times housed in the local jail because of the lack of other appropriate means to keep them and others safe—and many were treated in insane asylums (Dean, 1997). The United States Government Hospital for the Insane (USGHI; now known as St. Elizabeths Hospital) was created for military patients in the mid-1800s and eventually provided care for all government patients, including those who attempted to assassinate Presidents Andrew Jackson and Ronald Reagan (McGuire, 1990).

The Civil War saw the first documentation of substance use problems related to combat: abuse and addiction to alcohol, chloral hydrate, cocaine, morphine, and opium as well as substance withdrawal (Dean, 1997; Watanabe, Harig, Rock, & Koshes, 1994). Anecdotally, it appears that many of the chronic addiction problems among Civil War veterans were related to medical treatment for pain (Dean, 1997; see Chapter 10, this volume, for more information on substance abuse and the military).

WORLD WAR I

World War I (WWI) marked the official birth of military psychology in the United States. Specifically, in April 1917, Robert Yerkes, then the head of the American Psychological Association (APA), convened a group of psychologists, including James McKeen Cattell, G. Stanley Hall, Edward L. Thorndike, and John B. Watson. Their charter was to determine how psychology could help the war effort. The committee recommended that "psychologists volunteer for and be assigned to the work in which their service will be of the greatest use to the nation" (Yerkes, 1917). Committees were developed, ranging from the Committee on the Selection of Men for Tasks Requiring Special Skills to the Committee on Problems of Motivation in Connection with Military Service. On August 17, 1917, Yerkes was commissioned as a major in the Army (Uhlaner, 1967; Zeidner & Drucker, 1988), and by January 1918, 132 officers were commissioned for work in the Division of Psychology, Office of the Surgeon General (Zeidner & Drucker, 1988; see Figures 1.1 and 1.2). Their work signified the first concerted efforts to screen military recruits and included such notable statisticians as E. L. Thorndike, Louis Thurstone, and Arthur Otis (Driskell & Olmstead, 1989). WWI had such an impact on psychology that only one paper presented at the 1918 APA annual convention had nothing to do with the war (Gade & Drucker, 2000), and while there were only 200 members of APA at the time, 400 psychologists contributed to the war effort.

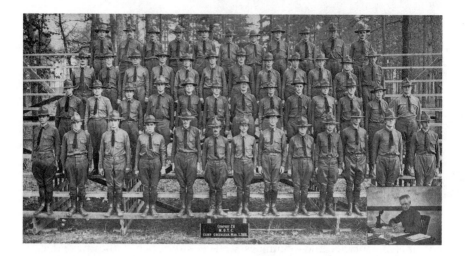

FIGURE 1.1. First company of commissioned psychologists, School for Military Psychology, Camp Greenleaf. (***denotes officer not a psychologist.) From left to right—front row: Wood, Roberts, Brueckner, Stone, Foster (instructor), Tyng (battalion major), Hunter, Hayes, ***, ***, Edwards, Stech, LaRue. Second row: ***, ***, Malmberg, Moore, Norton, Shumway, Arps, ***, ***, Stokes, Jones, Pedrick, Toll. Third row: Manuel, Bates, Miller, Chamberlain, Basset, Estabrook, Poffenberger, Benson, Trabue, Doll, Rowe, Elliott. Top row: Paterson, Dallenbach, Pittenger, Boring, Wylie, Bare, English, Sylvester, Morgan, Anderson, Houser. Maj. Yerkes is shown in the corner. Reprinted from Yerkes (1921).

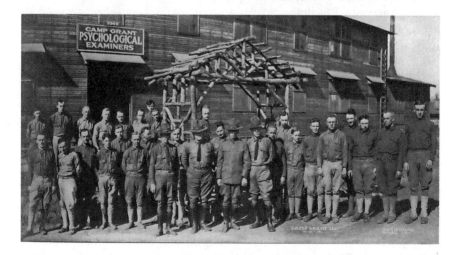

FIGURE 1.2. Supply company barracks assigned to psychological board at Camp Grant, showing typical psychological staff. Of the four officers in front, the captain at the left is the psychiatrist, and the three lieutenants (Sylvester, Benson, Terry) are psychologists. Reprinted from Yerkes (1921).

The Army alpha (for those who were literate in English; see Figure 1.3) and beta (for those who were not literate, who were literate in another language, and/or who failed the alpha) intelligence tests were developed and administered to 1,750,000 men during the war (Kevles, 1968). Of these men, 7,800 were recommended "for discharge by psychological examiners because of mental inferiority," 10,014 were recommended for assignment "to labor battalions because of low grade intelligence," and 9,487 were recommended for assignment to "development battalions, in order that they might be more carefully observed and given preliminary training to discover, if possible, ways of using them in the Army" (Yerkes, 1921, p. 99).

The Army alpha evolved into the Wechsler–Bellevue Scale, the precursor to the Wechsler Adult Intelligence Scale, which has become the most frequently used intelligence test today (Boake, 2002). Intelligence testing during WWI marked the first means of testing hundreds of individuals simultaneously and led Lewis Terman (1918) to emphasize the need for standardized administration of psychological tests. Intellectual testing was not the only focus during WWI. The Woodworth Personality Data Sheet, which became the model for subsequent personality assessments, was introduced at that time (Page, 1996), and Yerkes developed procedures to assess

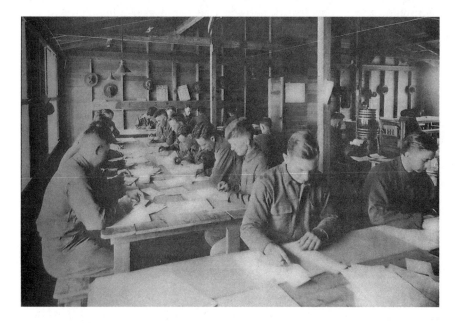

FIGURE 1.3. Scoring examination papers. The scorers are working at mess tables on examination alpha. Reprinted from Yerkes (1921).

and select individuals to become officers and undertake special assignments (Zeidner & Drucker, 1988).

The success of psychological testing in WWI was the impetus for the earliest recognition of psychology as a respected field. The success of group testing had significant implications for organizations like grade schools, universities, and licensing boards. These tests also kindled the interest of private industry in search of help from psychologists with such problems as employee absenteeism, employee turnover, and ways to increase industrial efficiency (Zeidner & Drucker, 1988).

Of particular note for today's war, WWI marked the creation of the specialty of neurosurgery and the means to save the lives of servicemen with head injuries. With these advances arose the field of cognitive rehabilitation, advocated heavily by Shepherd I. Franz, a psychologist at USGHI, whose efforts to create a rehabilitation research institute were unfortunately unsuccessful. However, Franz published manuals and books on cognitive assessment and "re-education" (Boake, 1989; Franz, 1923). Most military hospitals did provide rudimentary rehabilitation during WWI but were closed after the war because of lack of need.

Aviation psychology was born during WWI, and its major focus was the psychological screening of pilots in order to select those most likely to successfully complete training and avoid aviation accidents (Driskell & Olmstead, 1989). Early work showed that the best candidates possessed high levels of intelligence, emotional stability (i.e., low levels of excitability), perception of tilt, and mental alertness (Koonce, 1984). In addition to widespread intellectual testing, psychological screening and head injury rehabilitation, the clinical condition of war neurosis was identified (Young, 1999).

While in the United States psychiatrists filled the clinical role, in the United Kingdom army psychologists not only provided clinical care but did so in the combat zone, something U.S. military psychologists would not engage in until Korea (see The Korean War, p. 13). With the outbreak of WWI, British Army psychologists deployed to wartime France in 1914 in support of British troops. Operating from field hospitals and casualty clearing stations and, later, NYDN (Not Yet Diagnosed Neurological) hospitals, they saw large numbers of personnel suffering from shell-shock (Smith & Pear, 1917), disordered action of the heart (DAH), and related syndromes (Jones & Wessely, 2005). British psychologists also presided over the evacuation, to rear areas or to the United Kingdom, of military personnel who were deemed unfit for further combat, at least in the immediate future.

In Britain, a large number of hospitals were established, including Craiglockhart (made famous in novelist Pat Barker's Regeneration trilogy, as the hospital where the writers Siegfried Sassoon and Wilfred Owen were treated together by British Army psychologist W. H. Rivers; Shephard,

2000). Rivers and his colleague C.S. Myers were both medical practitioners who had taken up the new discipline of psychology, and both worked at Sir Frederick Bartlett's Department of Experimental Psychology at the University of Cambridge. Myers was to become Consultant Psychologist to the British Expeditionary Force and established four forward NYDN centers and, later, five forward DAH centers in France, which operated in addition to the hospitals in Britain (Greenberg, Hacker Hughes, & Earnshaw, 2011).

The first appropriate intervention for combat stress (i.e., shell-shock) was recognized, and the earliest cognitive restructuring techniques were documented well ahead of the development of formal cognitive theory (Howorth, 2000). Forward psychiatry was implemented, using the concept of PIE (proximity, immediacy, and expectation of recovery) and resulted in 40–80% of shell-shock cases returning to combat duty (Jones & Wessely, 2003). These early-intervention principles remain the foundation of combat stress intervention today and the practice of deployed combat stress units in all branches of service.

WWI also marked one of the first organized uses of chemical warfare: mustard gas (Harris, 2005). This gave rise to observations of "gas hysteria" and the recognition of a psychological response to threats of this nature. Lessons learned in WWI continue to guide mental health professionals in addressing the response to fears of and current terrorist threats to employ chemical and biological warfare.

In short, WWI was a time of major growth for the field of psychology, the successes of which continue to have a profound impact on psychology practice today. G. Stanley Hall (1919) foretold the future when he commented on the work of psychologists in WWI, noting that "only when the history of American psychology is recorded in large terms will we realize the full significance of the work."

WORLD WAR II

Between 1944 and 1946, the APA underwent significant reorganization when it merged with the American Association for Applied Psychology (AAAP). After this merger, the five sections of AAAP became charter divisions in the new APA, and included Division 19, the Division of Military Psychology (Gade & Drucker, 2000). In addition to stronger organizational foundations, World War II (WWII) saw an influx of esteemed German and Jewish psychologists to America, which strengthened the field of psychology in the United States significantly.

Psychologists were in high demand during WWII and worked in all branches of the military, as well as in such departments as the National

Research Council, Psychological Warfare Services, the Veterans Administration (VA), and the Department of Commerce (Gilgen, 1982). Work continued in psychometric testing, but a great diversification of developments and expansion in psychology occurred both during and immediately after the war. Boring (1945) published a comprehensive text on the application of psychology to the military, addressing such topics as adjustment to combat, personnel selection, morale, sexuality, and psychological warfare. He outlined seven fields of the "psychological business of the Army and Navy": observation, performance, selection, training, personal adjustment, social relations, and opinion and propaganda (p. 3). Books were also published for military members about the application of psychological principles to enhance performance (e.g., National Research Council, 1943; Shaffer, 1944) and to develop psychologically informed leadership abilities (Kraines, 1946) during the war. The Office of Strategic Services (OSS, now the Central Intelligence Agency) was developed, along with the first psychological selection program for individuals seeking positions as OSS operatives in espionage, counterespionage, and propaganda (Banks, 1995; OSS Assessment Staff, 1948), modeled after the selection procedures used by the German military for officers and leadership positions (Ansbacher, 1949). Individuals who helped to shape the field of psychology were once again employed by the military, including B. F. Skinner, who trained pigeons to guide missiles to targets prior to the existence of electronic guidance systems (Gilgen, 1982), and Griffin, who studied the realities of using bats to drop miniature explosives on Japan (Drumm & Ovre, 2011). Skinner did not deploy his trained pigeons because of moral objections, as the bombings were essentially suicide missions for the birds (Roscoe, 1997). Griffin faced hurdles given the load-bearing limitations of bats and a refocus of research efforts on the atomic bomb (Drumm & Ovre, 2011).

Screening for military service was improved, and in 1940 the Army General Classification Test (AGCT), developed by psychologists, was introduced as a means of measuring the aptitude of recruits and also of selecting men for specialist courses (Zeidner & Drucker, 1988) and for officer training (Harrell, 1992). The AGCT was taken by more than 12 million men for classification purposes and was valued over the intellectual testing format because of its minimization of verbal ability and the influence of formal education, its emphasis on spatial and quantitative reasoning, and its efficiency in administration (Harrell, 1992). After WWII, uniform aptitude testing in the military was mandated by the Selective Service Act of 1948, and in 1950 the Armed Forces Qualification Test (AFQT) was born. Although every service branch utilized the AFQT, each also continued to use their own screening procedures and instruments until 1968 (Defense Manpower Data Center, 1999).

Much of the improvement of classification and screening procedures was attributed to military psychologists' opportunity to test large groups of individuals from various geographical and cultural backgrounds. This observation and subsequent recognition that test results must be inter-preted differently depending on an individual's background were clearly documented during WWII, marking some of the first succinct reasoning for culturally fair psychological tests. An additional impact was the con-struction of abbreviated testing techniques, which could easily be applied in the civilian sector (Hunt & Stevenson, 1946). WWII also saw increased use of personality tests, and in 1943 the Army began using experimentally a newly published test, the Minnesota Multiphasic Personality Inventory, as a screening and selection instrument (Page, 1996; Uhlaner, 1967).

The increased emphasis on screening turned out to be a problem for those experiencing what was then identified as combat fatigue or com-bat exhaustion (combat stress). Because the thinking of the time was that screening would exclude those prone to the development of these problems, during WWII the United States did not initially utilize the lessons learned in WWI about combat stress reactions (i.e., the need for timely intervention near the frontline). Subsequently, little forward mental health (i.e., mental health providers in the combat zone) was practiced, favoring instead reli-ance on psychological screening to avoid negative psychological reactions to the war. In fact, in 1943, while the rejection rate based on psychological screening was three to four times that of WWI, the incidence of mental health disorders was three times that seen in WWI (Glass, 1969). Gen-eral George Marshall, in 1943, "observed that there were more individuals being discharged from the army for psychiatric reasons than the number of individuals being inducted into the army" (Allerton, 1969, p. 3). Between 1943 and 1945, 409,887 U.S. servicemen were hospitalized for combat fatigue in overseas Army hospitals: Of these, 127,660 were aeromedically evacuated to the United States (Tischler, 1969). One unfortunate result of the overemphasis on screening was that 40% of early discharges were attributed to combat fatigue (Neill, 1993), but it solidified the military's recognition of the need for battlefield interventions and preparation for the psychological toll of combat (U.S. Department of the Army, 1948). The overwhelming number of psychiatric casualties of WWII also confirmed the notion that combat stress reactions were generally normal responses to the emotional trauma and stressors of war as opposed to a defect of char-acter (Glass, 1969).

The United Kingdom recruited eight civilian psychologists to produce tests to aid in the selection of candidates for the Royal Navy (RN). As a second filter at the larger naval entry establishments, these psychologists administered short, graded, and easy-to-score tests comprising additional

tests of general intelligence, mathematical aptitude, and mechanical aptitude. At the end of 1943, the RN had a staff of 10 "industrial" psychologists and approximately 300 assistants, mainly Women's Royal Naval Service (WRNS), who were involved in the work of personnel selection.

In the British War Office, on the other hand, testers and nontechnical officers and noncommissioned officers (NCOs) were employed within
the Army's Directorate of Service Personnel, set up in July 1941 as part of
the Adjutant-General's Department. All 19 psychologists—14 men and 5
women—were uniformed officers. Additionally, there were a further 31
officers or NCO testers (26 men and 5 women), 584 nontechnical officers
(531 men and 53 women), and 697 NCOs (494 men and 203 women). The
tests included in the standard test battery comprised assessments of general intelligence, arithmetic, verbal and nonverbal skills, and "instructions"
(comprehension). Tests used for the selection for training in special trades
or duties included U.S. Army Morse Aptitude Tests for signalers; spelling,
shorthand, and typing tests for Auxiliary Territorial Service (ATS) clerks
and signalers; and assembly tests for drivers and mechanical trades. More
comprehensive testing was involved in officer selection, where psychologists collaborated with military officers and psychiatrists in the selection
of officer candidates and were concerned with formal psychological testing as well as the overall selection process. The formal tests involved not
only outdoor selection tasks, in which psychologists and psychiatrists collaborated on test design with the military staff of the War Office selection
boards (WOSB), but also a number of formal psychological tests, including intelligence tests, biographical questionnaires, projective tests, and a
more complicated version of the traditional Raven's Progressive Matrices
Test, together with tests of verbal intelligence and reasoning. Outside the
Adjutant-General's Department, the War Office also employed a small
number of men with psychological training at the Directorate of Scientific
Research and the Directorate of Biological Research within the War Office
Medical Department.

During the war multiple articles were published on malingering as a
means to avoid military service or discipline, then also referred to as gold-
bricking, faking, or malingery. The attitude toward malingerers at this time
was summed up by Hulett (1941): "It is indeed devastating to recognize as
we must, that all men are not possessed of manhood, and that the yellow
streak down the backs of some of our fellows is invisible to the unaided
human eye" (p. 138). Common methods of malingering were purported
to be the induction of symptoms with such substances as alcohol, epinephrine, sugar, and cathartics; claims of pain or other sensory problems
(e.g., blindness); claims of motor dysfunction; feigning of insanity; self-
mutilation; exaggeration of real symptoms; or refusing to seek treatment
for a curable condition (Campbell, 1943). Campbell noted that malingerers

had psychopathic personalities and had no place in the military, with the exception of "work battalions and [being] forced to serve under strict and uncompromising discipline" (p. 354); they were the "leading pension and compensation seekers" (p. 352). Bowers (1943) noted four types of individuals with suspicious symptoms: hysteria, inadequate personality, malingering, and mixed types. Ludwig (1944) advocated for the widespread use of sodium amytal for the differentiation between malingerers and bona fide patients. During WWII, the top five mental health diagnostic categories were neurosis, personality disorder, alcoholism, epilepsy, and insanity (Stearns & Schwab, 1943). Notably, the inadequacy of the existing mental health diagnostic system (Standard Nomenclature of Diseases and Operations) for military use during WWII was a significant impetus for the development of the *Diagnostic and Statistical Manual of Mental Disorders* (American Psychiatric Association, 1952).

Head injury rehabilitation reemerged on a large scale as well (Doherty & Runes, 1943), with many of the leading psychologists later gaining prominence in the field of neuropsychology (Boake, 1989; for further information, see Kennedy, Boake, & Moore, 2010). Unfortunately, once again, many of the rehabilitation centers were closed after the war, and the field did not emerge again until the late 1960s and early 1970s, in response to the increasing number of survivors of motor vehicle accidents (Boake, 1989).

Aviation psychology continued to evolve during WWII with the development of the U.S. Army Air Forces Aviation Psychology Program in 1941, the focus of which was to assist with the selection of aviation personnel (Driskell & Olmstead, 1989). In addition to the selection for such positions as pilots, navigators, and bombardiers, research was also conducted on the service member–equipment relationship, particularly with the new equipment that was developed at that time (Koonce, 1984). In 1947 the U.S. Air Force became a separate branch of the military, and industrial psychological research flourished in the new service (Hendrix, 2003). Within the British Air Ministry, there were 4 civilian advisors in psychology for training methods, 17 Women's Auxiliary Air Force (WAAF) aircrew selection officers, 14 ground crew selection officers, and nearly 100 junior technical assistants. Tests used included measures of general intelligence (including the Royal Air Force [RAF] GVK test of general, verbal, and spatial/practical intelligence) and mathematics (for all RAF and WAAF candidates), Morse aptitude, pilot aptitude and observer (radio) aptitude (for aircrew candidates) and fluency, technical information, Morse reading, and radar (for temperament). In addition to these duties, Air Ministry psychologists also collaborated on a number of research projects from 1937 onward, including tests of reaction time and deftness of speed of hands and feet (the Sensory Motor Apparatus to assess flying aptitude and the Angular

Perception Test to assess skills in making final approaches and landing aircraft). In addition, the Air Ministry, at the beginning of the war, had been using two tests: a group intelligence test prior to the selection board assessment and experimental preselection aptitude tests to try to determine the sort of flying for which a recruit would be best suited.

Across all three British services, psychologists were involved in the design and interpretation of a variety of questionnaires and interviews: the layout, arrangement, and display of operational equipment, particularly in RAF operations rooms but also with respect to, for example, the radius and position of turning handles in gunnery controls, as well as the design and use of a number of trainers and simulators for pilots, gunners and air gunners, and bomb aimers. Psychologists were also involved in work connected with a wide range of visual aspects of operational duties, including the use of goggles, instrument panel lighting, and night flying. Other more operational work involved advising in the special adaptation and modification of a variety of weapon systems. Job analyses and time and motion studies formed another aspect of wartime psychologists' work: for example, the job analyses of WRNS radio mechanics, air mechanics, and torpedo mechanics for the admiralty and the organization of WOSBs for potential ATS officers for the War Ministry; time and motion studies of gun laying and gun drills; and studies of extreme climatic conditions in tropical and Arctic conditions (Hacker Hughes, 2007).

Following WWII, the field of aviation psychology grew dramatically, affecting practices of civilian airlines and creating new roles for aviation psychologists. These psychologists are now involved in a wide range of activities, including research and identification of individuals involved in terrorist activities, aircraft accident investigations (Koonce, 1984), assessment and selection of flight personnel, performing aeromedical psychological evaluations, and continuing research into human factors issues.

WWII was also the first and only time that nuclear weapons were used. Survivors developed both acute and chronic psychological reactions, including withdrawal, severe fear reactions, psychosomatic symptoms, and posttraumatic stress disorder (PTSD; Salter, 2001). Beyond the effect of the bombings on the people of Japan, the images from Hiroshima and Nagasaki in 1945 continue to instill fear into societies threatened with such use today. Concerns mount about the capacity of terrorists to obtain and use these weapons (Knudson, 2001). In a similar vein, WWII was known for Japanese suicide bombers, or kamikaze pilots. Kamikaze attacks accounted for a large proportion of the sailors who were wounded in action, second only to attacks that involved multiple weapons (Blood, 1992). The threat of suicide bombers has arisen as a heightened concern, and some of the lessons learned in WWII are applicable to this modern-day weapon (see Chapter 13, this volume).

In the United States, military clinical psychology emerged during WWII, with the first military psychologists assigned to hospitals (McGuire, 1990; Uhlaner, 1967). Following the war, the growth of clinical psychology in the military continued. Because there were too few physicians and psychiatrists to meet the emotional needs of veterans, psychologists provided both group and individual therapy in VA facilities (Cranston, 1986). In 1946 the first psychology internship programs were established, enrolling 200 interns within the VA system. These efforts resulted in increased acceptance of psychologists, not just as researchers and experts in assessment but also as mental health providers (Phares & Trull, 1997). As after WWI, psychologists were demobilized following WWII; however, in 1947 they obtained permanent active-duty status (McGuire, 1990; Uhlaner, 1967). Two years later, the first military clinical psychology internship programs were established in the Army, one of which was at the Walter Reed General Hospital in Washington, DC.

THE KOREAN WAR

During the Korean War psychologists served in several new positions: in service overseas, in combat zones, and on hospital ships (McGuire, 1990). The war saw significant use of torture, as well as the execution of U.S. prisoners of war, and gave rise to the concept of brainwashing (Ursano & Rundell, 1995). U.S. troops were exposed to forced marches, severe malnutrition, inhumane treatment, and continuous propaganda and "reeducation" on communism (Ritchie, 2002). The Korean experience prompted the military to make significant changes in survival schools, or training programs to help service members who are captured as prisoners of war. Repatriated prisoners of war from the Korean conflict are credited for the inception of the survival, evasion, resistance, and escape (SERE) model of training currently provided to U.S. service members whose duties place them at high risk of enemy capture (e.g., special forces, aviation personnel). The SERE training paradigm and psychology's role therein are covered in depth in Chapter 12 (this volume), and information is presented about prisoners of war from WWII, Korea, and Vietnam (see also Moore, 2010).

Unfortunately, early in the war the principle of treating combat stress near the frontline to enable military members to return to duty was not possible to implement because of the abrupt start of the conflict and the lack of prepared support units (McGuire, 1990). As a result, 250 troops per 1,000 were declared psychological casualties. However, the lessons of WWII regarding the need for mental health providers in the combat zone were not forgotten (Glass, 1969). Later in the war, mental health providers were deployed, and 80% (Ritchie, 2003) to 90% (Jones, 1995) of combat fatigue cases fully returned to duty. After the first year of combat in Korea, a rotation policy of 9 months in combat was implemented, which also helped to significantly reduce the number of psychiatric casualties (Glass, 1969).

Psychology's role in testing did not diminish during the Korean War. The Army and Air Force collaborated on a technical manual outlining the roles of the military psychologist and proper use of psychological tests (U.S. Departments of the Army and the Air Force, 1951), with such distinguished contributors as David Wechsler and Paul Meehl (Uhlaner, 1967). Instruments created to select individuals for specific jobs and officer programs continued to be developed.

Following the Korean War, the Army began to devote significant resources to the study of motivation, leadership, morale, and psychological warfare (Uhlaner, 1967), and the concept of human systems related to military functioning increased in popularity (Zeidner & Drucker, 1988). The Air Force and Navy also created research centers for the study of what was then called human engineering. The goal of increasing the performance of military personnel given different equipment, various physical states (e.g., fatigue), and various environments gave rise to increased research in human factors engineering (Roscoe, 1997; Uhlaner, 1967).

THE VIETNAM WAR

After the Korean War, the U.S. Air Force implemented the Airman Qualifying Examination in 1958 for administration to high school students. Shortly thereafter, the Army and Navy developed their own group ability tests, and ultimately in 1968 the Armed Services Vocational Aptitude Battery (ASVAB) was implemented to make a truly uniform aptitude tool (Defense Manpower Data Center, 1999). The ASVAB has become an integral screening and aptitude tool for military recruits, and it has been regularly used by military neuropsychologists over the years for the assessment of head-injured service members, as its composite score is a reliable indicator of premorbid intellectual functioning (Kennedy, Kupke, & Smith, 2000; Welsh, Kucinkas, & Curran, 1990).

As in Korea, psychologists served in combat zones during Vietnam. Forward mental health was practiced from the beginning of the war, and low levels of traditional combat stress were seen. Compared with the psychiatric casualty rates of WWII (28–101 per 1,000 troops per year) and Korea (37 per 1,000 troops per year), troops in Vietnam exhibited very low rates, 10–12 per 1,000 troops per year (Allerton, 1969). As in no other conflict before or since, however, there was an extraordinary amount of substance abuse (see Chapter 10, this volume). Also, a higher proportion of character disorders were diagnosed during the war, possibly related to the characteristics of individuals who could not avoid the draft. In other words, those with more resources were able to obtain education deferments or other exemptions to avoid military service (McGuire, 1990). In addition, the spirit of the times in the United States was highly tolerant of drug use, and this probably affected those serving in Vietnam as well. Because of the large numbers of troops who were abusing substances and had to be medically evacuated from the theater, mandatory drug testing was implemented and opportunities for alcohol and drug rehabilitation were increased.

In comparison to U.S. methods, the Vietnamese army also implemented psychiatric services for its troops. The practice of mental health care was still in its infancy at the time of the war, and local medical providers were ill prepared for psychiatric casualties. During the war, the Vietnamese army utilized one hospital, the Psychiatric Service of Cong Hoa General Hospital, to provide care for its servicemen. This hospital was staffed by one psychiatrist, one internist, one health technician, one nurse, two corpsmen, and two civilians who worked as guard and orderly. The psychiatric service had 80 beds and regularly maintained 80–100 inpatients during the war. In addition, 10–15 outpatients were seen daily. Treatments consisted of psychopharmacology (e.g., chlorpromazine, thioridazine, diazepam), electric shock, and very limited supportive therapy to select patients (Nguyen, 1969). Although rates for admission remained low in consideration of the total size of the Vietnamese army (which grew from 150,000 early in the war to 700,000 by 1967), this is partially hypothesized to be due to the limited resources for treatment (and documentation), shortage of personnel, transportation problems, misattribution of the origin of symptoms, and cultural differences in the conceptualization of some issues (e.g., suicidal thoughts and actions). Although barriers to care were significant, Nguyen (1969) hypothesized that some character traits of the Vietnamese people as a group may have made them less susceptible to the development of combat neuroses, namely protective personality characteristics fostered by strong family ties and loyalties, lack of awareness of psychiatric symptoms, and attitudes toward those who adopted a sick role.

Vietnam was a significantly complex war, involving the use of weapons technologies not seen before that could inflict significant destruction, even on the level of the individual soldier (Zeidner & Drucker, 1988). American military members faced a well-trained force and were confronted with challenging jungle warfare as well as horrific prisoner of war experiences (see Moore, 2010). Military rotation policies at the time dictated specific tour lengths for individuals as opposed to rotations of entire units, resulting in poor unit cohesion because of the constant arrivals and departures of personnel (Zeidner & Drucker, 1988). Compounding these problems, the attitude on the home front regarding the utility of the war was largely unsupportive of the troops. The psychological impact of all these factors is hypothesized to have resulted in high rates of PTSD, with many surviving veterans still suffering symptoms today.

Following Vietnam, the military recognized the need for a formal response to noncombat critical incidents, such as the deaths of service members from training accidents or suicide. In 1978 the Portsmouth Naval Hospital Psychiatry Department organized a Special Psychiatric Rapid Intervention Team, consisting of psychologists, psychiatrists, chaplains, nurses, and corpsmen (McCaughey, 1987), to respond to such critical incidents as training accidents, suicides, natural disasters, and bombings (for modern disaster response, see Chapter 7, this volume).

OPERATIONS DESERT SHIELD AND DESERT STORM

Military personnel in Operations Desert Shield and Desert Storm were exposed to multiple combat stressors: greater numbers of enemy forces, possible use of chemical and biological weapons, environmental challenges (i.e., desert exposure, sandstorms), lethal animal life, inadequate or insufficient hygiene opportunities, and a culture that did not accept American values (Martin, Sparacino, & Belenky, 1996). Although there was great capacity for significant stress casualties, the limited number of wounded and killed American troops and the availability of forward mental health support resulted in relatively few combat stress casualties; however, rates of PTSD have increased over time in these veterans. In addition to forward mental health support on the ground during the Persian Gulf War, for the first time a psychologist was deployed on a Navy aircraft carrier, the USS *John F. Kennedy,* which subsequently had no incidence of medical evacuation for mental health reasons (Wood, Koffman, & Arita, 2003).

Despite good mental health support, Gulf War syndrome or Gulf War illness, an ambiguous conglomeration of physical and psychological symptoms, was unique to the Persian Gulf War. Years of research have not been able to characterize these presenting problems as a specific syndrome with specific symptoms (Bieliauskas & Turner, 2000; Everitt, Ismail, David, & Wessely, 2002). Gulf War syndrome was hypothesized to originate from vaccinations, exposure to toxic substances (e.g., smoke from burning oil wells), and psychological trauma. Years of studying Gulf War veterans have largely led to the conclusion that, although risk factors for the syndrome were inoculations and exposures to noxious chemicals and psychological trauma, the persistence of the syndrome is the result of previous psychological distress and individual veterans' attribution of their symptoms (i.e., the belief that they were exposed to toxic agents; Hotopf, David, Hull, Nikalaou, Unwin, & Wessely, 2004; Stuart, Ursano, Fullerton, Norwood, & Murray, 2003). Despite the lack of a clear definition of Gulf War syndrome, veterans who have unexplained symptoms that began during or after the war are given financial and health benefits (Campion, 1996), and research into this issue continues.

PEACEKEEPING OPERATIONS
(MILITARY OPERATIONS OTHER THAN WAR)

Peacekeeping missions have their own unique characteristics and impact on military personnel. Stress control units have been regularly utilized for those deployed for peacekeeping operations since Operation Restore Hope in Somalia in 1992 (Bacon & Staudenmeier, 2003), given that peacekeeping forces often face an unfriendly populace, come under fire, live in unhygienic conditions, and are separated from their families (Hall, Cipriano, & Bicknell, 1997). In addition, peacekeeping missions put more strain on individuals who may be vulnerable, have a preexisting mental health condition, abuse alcohol, or are experiencing relationship problems. These have been deemed risk factors for suicide in peacekeepers specifically (Wong et al., 2001).

Operation Uphold Democracy in Haiti saw significant stress among U.S. troops, including three suicides in the first 30 days of the mission (Hall, 1996). This reinforced the need for frontline mental health providers to administer preventive and early intervention measures for military personnel supporting peacekeeping missions (Hall et al., 1997). With operational stress support, 94% of soldiers presenting with psychological symptoms during Operation Uphold Democracy were returned to full duty without the need for medical evacuation (Hall, 1996).

Operation Joint Endeavor in Bosnia saw an unprecedented number of military mental health professionals on hand for suicide prevention, stress management, critical incident debriefings, and clinical care in country (Pincus & Benedek, 1998). Mental health providers made advances during this mission in learning to increase awareness of available services and in destigmatizing help-seeking behavior by offering a comprehensive outreach program (Bacon & Staudenmeier, 2003).

RECENT DEVELOPMENTS

Military psychologists continue to make history. Today's war has created an immediate need for better understanding of combat stress in the context of modern warfare. The pervasive use of improvised explosive devices and rocket and mortar attacks is designed to cause psychological injuries as well as physical wounds. The frequent blasts and explosions have once again brought up the issue of blast concussion, first examined in WWI. Across the services, programs are in place to educate service members on blast concussion and combat stress, and research is beginning to emerge. In addition, prevention, diagnosis, and treatment are integrated into post-deployment health readiness programs throughout the military. Military neuropsychologists have made major contributions in establishing guidelines for assessment and treatment of blast concussion.

Psychologists also continue to expand their roles, including support for conventional and special operations. As early as October 2001, psychologists were deployed to main and forward-staging bases supporting Operation Enduring Freedom (OEF). In addition, psychologists have served at forward-fire bases, providing expeditionary support to soldiers and Marines and consultation for commanders in both OEF and Operation Iraqi Freedom (OIF). Psychologists have also treated enemy combatants through the Global War on Terror, both in theater and in the detention facility at Guantanamo Bay (see Chapter 14, this volume).

Operationally, military psychologists continue to provide integral support in repatriation operations, selection and assessment for special operations, hostage negotiation, and human factors research, and roles have expanded dramatically in counterintelligence, counterterrorism, and interrogation support.

Other advances include the inception of prescription privileges for psychologists starting in 1994, when the first trial psychopharmacology fellows graduated from training (Sammons, Levant, & Paige, 2003), to 2005, when the psychopharmacology fellowship was established at the Tripler Army Medical Center in Hawaii. The military's success in training psychologists as prescribers has served as a model for other psychologists (Dittman, 2003). Two states (New Mexico and Louisiana) and one U.S. territory (Guam) have enacted laws granting prescribing privileges to appropriately trained psychologists.

Psychologists have been permanent ship's company on aircraft carriers since 1998, and the Psychology at Sea program has been successful (Wood et al., 2003). Service aboard these ships can be mentally stressful to the crew and is at times referred to as working "on top of a nuclear reactor and under an airport." Each carrier is assigned one psychologist, who serves not only the carrier but also the battle group that accompanies it, comprising a total of approximately 12,000 people. As the sole mental health provider, with assistance from a neuropsychiatric technician and one or two substance abuse counselors, psychologists have had to move away from traditional forms of therapy. The focus is on prevention, interventions that involve the individual's chain of command, and truly creative means of addressing the needs of such a large and unique population. This very successful model of expeditionary/embedded psychology has been followed by Operational Stress Control & Readiness providers who deploy in the Marine Corps with assigned units. This new mode of battlefield care is tackling stigma and shows promise in the arenas of problem prevention and early detection.

SUMMARY

The history of military psychology, although brief, is extensive and ongoing. Not only has the field of psychology had an extraordinary impact on the military, but the developments that have grown out of the various wars and the needs of the military have directly affected the practice of psychology. Military mental health providers continue to make history today in their support of the war efforts in Afghanistan, in their contributions to national security, and in improving services for active-duty members and their families everywhere. The following chapters focus on these efforts and subsequent developments and military psychologists' increasing roles in clinical, expeditionary, and operational psychology. Lessons learned today will certainly be the next chapter in the history of not only military psychology but also psychology as we know it across the world.

REFERENCES

Allerton, W. S. (1969). Army psychiatry in Viet Nam. In P. G. Bourne (Ed.), *The psychology and physiology of stress: With reference to special studies of the Viet Nam War* (pp. 1–17). New York: Academic Press.

American Psychiatric Association. (1952). *Diagnostic and statistical manual of mental disorders*. Washington, DC: Author.

Ansbacher, H. L. (1949). Lasting and passing aspects of German military psychology. *Sociometry, 12,* 301–312.

Bacon, B. L., & Staudenmeier, J. J. (2003). A historical overview of combat stress control units of the U.S. Army. *Military Medicine, 168,* 689–693.

Banks, L. M. (1995). *The Office of Strategic Services psychological selection program.* Unpublished master's thesis, U.S. Army Command and General Staff College.

Bieliauskas, L. A., & Turner, R. S. (2000). What Persian Gulf War syndrome? *The Clinical Neuropsychologist, 14,* 341–343.

Blood, C. G. (1992). Analyses of battle casualties by weapon type aboard U.S. Navy warships. *Military Medicine, 157,* 124–130.

Boake, C. (1989). A history of cognitive rehabilitation of head-injured patients, 1915–1980. *Journal of Head Trauma Rehabilitation, 4,* 1–8.

Boake, C. (2002). From the Binet–Simon to the Wechsler–Bellevue: Tracing the history of intelligence testing. *Journal of Clinical and Experimental Neuropsychology, 24,* 383–405.

Boring, E. G. (1945). *Psychology for the armed forces.* Washington, DC: National Research Council.

Bowers, W. F. (1943). Hysteria and malingering on the surgical service. *The Military Surgeon, 92,* 506–511.

Campbell, M. M. (1943). Malingery in relation to psychopathy in military psychiatry. *Northwest Medicine, 42,* 349–354.

Campion, E. (1996). Disease and suspicion after the Persian Gulf War. *New England Journal of Medicine, 335,* 1525–1527.

Cranston, A. (1986). Psychology in the Veterans Administration: A storied history, a vital future. *American Psychologist, 41,* 990–995.

Dean, E. T., Jr. (1997). *Shook over hell: Post-traumatic stress, Vietnam, and the Civil War.* Cambridge, MA: Harvard University Press.

Defense Manpower Data Center. (1999). *Technical manual for the ASVAB 18/19 career exploration program* (rev. ed.). North Chicago: HQ USMEPCOM.

Dittman, M. (2003). Psychology's first prescribers. *Monitor on Psychology, 34,* 36.

Doherty, W. B., & Runes, D. D. (1943). *Rehabilitation of the war injured: A symposium.* New York: Philosophical Library.

Driskell, J. E., & Olmstead, B. (1989). Psychology and the military: Research applications and trends. *American Psychologist, 44,* 43–54.

Drumm, P., & Ovre, C. (2011). A batman to the rescue. *Monitor on Psychology, 42,* 24–26.

Everitt, B., Ismail, K., David, A. S., & Wessely, S. (2002). Searching for a Gulf War syndrome using cluster analysis. *Psychological Medicine, 32,* 1371–1378.

Franz, S. I. (1923). *Nervous and mental re-education.* New York: Macmillan.

Gade, P. A., & Drucker, A. J. (2000). A history of Division 19 (Military Psychology). In D. A. Dewsbury (Ed.), *Unification through division: Histories of the divisions of the American Psychological Association* (Vol. V, pp. 9–32). Washington, DC: American Psychological Association.

Gilgen, A. R. (1982). *American psychology since World War II.* Westport, CT: Greenwood Press.

Glass, A. J. (1969). Introduction. In P. G. Bourne (Ed.), *The psychology and physiology of stress: With reference to special studies of the Viet Nam War* (pp. xiii–xxx). New York: Academic Press.

Greenberg, N., Hacker Hughes, J. G. H. Earnshaw, N. M., & Wessely, S. (2011). Mental healthcare in the United Kingdom Armed Forces. In E. C Ritchie (Ed.), *Textbook of military medicine* (pp. 657–665). Washington, DC: Department of the Army, Office of the Surgeon General, Borden Institute.

Hacker Hughes, J. G. H. (2007). *British naval psychology 1937–1947: Round pegs into square holes.* Unpublished master's thesis, University of London.

Hall, D. P. (1996). Stress, suicide, and military service during Operation Uphold Democracy. *Military Medicine, 161,* 159–162.

Hall, D. P., Cipriano, E. D., & Bicknell, G. (1997). Preventive mental health interventions in peacekeeping missions to Somalia and Haiti. *Military Medicine, 162*, 41–43.

Hall, G. S. (1919). Some relations between the war and psychology. *American Journal of Psychology, 30*, 211–223.

Harrell, T. W. (1992). Some history of the Army General Classification Test. *Journal of Applied Psychology, 77*, 875–878.

Harris, J. C. (2005). Gassed. *Archives of General Psychiatry, 62*, 15–17.

Hendrix, W. H. (2003). Psychological fly-by: A brief history of industrial psychology in the US Air Force. *American Psychological Society Observer, 16*. Retrieved May 20, 2012, from *www.psychologicalscience.org/observer/getArticle.cfm?id=1451*.

Hotopf, M., David, A., Hull, L., Nikalaou, V., Unwin, C., & Wessely, S. (2004). Risk factors for continued illness among Gulf War veterans: A cohort study. *Psychological Medicine, 34*, 747–754.

Howorth, P. (2000). The treatment of shell-shock: Cognitive theory before its time. *Psychiatric Bulletin, 24*, 225–227.

Hulett, A. G. (1941). Malingering—A study. *The Military Surgeon, 89*, 129–139.

Hunt, W. A., & Stevenson, I. (1946). Psychological testing in military clinical psychology: I. Intelligence testing. *Psychological Review, 53*, 25–35.

Johnson, R. D. (1997). *Seeds of victory: Psychological warfare and propaganda.* Atglen, PA: Schiffer.

Joint Chiefs of Staff. (2003). *Doctrine for joint psychological operations.* Washington, DC: Author.

Jones, E., & Wessely, S. (2003). "Forward psychiatry" in the military: Its origins and effectiveness. *Journal of Traumatic Stress, 16*, 411–419.

Jones, E., & Wessely, S. (2005). *Shell shock to PTSD: Military psychiatry from 1900 to the Gulf War.* New York: Psychology Press.

Jones, F. D. (1995). Psychiatric lessons of war. In R. Zattchuk & R. F. Bellamy (Eds.), *Textbook of military medicine: War psychiatry* (pp. 1–33). Washington, DC: Office of the Surgeon General, U.S. Department of the Army.

Kennedy, C. H., Boake, C., & Moore, J. L. (2010). A history and introduction to military neuropsychology. In C. H. Kennedy & J. L. Moore (Eds.), *Military neuropsychology* (pp. 1–28). New York: Springer.

Kennedy, C. H., Kupke, T., & Smith, R. (2000). A neuropsychological investigation of the Armed Service Vocational Aptitude Battery (ASVAB). *Archives of Clinical Neuropsychology, 15*, 696–697.

Kevles, D. J. (1968). Testing the Army's intelligence: Psychologists and the military in World War I. *Journal of American History, 55*, 565–581.

Knudson, G. B. (2001). Nuclear, biological, and chemical training in the U.S. Army Reserves: Mitigating psychological consequences of weapons of mass destruction. *Military Medicine, 166*, 63–65.

Koonce, J. M. (1984). A brief history of aviation psychology. *Human Factors, 26*, 499–508.

Kraines, S. H. (1946). *Managing men: Preventive psychiatry.* Denver: Hirschfeld Press.

Lande, R. G. (1997). The history of forensic psychiatry in the U.S. military. In R.

G. Lande & D. T. Armitage (Eds.), *Principles and practice of military forensic psychiatry* (pp. 3–27). Springfield, IL: Charles C Thomas.

Ludwig, A. O. (1944). Clinical features and diagnosis of malingering in military personnel: Use of barbiturate narcosis as an aid in detection. *War Medicine, 5,* 378–382.

Martin, J. A., Sparacino, L. R., & Belenky, G. (1996). *The Gulf War and mental health.* Westport, CT: Praeger.

McCaughey, B. G. (1987). U.S. Navy Special Psychiatric Rapid Intervention Team (SPRINT). *Military Medicine, 152,* 133–135.

McGuire, F. L. (1990). *Psychology aweigh! A history of clinical psychology in the United States Navy, 1900–1988.* Washington, DC: American Psychological Association.

Moore, J. L. (2010). The neuropsychological functioning of prisoners of war following repatriation. In C. H. Kennedy & J. L. Moore (Eds.), *Military neuropsychology* (pp. 267–295). New York: Springer.

National Research Council. (1943). *Psychology for the fighting man.* Washington, DC: Penguin.

Neill, J. R. (1993). How psychiatric symptoms varied in World War I and II. *Military Medicine, 158,* 149–151.

Nguyen, D. S. (1969). Psychiatry in the army of the republic of Viet Nam. In P. G. Bourne (Ed.), *The psychology and physiology of stress: With reference to special studies of the Viet Nam War* (pp. 45–73). New York: Academic Press.

OSS Assessment Staff. (1948). *Assessment of men.* New York: Rinehart.

Page, G. D. (1996). Clinical psychology in the military: Developments and issues. *Clinical Psychology Review, 16,* 383–396.

Phares, E. J., & Trull, T. J. (1997). *Clinical psychology: Concepts, methods, and profession* (5th ed.). Pacific Grove, CA: Brooks/Cole.

Pincus, S. H., & Benedek, D. M. (1998). Operational stress control in the former Yugoslavia: A joint endeavor. *Military Medicine, 163,* 358–362.

Ritchie, E. C. (2002). Psychiatry in the Korean War: Perils, PIES, and prisoners of war. *Military Medicine, 167,* 898–903.

Ritchie, E. C. (2003). Psychiatric evaluation and treatment central to medicine in the US military. *Psychiatric Annals, 33,* 710–715.

Roscoe, S. N. (1997). The adolescence of engineering psychology. *Human Factors History Monograph Series,* 1. Retrieved September 14, 2005, from *www.hfes.org/PublicationMaintenance/FeaturedDocuments/27/adolescencehtml.html.*

Salter, C. A. (2001). Psychological effects of nuclear and radiological warfare. *Military Medicine, 166,* 17–18.

Sammons, M. T., Levant, R. F., & Paige, R. U. (2003). *Prescriptive authority for psychologists: A history and guide.* Washington, DC: American Psychological Association.

Shaffer, L. F. (1944). *The psychology of adjustment: An objective approach to mental hygiene.* Washington, DC: Houghton Mifflin, for the United States Armed Forces Institute.

Shephard, B. (2000). *A war of nerves: Soldiers and psychiatrists 1914–1994.* London: Jonathan Cape.

Shorter, E. (1997). *A history of psychiatry.* New York: Wiley.

Smith, G. E., & Pear, T. H. (1917). *Shell shock and its lessons.* Manchester, UK: Manchester at the University Press.

Stearns, A. W., & Schwab, R. S. (1943). Five hundred neuro-psychiatric casualties at a naval hospital. *Journal of the Maine Medical Association, 34,* 81–89.

Stuart, J. A., Ursano, R. J., Fullerton, C. S., Norwood, A. E., & Murray, K. (2003). Belief in exposure to terrorist agents: Reported exposure to nerve or mustard gas by Gulf War veterans. *Journal of Nervous and Mental Disease, 191,* 431–436.

Terman, L. M. (1918). The use of intelligence tests in the Army. *Psychological Bulletin, 15,* 177–187.

Tischler, G. L. (1969). Patterns of psychiatric attrition and of behavior in a combat zone. In P. G. Bourne (Ed.), *The psychology and physiology of stress: With reference to special studies of the Viet Nam War* (pp. 19–44). New York: Academic Press.

Uhlaner, J. E. (1967, September). *Chronology of military psychology in the Army.* Paper presented at the 75th annual convention of the American Psychological Association, Washington, DC.

Ursano, R. J., & Rundell, J. R. (1995). The prisoner of war. In R. Zajtchuk & R. F. Bellamy (Eds.), *Textbook of military medicine: War psychiatry* (pp. 431–455). Washington, DC: Office of the Surgeon General, U.S. Department of the Army.

U.S. Department of the Army. (1948). *Military leadership psychology and personnel management* (an extract from the *Senior ROTC Manual,* Vol. II). Washington, DC: Author.

U.S. Departments of the Army and the Air Force. (1951). *Military clinical psychology, technical manual, TM 8-242, Air Force manual, 1600-45.* Washington, DC: Author.

Walters, H. C. (1968). *Military psychology: Its use in modern war and indirect conflict.* Dubuque, IA: Wm. C. Brown.

Watanabe, H. K., Harig, P. T., Rock, N. L., & Koshes, R. J. (1994). Alcohol and drug abuse and dependence. In R. Zajtchuk & R. F. Bellamy (Eds.), *Textbook of military medicine: Military psychiatry: Preparing in peace for war* (pp. 61–90). Washington, DC: Office of the Surgeon General, U.S. Department of the Army.

Welsh, J. R., Kucinkas, S. K., & Curran, L. T. (1990). *Armed Services Vocational Aptitude Battery (ASVAB): Integrative review of reliability studies.* Brooks Air Force Base, TX: Air Force Systems Command.

Wong, A., Escobar, M., Lesage, A., Loyer, M., Vanier, C., & Sakinofsky, I. (2001). Are UN peacekeepers at risk for suicide? *Suicide and Life-Threatening Behavior, 31,* 103–112.

Wood, D. P., Koffman, R. L., & Arita, A. A. (2003). Psychiatric medevacs during a 6-month aircraft carrier battle group deployment to the Persian Gulf: A Navy force health protection preliminary report. *Military Medicine, 168,* 43–47.

Yerkes, R. M. (1917). Psychology and national service. *Journal of Applied Psychology, 1,* 301–304.

Yerkes, R. M. (Ed.). (1921). *Memoirs of the National Academy of Sciences: Psychological examining in the United States Army* (Vol. XV). Washington, DC: U.S. Government Printing Office.

Young, A. (1999). W. H. R. Rivers and the war neuroses. *Journal of the History of the Behavioral Sciences, 35,* 359–378.

Zeidner, J., & Drucker, A. J. (1988). *Behavioral science in the Army: A corporate history of the Army Research Institute.* Washington, DC: Army Research Institute for the Behavioral and Social Sciences.

CHAPTER 2

Fitness-for-Duty Evaluations

Mark C. Monahan
James M. Keener

Clinical military psychologists assess a service member's fitness for duty each time they conduct a psychological evaluation, whether in a deployed or an expeditionary setting, at a stateside military treatment facility (MTF), or in an outpatient clinic. Based on U.S. Department of Defense (DoD) terminology, fitness for duty is defined as a service member's ability to perform the duties of his or her office, grade, rank, or rating.

Military psychologists make an initial assessment of the member's fitness for duty and write a narrative report. On the basis of this evaluation, they determine whether the service member is fit and suitable for full duty or whether further review is needed. To find a service member unfit for duty, the military uses a formal review process that involves a Medical Evaluation Board (MEB) and a Physical Evaluation Board (PEB). Suitability for further service is determined at the command level and refers to issues of development and personality. This chapter guides the reader through the fitness and suitability-for-duty evaluation process.

CONDUCTING A FITNESS-FOR-DUTY EVALUATION

Fitness-for-duty evaluations can arise from one of three sources: self-referral, referral from other medical providers, and command referral. Initially, we discuss a nonemergent fitness-for-duty evaluation (self-referral and voluntary medical referral) and then focus on the special requirements of a command-directed evaluation (CDE). It should be noted that the different branches of service have somewhat differing administrative requirements and lingo; however, the components of the fitness-for-duty evaluation are the same across all.

It is generally accepted that a service member rarely presents to a mental health provider as a first response in coping with psychological problems. Friends, family members, and sometimes chaplains are the first-line resources for emotional support. Most often then, all other self-help approaches have been tried without adequate success before mental health professionals are approached. Therefore, when a service member comes to a mental health clinic, he or she usually presents with problems that significantly affect quality of life. Most often, the individual is experiencing problems in relationships, self-image, and performance of duties. Although it is usually the individual who decides to seek help, this decision is often influenced by the advice of friends, family members, coworkers, or supervisors; it may be generally recognized that the individual's level of functioning has declined. Therefore, it is necessary for the military psychologist to determine whether the decline in functioning has reached a level at which the service member can no longer adequately perform his or her assigned military duties (i.e., determine fitness for duty).

To determine whether the service member can adequately perform his or her assigned duties, the military psychologist must first understand what the individual's job responsibilities involve. Obviously, the duty requirements for a junior enlisted sailor with little time in service and no leadership responsibilities are not commensurate with those of senior enlisted and officers. Likewise, the duty requirements of a Navy SEAL, for example, will be very different from those of a service member whose position is primarily administrative. For this reason, certain rates (job specialties), military occupational specialties (MOS), and special duty assignments require specialized screening and consideration when determining fitness or suitability. An explanation of special screenings for several specialized communities is provided later in this chapter. Also see Chapter 3, this volume, for information on assessing and selecting personnel for high-risk jobs.

The process for assessing a service member's fitness for duty requires a comprehensive evaluation of his or her situation. The primary instruments for this evaluation are the clinical interview and a review of pertinent history and collateral information. In addition to the careful history obtained by interviewing the patient, the military psychologist will also review the member's service and medical records and obtain a history from his or her collateral sources.

The military service record contains details about the service member's training, performance of duties, educational history, military award history, Armed Services Vocational Aptitude Battery (ASVAB) scores, enlistment waivers, and disciplinary issues. The medical record details medical issues beginning with the service member's entry into the military and all subsequent contacts in the military healthcare system, including mental health. Importantly, medical records originating in the combat zone are increasingly becoming available for review. In routine mental health evaluations, if given permission to contact supervisors in the chain of command, the military psychologist is better able to assess how the individual's mental health problems are affecting his or her ability to perform assigned duties (for information on confidentiality and the military, see Chapter 14, this volume). Further, if given permission to contact family members, the psychologist is able to gain a better understanding of the service member's preservice personality, the family's perception of any changes, and general functioning, contrasting information to verify the accuracy of the interview data and gathering details regarding developmental and preservice influences and behaviors. Tapping these valuable sources of information can prove challenging, however; despite efforts to destigmatize mental health services, many service members are still reluctant to allow their mental health provider to contact family, friends, and/or the chain of command.

It has been our experience that routine evaluations will usually find the service member fit for full duty. However, when the psychologist finds the individual unable to adequately perform assigned duties, the psychologist must determine whether a course of treatment is likely to return the individual to full-duty status within a reasonable period (e.g., 6–12 months). In the U.S. Navy, the individual would be placed on a 6-month limited-duty (LIMDU) board, also referred to as temporary limited duty (TLD), if a course of treatment is expected to result in unrestricted return to duty. LIMDU is determined by the actions of the MEB and is an official documented period of restricted duty during which the service member receives ongoing treatment (U.S. Department of the Navy, 2010). The U.S. Army and the U.S. Air Force use a physical profile serial report in place of a LIMDU board. With few exceptions, a service member may be placed on a maximum of two periods of limited duty, not to exceed a total of 12 months during his or her career. Because of this limitation, it is incumbent upon the mental health professional to monitor the member's progress closely and facilitate return to full duty as soon as he or she is ready. Returning a service member to full duty requires approval from a convening authority; however, an MEB does not need to be convened. If LIMDU does not return the service member to full duty within the allowed time frame or the illness is sufficiently severe and chronic (e.g., schizophrenia) such that the member is not expected to return to unrestricted duty, then he or she is referred to an MEB.

The U.S. Army and U.S. Air Force are guided in the fitness-for-duty process by their own instructions. Although similar to U.S. Navy guidelines, there are subtle differences to address mission-specific requirements. The reader is invited to review the branch-specific instructions for MEBs referenced in the following sections.

MEDICAL EVALUATION BOARD

By DoD Instruction (DoDI) 1332.38 (DoD, 1996) the service member must be referred to an MEB if his or her medical condition has prevented return to full duty for 12 months. This process begins with a licensed psychologist, psychiatrist, or doctorate-level social worker submitting a narrative report to the board (for an example, see Appendix 2.1). A narrative report from a psychologist or social worker must be co-signed by at least two psychiatrists. (Note, however, that the requirement for psychiatrists' cosigning psychologist's submissions to the MEB has recently been removed by the DoD [Under Secretary of Defense, 2011], and individual service policies are currently under review by the branch secretaries). MEBs are conducted at military MTFs; the commander of the facility is the convening authority. However, signatory authority can, and often is, delegated to the MEB. An MEB consists of two officers of any medical specialty. Rarely is psychiatry one of those specialties; therefore, the narrative report should be written in a manner that physicians from other specialties can understand, without jargon or overly specialized terminology. The MEB does not make the final determination on fitness for duty; this is determined by the PEB, later in the process. The Army initiates an MEB under the provisions of Army Regulation 40-400, and the Air Force initiates an MEB under the provisions of Air Force Instruction 36-3212 (Secretary of the Air Force, 2006e). Under the provisions of Title 10, U.S.C., Chapter 61, branch secretaries of the military are given the authority to separate members found unfit for duty.

The MEB considers several sources when making a determination: the provider's narrative summary, a nonmedical assessment by the member's command, a physical examination, and a line-of-duty determination, if needed. A line-of-duty determination is necessary if there is a question about the member's duty status at the time of an injury or disease or if the condition was caused by "gross negligence, intentional misconduct, or willful neglect" (NAVMED P-117; U.S. Department of the Navy, 2005). A nonmedical assessment provides the board with critical information regarding the member's performance of assigned duties at the work site, supervisors' behavioral observations, and possible psychosocial factors. The MEB makes its determinations based on the diagnosis, prognosis for return to full duty, need for further treatment, and medical recommendations. If the MEB determines that the service member is unable to adequately perform his or her duties, it will refer the case to a PEB. The member can file an appeal if he or she does not agree with the findings of the MEB. This specific appeals process is discussed in more detail in the next section.

PHYSICAL EVALUATION BOARD

By instruction, referrals to the PEB can only come from two sources: LIMDU reports submitted by the service headquarters for PEB evaluation and MEB reports submitted by the MTFs. When reviewing cases based on mental illness, the PEB requires the diagnosis of a clinical psychiatric disorder or other psychiatric condition that may be a focus of clinical attention (SECNAVINST 1850.4E; Secretary of the Navy, 2002). The narrative summary must include a five-axes diagnosis as delineated in the American Psychiatric Association's *Diagnostic and Statistical Manual of Mental Disorders* (fourth edition, text revision; American Psychiatric Association, 2000). Each branch of service has its own specific guidelines for fitness-for-duty evaluations, although the basics are very similar (Secretary of the Air Force, 2006a, 2006b, 2006c, 2006d; Secretary of the Army, 2006, 2007; Secretary of the Navy, 2002, 2005). In the Navy, for example, a PEB is convened under the authority of the Secretary of the Navy. A PEB is composed of a presiding officer, a line officer 05 or above, from either the Navy or the Marine Corps; a second-line officer, 05 or above, from either the Navy or the Marine Corps; and a medical officer, 05 or above. For reservists, at least one line officer on the board must be a reservist. As in the MEB process, the medical officer who reviews mental health reports may practice any type of medical specialty.

An informal PEB screens all new cases and performs the initial disability evaluation based on a documentary review. If the service member is found fit for full duty but disagrees with the finding, then he or she can request a formal PEB if the request can be substantiated with new information not already reviewed by the board. When found unfit by the informal PEB, the member has 15 days to decide either to accept the findings or to request a hearing by the formal PEB. If a formal PEB is requested, the case will be reexamined. The member will have the opportunity to meet with the board and present additional material to support his or her position, and may be represented by counsel. A judge advocate general (JAG) officer will be provided at no cost, or a civilian attorney is allowed at the member's expense. The case will be decided on the basis of new evidence in addition to previously documented evidence.

A PEB will not consider a case if the member is being processed for misconduct that may result in punitive discharge. In such a situation, the board will be postponed until disciplinary issues are resolved. If the member is discharged for misconduct, the PEB's actions to that point will be filed in the member's medical records and the PEB process will be terminated.

Certain diagnoses lead to an administrative separation rather than the PEB process. These include personality disorders, learning disorders, attention-deficit/hyperactivity disorder (ADHD), and borderline intellectual functioning. These conditions existed prior to service (EPTS). When a service member is deemed unable to perform assigned duties because of one of these conditions, he or she is considered for an administrative separation as "unsuitable" rather than a medical separation (PEB) as "unfit." Guidance for administrative separations for these conditions can be found in DoDI 1332.14 (DoD, 2008). In our experience, although it is not unusual to receive a consult to rule out borderline intellectual functioning, it is very unusual to find an active-duty member with an IQ below 85. The ASVAB (DoD, 1984) and other entry-level screening tools appear to be adequate methods of avoiding such cases. Learning disorders and ADHD, however, are not uncommon in the military, although the more severe cases are often caught in the screening process (Hess, Kennedy, Hardin, & Kupke, 2010). The diagnosis of a learning disorder or ADHD will not automatically lead to discharge; these conditions lead to discharge only if they affect the member to the degree that he or she cannot adequately perform assigned duties. However, some medications prescribed for the treatment of ADHD (e.g., stimulants) can disqualify an individual in certain military communities (e.g., special operations forces, aviation, nuclear power). Personality disorders are addressed in detail in the Suitability Evaluations section later in this chapter.

COMPETENCY EVALUATIONS

All service members are presumed competent to manage their own affairs and are responsible for their actions (SECNAVINST 1850.4E; Secretary of the Navy, 2002). Per instruction, clear and convincing evidence is required to overcome this presumption. When mental competency is in question, a competency board is convened. The board consists of three physicians, one of whom must be a psychiatrist. The board will determine the need for a trustee to manage the member's pay and allowances. The physicians on the board must be members of the Navy, Army, or Air Force or must be employed by one of these services, the U.S. Department of Health and Human Services, or the U.S. Department of Veterans Affairs, in accordance with (f) (MANMED) chapter 18 and 37 U.S.C. 602.

COMMAND-DIRECTED EVALUATIONS

CDEs are performed when a commanding officer (CO) becomes concerned about the emotional state and subsequent fitness for duty of a service member under his or her command. This process should also be followed when a medical provider outside of the service member's chain of command has determined a mental health referral is needed but the service member will not consent (DoD 1997a, 1997b). It should be noted that evaluations arising from family advocacy cases (e.g., domestic violence) or alcohol problems are covered under different instructions and are not considered CDEs. Emergent considerations are presented in the next section.

Conducting a CDE involves the following sequence of steps:

• *Step 1:* The CO must consult with a mental health care provider, who is a psychologist, psychiatrist, or doctorate-level social worker, to discuss the service member's actions and behaviors. If a mental health care provider is not available, the CO may consult with a physician or, if a physician is not present, another senior privileged provider. The mental health provider will provide guidance and recommendations about whether an evaluation should be conducted and whether the evaluation should be done on a routine or emergency basis.

• *Step 2:* The CO must provide a written letter at least 2 business days before the evaluation date. The letter must include a brief factual description of the behaviors or communications that led the CO to make the referral; the name of the mental health provider with whom the CO consulted before making the referral; notification of the service member's rights per reference (DoD Directive 7050.06; DoD, 2000); the date, time, and place of the scheduled mental health evaluation; and the name and rank of the provider whom the service member will meet. The service member will be provided the titles and telephone numbers of other authorities, including attorneys, the inspector general, and chaplains, who can provide assistance if he or she questions the necessity for the referral or the name and signature of the CO.

• *Step 3:* The service member must acknowledge having been advised of the reasons for the referral and of their rights by signing the letter. If the member refuses to sign the letter, the CO should document the refusal on the letter, in addition to any reasons the member may have given for not signing. Refusal by the service member to sign the letter does not stop the evaluation.

• *Step 4:* A copy of the signed letter is provided to the service member, and a copy is kept by the mental health provider who will conduct the evaluation.

• *Step 5:* The mental health provider ensures that all procedures are followed per DoD Directive 6490.1 (DoD, 1997b). The mental health provider reviews all signed letters. If not considered appropriate, the provider will contact the referring command to clarify questions and resolve concerns. If the referral still does not meet necessary guidelines, this should be discussed with the provider's chain of command.

• *Step 6:* The provider meets with the service member for the evaluation and, before starting, explains the purpose, nature, and possible consequences of the evaluation. The service member must be informed that the findings of the evaluation are not confidential. If the provider has also been giving therapy to the service member, the potential conflict of duties should be discussed with the patient (dual/mixed agency is discussed in more detail in Chapter 14, this volume). Following the evaluation, the provider forwards a letter to the service member's CO to inform him or her of the results and gives recommendations.

EMERGENCY FITNESS-FOR-DUTY EVALUATIONS

When it is feared that the member poses a danger to him- or herself or others or is grossly impaired and unable to make rational decisions, emergency procedures should be followed. (See Chapter 9, this volume, for more information about suicide in the military.) Gross impairment can be the result of severe mental illness when the service member is unable to distinguish between reality and fantasy or to use good judgment in making reasoned decisions. The priority is to ensure the safety of the service member and others. Therefore, if the provider determines that the situation constitutes the need for an emergency evaluation, the steps required before a CDE can be postponed.

Even if the situation constitutes an emergency, it is still expected that the CO will make every effort to consult with a mental health provider before sending the individual, but it is understood that the CO's first priority is to protect the individual and others from harm without delay. If unable to contact a mental health provider for consultation, the letter from the CO explaining the reasons for the referral and his or her concerns is forwarded to the provider as soon as possible. Likewise, the CO will provide a copy of the letter and a statement of rights to the service member as soon as practicable.

The mental health provider will conduct a risk assessment and determine whether the situation is a true emergency. The provider will contact the referring command for further details and support for the evaluation. If deemed improper, the provider will report the situation to his or her medical facility's chain of command. Out of safety concerns, if the provider deems it a true emergency, the evaluation will go forward regardless of procedural concerns. Following the evaluation, the provider will forward a letter to the service member's CO to inform the CO of the results of the mental health evaluation and provide recommendations.

SUITABILITY EVALUATIONS

Mental health separations from the military based on unsuitability are most often due to personality disorders. For a service member to be found unsuitable, the personality disorder must impair his or her ability to perform assigned duties and to work with and take guidance from others. Being unable to do so can result in adjustment difficulties, disciplinary issues, and inadequate performance of assigned duties. When the personality disorder is severe, the individual may become a threat to his or her own safety or the safety of others. Before a service member can be separated as unsuitable because of inadequate performance of assigned duties, his or her command must have officially counseled the member about his or her deficiencies and made efforts to help correct them. If the member has demonstrated a pattern of misconduct that would lead to separation for violations under the Uniform Code of Military Justice (UCMJ), a separation for misconduct should be pursued rather than a separation for behaviors associated with a personality disorder. As in fitness-for-duty evaluations, the military psychologist must make the determination that mental health treatment will not adequately change the member's suitability status. In other words, when finding a member unsuitable, the psychologist is saying that the service member and the military would be best served if the member left the service.

When a military psychologist finds a service member unsuitable for military service because of a personality disorder, an administrative separation is recommended. This is only a recommendation made by the mental health professional. In most cases, the member's CO has the separation authority and ultimately makes the decision. If the service member has served in a combat zone, then only a CO with general court-martial convening authority or Navy personnel command has authority for administrative separation based on a personality disorder (MILPERSMAN 1910-122; U.S. Department of the Navy, 2009). A service member diagnosed with posttraumatic stress disorder (PTSD) or mild traumatic brain injury (mTBI/concussion) may not be separated based on a personality disorder. This policy was instituted to protect combat veterans from the possibility of being misdiagnosed with a personality disorder when they exhibit behavioral problems secondary to combat stress or concussive injuries.

For a full review and guidance regarding the conditions that may lead to an administrative separation, the reader is referred to SECNAVINST 1850.4E (Secretary of the Navy, 2002). The following mental disorders may lead to administrative separation:

- Uncomplicated alcoholism or other substance use disorder
- Personality disorders, unless diagnosed with PTSD or a TBI
- Dyslexia and other learning disorders
- Phobic fear of air, sea, and submarine modes of transportation
- Borderline intellectual functioning or mental retardation
- Adjustment disorders, unless diagnosed with PTSD or a TBI
- Impulse control disorders
- Sexual paraphilias
- Factitious disorder
- Sleepwalking and/or somnambulism
- Incapacitating fear of flying

Although homosexuality is not a "mental disorder," based on our experience, it was not uncommon for a military psychologist to be consulted on questions involving homosexuality. The best response was always to educate the referring source that homosexuality is not a mental disorder and that it is a legal issue within the military and not a mental health matter. The "Don't Ask, Don't Tell" policy was officially repealed on September 20, 2011. Sexual orientation is no longer a factor in "accession, promotion, separation, or other personnel decision-making" (U.S. Department of Defense, 2011).

FITNESS FOR ENLISTMENT AND ENTRY INTO MILITARY SERVICE

Fitness for military service is assessed for every person who desires enlistment or commissioning. The DoD sets common physical and psychological standards, which are assessed prior to taking the oath of enlistment or the oath of office. Once prospective applicants have consulted with a recruiter and then choose to join the service, they are taken to a local Military Entrance Processing Station (MEPS), where they undergo a variety of assessments, including an intensive physical exam. At MEPS prospective service members are medically screened and a comprehensive review of their past record is completed. Candidates who have a history of a mental health condition may be seen by a psychologist or psychiatrist at MEPS to assist in determining their fitness for military service. DoD (2010b) has established a policy that clearly identifies medical standards for appointment, enlistment, or induction in the military service. These medical and mental health standards are comprehensive. Prospective service members are found fit for enlistment or commissioning once they have met these medical standards. While a condition may be disqualifying according to the DoD, it is important to note that service-specific waivers can be requested in some cases where the prospective service member does not meet the minimum standards of enlistment.

These medical standards are important points of reference for mental health professionals working at MEPS and or at mental health clinics attached to a recruit training command, such as the Navy Recruit Training Command outside Chicago or the Marine Corps Recruit Depot at Parris Island or San Diego. At these recruit training commands, mental health professionals perform fitness-for-duty evaluations on a regular basis. It is possible that during training a recruit will disclose a history of a psychological condition that was not previously disclosed and that is not appropriate for military service. Based on a comprehensive clinical interview and a review of available records, a decision will need to be made regarding whether the recruit's condition existed prior to enlistment (EPTE) and whether the recruit can continue to train. If the recruit is found not fit for continued training, a recommendation is made to the recruit's command for an entry-level separation (ELS) for an EPTE condition. A service member is eligible for an ELS if he or she has been in the service for less than 180 days.

These standards do not offer fitness-for-duty guidance on the numerous special or arduous duties that are available to some service members (e.g., aviation, special operations, submarine, intelligence). There are myriad specialized duties within the military in which initial or ongoing psychological evaluations are conducted. Knowledge of the specific rules and regulations impacting service members is crucial for mental health professionals who are routinely called upon to consult, evaluate, and treat service members from a variety of communities.

OVERSEAS SCREENINGS

In 2010 the DoD released its annual base structure report, which indicated that there are 662 military installations located overseas (DoD, 2010a). According to the report, an additional 88 bases are located in overseas U.S. territories. These bases are outside of the continental United States (OCONUS) and are often occupied by uniformed service members who, in some cases, are accompanied by their families. The size, structure, and mission of these bases vary considerably, as do the medical and mental health resources available. At some of the smaller locations, treatment options may be limited. To determine medical and psychological fitness for overseas duty, the service member and accompanying family members must complete an overseas screening (OSS). While each service varies slightly in how they complete an OSS, the general process and structure are similar across branches. In the Navy, the medical evaluation conducted as part of the OSS is called a "suitability screening." A suitability screening is designed to determine suitability for service in overseas or remote duty assignments. This screening is conducted by a medical provider at the service member's transferring command, whose goal is to identify medical, psychological, dental, and educational problems that may be duty limiting.

Mental health professionals may be asked to complete a supplemental evaluation as part of the suitability screening to determine whether a psychological condition or educational need (e.g., individualized education program) is present and what treatment or services are recommended. If a need for ongoing mental health services is identified, information from the evaluation is sent to the gaining command, who determines whether the necessary treatment options are available at that command. If the recommended treatment options are not available, it may be determined that the service or family member is not suitable for the new duty station, and new orders may need to be issued.

SUBMARINE DUTY

The environment and mission of a submarine are unique: Serving on a submarine can be an extremely difficult and arduous duty, marked by long periods of limited contact with family and friends, a high operational tempo, and intense cognitive demands. While onboard care is available for many physical complaints and illnesses through a dedicated independent duty corpsman (IDC), mental health professionals are not assigned to submarines. Because of the lack of available mental health resources and the demanding nature of submarine duty, rigorous psychological standards must be met before a sailor can serve aboard a submarine.

Once sailors complete recruit training, their path to service aboard a submarine is voluntary and varies depending on their chosen rate. If their rate will require them to perform a support function aboard the submarine, such as in the case of a culinary specialist (CS) or yeoman (YN), they will first learn about the technical aspects of their rate at "A" School. Once they complete their technical training at "A" School, they will attend Basic Enlisted Submarine School (BESS), where they will learn about the basic operations of the submarine. If their rate will require them to perform more technical duties, such as machinist's mate (MM), electronics technician (ET), or electrician's mate (EM), then they will attend BESS shortly after completing recruit training. After completing BESS, they will attend A School, where they will gain the technical knowledge of their rate.

Prospective submariner candidates are assessed during training at BESS for psychiatric suitability using the Subscreen and if necessary a follow-up evaluation with a psychologist or psychiatrist. The Subscreen is a 240-item self-report measure of mental health functioning, motivation, and adaptability that has been shown to be a useful and valid measure in identifying attrition for psychiatric reasons during BESS (Schlichting, 1993). Research has shown that the use of the Subscreen has led to disqualification of approximately 3% of BESS candidates for unsuitability for submarine duty (Daniel, 2006). The SubMarine Attrition Test (SMART) is a subset of the Subscreen used to determine those who are at a high risk of attrition for negative causes. Scores on the SMART correlate with the probability that the BESS candidate will be successful in the fleet during his or her first enlistment (Bing, Horn, Crisman, & Gudewicz, 2005).

Once a submariner has completed the required training, has been found physically and psychologically fit for submarine duty, and has been granted the required security clearance, there are strict regulations that determine continued fitness for duty. According to the U.S. Department of the Navy (2010), "Psychological fitness for submarine duty must be carefully and continuously evaluated in all submarine personnel. It is imperative that individuals working in this program have a very high degree of reliability, alertness, and good judgment" (p. 15-93a). There are a litany of psychiatric conditions that are disqualifying for continued submarine service, including psychotic disorders, anxiety and mood disorders, somatoform disorders, dissociative disorders, eating disorders, impulse control disorders, and severe personality disorders. Some psychiatric conditions are not disqualifying from service, including adjustment disorders and bereavement, if they resolve within 30 days. For conditions lasting longer than 30 days, a waiver can be requested by the submariner's underwater medical officer (UMO) in consultation with the treating psychologist or psychiatrist. Mental health professionals who have contact with submariners should closely consult with UMOs and IDCs because they can provide further guidance on fitness-for-duty issues arising with this unique population.

NUCLEAR FIELD DUTY

Nuclear Field duty is a specialized Navy program open to officers and certain enlisted ratings and involves work in the Naval Nuclear Propulsion Program. Enlisted sailors work in the nuclear field as MM(N), ET(N), and EM(N) and perform a variety of highly skilled duties. These sailors work on nuclear propulsion plants and operate reactor control, propulsion, and power generation systems. Nuclear Field duty is highly competitive and requires a great deal of motivation, a clean service record, and a strong academic background. Sailors selected for Nuclear Field duty are sent to the Naval Nuclear Power Training Command in South Carolina. Upon graduation from this academically rigorous training program, sailors are sent to Nuclear Prototype School, where their education continues in an environment similar to that of their work in the fleet. After completing this program, they are sent to a variety of duty stations, including the surface fleet aboard one of the 11 nuclear-powered aircraft carriers or one of the numerous nuclear-powered submarines.

Mental health professionals stationed aboard aircraft carriers and those attached to clinics serving sailors from nuclear submarines may encounter service members who are qualified to work in Nuclear Field duty after a self-referral, a CDE, or a referral from the service member's medical provider related to a periodic medical exam. Service members who are qualified for Nuclear Field duty receive periodic medical exams, during which, according to the U.S. Department of the Navy (2010), the medical provider will "pay special attention to the mental status, psychiatric, and neurological components of the examination, and will review the entire health record for evidence of past impairment" (p. 15-79). Mental health professionals who encounter Nuclear Field-qualified personnel should work closely with these service members' radiation health officer (RHO), UMO, or IDC, because there are numerous psychological and neurological conditions that are disqualifying from duty. A fitness-for-duty evaluation should be comprehensive, and evaluators should pay special attention to current mental health symptoms and a history of impulsivity, evidence of poor judgment, poor interpersonal skills, and anxiety or mood symptoms impacting ability to function in a high-stress environment.

MENTAL HEALTH EVALUATIONS IN A COMBAT ENVIRONMENT

Mental health professionals working in combat zones will often find themselves assisting service members with managing the challenges of separation from family and friends while simultaneously managing the day-to-day operational demands unique to a combat environment. Combat troops are exposed to experiences difficult for those outside the combat zone to fully grasp. Service members' safety is of the upmost importance, and safety is paramount in an environment where all service members, including the psychologist, have access to one or multiple weapons.

Despite the obvious challenges of serving in an operational setting, the fitness-for-duty process remains essentially the same. Over the past decade, military mental health personnel, both officers and enlisted, from all branches of service have been routinely deployed to combat zones to support combat troops during Operation Iraqi Freedom and Operation Enduring Freedom. Fitness-for-duty evaluations in a combat zone must take into consideration the specific duty requirements of the patient. Some combat troops go on combat missions almost every day, while others remain mostly "within the wire" in combat support positions. From a mental health perspective, deployed military psychologists must help make a determination regarding the service member's ability to function within this unique environment. They will work closely with the service member and his or her command unit to ensure the member can safely remain on full duty. Requirements for CDEs remain the same. Recommendations to the service member's commander may include keeping the service member behind the wire for a specified period so he or she can get needed sleep, hot food, and a chance to receive mental health services. The goal is to return the service member to normal operations as soon as possible. Depending on the mission of the service member's command, the specified period away from combat operations may be extended for days or even weeks. However, based on our experience, if the service member does not benefit significantly from a brief mental health intervention, then he or she will be evacuated from theater to the continental U.S. (CONUS), where there are greater resources for further evaluation and treatment. In cases in which the service member is considered a danger to self or others, the evacuation is expedited.

SUMMARY

Psychologists working with service members regularly evaluate and make recommendations related to fitness for duty at the initial point of enlistment into the service, during recruit training, during selection for special communities, at any time that commanding officers are concerned for a service member's welfare, and at additional points throughout a service member's career. Fitness-for-duty evaluations are a critical responsibility that active-duty and civilian psychologists are routinely asked to perform. Psychologists working within military institutions should be well versed and knowledgeable about the various occupational settings and specialties, the service-specific requirements for these specialties, and the instructions that guide these evaluations. Conducting these multifaceted and at times complex evaluations allows psychologists to make an impact on the lives of individual service members and the fighting force as a whole by identifying those members who are fit and suitable for various occupations, evaluating where psychological interventions may be beneficial, and helping them return to productive service whenever possible.

REFERENCES

American Psychiatric Association. (2000). *Diagnostic and statistical manual of mental disorders* (4th ed., text rev.). Washington, DC: Author.

Bing, M., Horn, W., Crisman, K., & Gudewicz, T. (2005). *Test and evaluation of the Submarine Attrition Risk Test* (SMART, formerly known as the Submarine Attrition Risk Scale, or SARS) (Protocol Number NSMRL.2004.005). Groton, CT: Naval Submarine Medical Research Laboratory.

Daniel, J. C. (2006). *Leveraging biomedical knowledge to enhance homeland defense, submarine medicine and warfighter performance at Naval Submarine Medical Research Laboratory.* Groton, CT: Naval Submarine Medical Research Laboratory.

Hess, D. W., Kennedy, C. H., Hardin, R. A., & Kupke, T. (2010). Attention deficit/hyperactivity disorder and learning disorders. In C. Kennedy & J. Moore (Eds.), *Military neuropsychology* (pp. 199–226). New York: Springer.

Schlichting, C. L. (1993). *Psychiatric screening for the submarine service: Enlisted personnel.* Groton, CT: Naval Submarine Medical Research Laboratory.

Secretary of the Air Force. (2006a). *Medical examinations and standards: Volume 1. General provisions* (Air Force Instruction 48-123). Washington, DC: Author.

Secretary of the Air Force. (2006b). *Medical examinations and standards: Volume 2. Accession, retention, and administration* (Air Force Instruction 48-123). Washington, DC: Author.

Secretary of the Air Force. (2006c). *Medical examinations and standards: Volume 3. Flying and special operational duty* (Air Force Instruction 48-123). Washington, DC: Author.

Secretary of the Air Force. (2006d). *Medical examinations and standards: Volume 4. Special standards and requirements* (Air Force Instruction 48-123, Vol. 4). Washington, DC: Author.

Secretary of the Air Force. (2006e). *Physical evaluation for retention, retirement and separation* (Air Force Instruction 36-3212). Washington, DC: Author.

Secretary of the Army. (2006). *Physical evaluation for retention, retirement, and separation* (Army Regulation 635-40). Washington, DC: Author.

Secretary of the Army. (2007). *Standards of medical fitness* (Army Regulation 40-501). Washington, DC: Author.

Secretary of the Navy. (1999). *Mental health evaluations of members of the armed forces* (SECNAVINST 6320.24A). Washington, DC: Author.

Secretary of the Navy. (2002). *Department of the Navy disability determination manual* (SENINST 1850.4E). Washington, DC: Author.

Secretary of the Navy. (2005). *Manual of the medical department U.S. Navy* (NAVMED P-117). Washington, DC: Author.

U.S. Department of Defense. (1984). *Test manual for the Armed Services Vocational Aptitude Battery.* North Chicago: U.S. Military Entrance Processing Command.

U.S. Department of Defense. (1996). *Physical disability evaluation* (DoD Instruction 1332.32). Washington, DC: Author.

U.S. Department of Defense. (1997a). *Requirements for mental health evaluations of members of the armed forces* (DoD Instruction 6490.4). Washington, DC: Author.

U.S. Department of Defense. (1997b). *Mental health evaluations of members of the armed forces* (DoD Instruction 6490.1). Washington DC: Author.

U.S. Department of Defense. (2000). *Military whistleblower protection* (Directive 7050.6). Washington, DC: Author.

U.S. Department of Defense. (2008). *Enlisted administrative separations* (DoD Instruction 1332.14). Washington, DC: Author.

U.S. Department of Defense. (2010a). *Base structure report: Fiscal year 2010 baseline.* Retrieved March 6, 2011, from *www.acq.osd.mil/ie/download/bsr/bsr-2010baseline.pdf.*

U.S. Department of Defense. (2010b). *Medical standards for appointment, enlistment, or induction in the military services* (DoD Instruction 6130.03). Washington, DC: Author.

U.S. Department of Defense. (2011). *Memorandum of the Under Secretary of Defense: Repeal of "Don't Ask, Don't Tell."* Washington, DC: Author.

U.S. Department of the Navy. (2005). *Manual of the medical department* (NAVMED P-117). Washington, DC: Author.

U.S. Department of the Navy. (2008). *Naval Military Personnel Manual.* Article 1910-122: *Separation by reason of convenience of the government—personality disorder(s).* (CH 28). Washington, DC: Author.

U.S. Department of the Navy. (2010). *Change 136: Manual of the medical department* (NAVMED P-117). Washington, DC: Author.

APPENDIX 2.1. Report to Medical Evaluation Board

All characters appearing in this work are fictitious. Any resemblance to real persons, living or dead, is purely coincidental.

Date and Time: 26 September 2011

Service Member's Name: Sergeant First Class (SFC) Joe Example

Reason for Convening of the MEB (*physician directed or command directed*):

SFC Joe Example is being recommended for a Medical Evaluation Board by Dr. Maria Williams because of a history of posttraumatic stress disorder (PTSD) and dysthymic disorder.

Nature of the Evaluation (*voluntary or command-directed mental health evaluation*):

SFC Example was initially evaluated on 14 July 2010 by Dr. Williams on a self-referral basis, and per his report there was no pressure or command coercion to attend the evaluation or any of his subsequent follow-up appointments.

Sources of Information (*initial assessment; number of follow-up sessions; review of inpatient and outpatient treatment records; interview with collateral sources; interview with command sources; psychological assessments*):

The information for this current report was received from SFC Example and from a review of his outpatient medical records.

Identifying Information (*age; marital status; ethnicity*):

SFC Example is a 32-year-old, married, Caucasian and Hispanic male with approximately 10 years and 2 months of continuous active-duty serving with the U.S. Army. SFC Example's military occupational specialty (MOS) is military police (MP, 31B), and his current home duty station is Any Base, USA. SFC Example reported that he has deployed three times to an imminent-danger pay area.

Military Status and Military History (*date of first and most recent entry into service; estimated termination of service [i.e., EAOS/EAS]; duty status: active duty or reservist; time in service; military occupational specialty [MOS]; dates and locations of deployments; pertinent history of improvised explosive device [IED] or other blast exposure; motor vehicle accidents; vehicle rollovers; significant mortar indirect fire; or rocket attacks that landed close to the service member; taking small-arms fire; seeing fellow service members who were injured or killed; treating wounded; attending to service members who were killed in action [KIA]; being injured in combat; awards received; pending disciplinary action and punishments; past disciplinary actions and punishments*):

SFC Example reported that he enlisted in the U.S. Army in 1999 because he wanted to serve his country and learn a valuable skill. All of his time served has been on

42

active duty. He has served on three combat deployments, all in support of Operation Iraqi Freedom (OIF; 2004–2005, 2006–2007 and 2009–2010). He endorsed numerous examples of small-arms engagements, seeing fellow service members who were injured and killed, treating wounded, and attending to service members KIA during each of his deployments. He denied a history of IED blast exposure, motor vehicle accidents in theater, HMMWV rollovers, significant mortar (IDF) or rocket attacks that landed close to him, or being injured in combat. SFC Example stated that he has performed well in his military career thus far, has never received a nonjudicial punishment or other disciplinary action, and until recently has typically gotten along well with peers and superiors. He has been awarded three Army Commendation Medals, one Army Achievement Medal, an Iraqi Campaign Medal, and a Global War on Terror Service Medal. SFC Example is pending end of obligated service in 2014, and per his report he hopes to attend college and study international finance.

Chief Complaint at Intake (*chief complaint at time of initial outpatient visit or inpatient hospitalization in the service member's own words*):

"Deployment stress"

History of Present Illness (*circumstances surrounding initial presentation of symptoms/stressors; current and past symptoms; frequency of symptoms; duration of symptoms*):

SFC Example was initially evaluated on 14 July 2010 when he presented on a walk-in basis to the Behavioral Health Clinic. SFC Example's chief complaint during that evaluation was "deployment stress" and he described numerous symptoms of anxiety and depression. During the initial evaluation, SFC Example stated that he had been feeling increasingly anxious and depressed since returning from a 12-month deployment in support of OIF in early 2010. SFC Example stated that his wife complained that he was "jumpy," on guard, and irritable, and that members of his extended family were concerned about his visible change in mood and behaviors. He stated that he was often on guard and fearful that he would be attacked. SFC Example also stated that he felt distant and detached from his wife and two young sons. He described trouble connecting with his wife and children and noted that he would often feel guilty for wanting to isolate himself from his family. Other symptoms endorsed included trouble falling asleep, nightmares (three to four per week), experiencing moments in which he would "zone out" and remember his deployment experiences, difficulties concentrating, avoidance of large crowds (including busy restaurants, classrooms, amusement parks, and church), avoidance of talking about his deployment experiences, and avoidance of driving on busy streets. He also noted periods of a depressed mood, never lasting more than 2 days at a time. He denied symptoms consistent with a mood disorder, mania, or psychosis during his initial presentation.

Present Condition/Review of Symptoms and Current Functional Status (*current psychiatric symptoms; required treatment; service member's ability to perform required duties; compliance with treatment*):

SFC Example completed a course of outpatient individual psychotherapy targeting symptoms of PTSD, monthly medication management appointments, and an intensive outpatient treatment program specifically for PTSD. A significant improvement was seen in his ability to manage his irritable moods and connect with family. However, he continues to complain of difficulties falling and staying asleep, nightmares, increased anxiety, increased arousal, difficulties with sustained attention and concentration, avoidance of thinking and speaking about his deployment experiences, avoidance of large crowds, and feeling fearful and on guard. These symptoms have impacted his occupational functioning, because he cannot perform the typical duties of an MP or standard administrative duties without extreme difficulties. His symptoms have also greatly impacted his social functioning; he has noted declines in his relationships with his extended family and friends, mainly attributed to his fearfulness and symptoms of avoidance. He has been compliant thus far with his treatment regimen, although avoidance of initial treatment was seen, and he has stated multiple times that he does want to continue with treatment. Future treatment recommendations include continued outpatient psychotherapy and medication management.

Mental Health History (*history of mental health diagnoses; history of mental health treatment; past hospital course; history of suicidal and/or homicidal ideations, intentions, urges, or plans; past disability rating; supporting data*):

SFC Example denied a significant history of diagnoses or treatment for mental health illnesses prior to July 2010 when he presented to the Behavioral Health Clinic. Supporting documents indicate that he has never been given a prior disability rating and per his report he has never sought treatment through the Veterans Administration (VA) system. SFC Example reported that he has never participated in individual psychotherapy as an adult but at age 7 he saw a child psychologist for three sessions. SFC Example reported that his mother wanted him to see a child psychologist to process some of his feelings following his parents' divorce. Records from this psychologist were unavailable. SFC Example stated that he has never had a mental health hospitalization. He went on to deny a history of suicidal ideations, intentions, plans, urges, or attempts. He further denied a history of homicidal ideations, intentions, urges, or plans.

Family Psychiatric History: (*family history of mental health diagnoses; family history of mental health treatment; family history of suicidal behaviors*):

SFC Example stated that his biological grandmother drank excessively throughout her adult years, and he described memories of seeing her intoxicated at family functions. He was unclear whether she ever received treatment for substance abuse. SFC Example denied any further history of mental illness or treatment for mental illness in his family. SFC Example also denied a family history of suicide and a family history of hospitalizations for mental health reasons.

Psychosocial History (*information related to birth and childhood; relevant childhood events [including abuse]; current relationships with parents and siblings; cur-*

rent sources of social support; current living arrangements, current information related to functioning in relationships):

SFC Example was born in Europe and raised throughout the northeastern United States. He is the youngest of five children. He described his childhood as "wonderful" until his parents divorced when he was 7 years old. He denied a history of physical, verbal, or sexual abuse as a child; however, he noted that he was often exposed to verbal arguments between his parents centered on their difficult financial situation. SFC Example described his father as a successful international salesman who often spent money on expensive cars, and his mother was a Spanish teacher who tutored middle school children. SFC Example noted that his parents had joint physical custody after their divorce; however, he spent most of his time with his mother because of his father's busy travel schedule. He noted that he performed well throughout grade school and into high school with the exception of the year that his parents divorced. SFC Example noted that his grades slipped and his teachers complained that he was preoccupied, which prompted his mother to consult with his pediatrician, who subsequently referred him to a child psychologist. SFC Example graduated from high school on time with a 3.65 grade point average (GPA), and he participated in band, drama club, and field hockey. He denied any behavioral difficulties during high school and noted that he got along well with classmates, teachers, and coaches. After high school graduation, he applied to three local universities and decided to enroll in Any Town University to study finance and play field hockey. He met his future wife during his first year of college and was married 8 months later. He completed 1½ years of college, obtaining a 3.0 GPA and making the field hockey team, before he was forced to leave school because his father could no longer afford the high tuition. At the urging of his field hockey coach, he spoke with an Army recruiter. He is currently married and has twin sons (6 years of age). His social support network includes his wife, Army buddies, siblings, and mother. He noted that during the past year he has been withdrawing from others and now only speaks with his friends and family when they stop in to his home unannounced. He stated that he has more than 16 voicemails from friends and family on his cell phone, which he has not returned. He also noted that his young sons complain that he no longer plays with them and his wife complains that he will not attend social functions with other families.

Legal History (*History of police contact and arrests*):

SFC Example stated that he has never been arrested. He did report that two months ago he received a ticket for failing to stop at a stop sign while driving home from work. He stated that he was distracted and wasn't paying attention when he ran the stop sign. He denied any other police contact, which is consistent with his command's report.

Substance Use/Abuse (*alcohol: include age of first use, past heavy use, current frequency and duration of use, and symptoms consistent with abuse or dependence; illicit drugs: include age of first use, past heavy use, current frequency and duration of use, and symptoms consistent with abuse or dependence; supplements,* *including workout supplements and energy drinks; caffeine; nicotine; misuse of over-the-counter [OTC] medications*):

- *Alcohol:* SFC Example noted that he first drank alcohol at the age of 18 while at a school party. He reportedly drinks two alcoholic beverages one to two times per week. He denied a history of heavy alcohol use and stated that seeing his grandmother's drinking was influential and taught him to avoid heavy alcohol use. He denied ever experiencing symptoms consistent with alcohol withdrawal or symptoms consistent with alcohol abuse or dependence.
- *Illicit drugs:* SFC Example stated that he smoked marijuana approximately six times with members of his field hockey team during his sophomore year of high school. He denied any further history of illicit drug use.
- *Supplements:* He denied current supplement use.
- *Caffeine:* He reported that he currently drinks six to seven cups of coffee per day. He stated that he drinks coffee because he believes that it will help him stay awake and "get through the day" without dozing off. He noted that he has also tried various energy drinks to help him stay awake throughout the day.
- *Nicotine:* SFC Example reported that he currently does not smoke cigarettes; however, he has tried chewing tobacco and uses one can of chewing tobacco per month.

Current Medications:

SFC Example is currently prescribed fluoxetine hydrochloride, 40 mg per day. He has previously been prescribed Citalopram and Zolpidem in the past, both of which have been discontinued.

Medical History (*current treatment for significant medical illnesses; history of major medical illnesses or treatment; history of head traumas or injuries; past disability rating*):

SFC Example is currently not receiving any treatment for significant medical illnesses. He does have a history of a tonsillectomy at the age of 13 and a surgery to repair a fractured right orbit after he was punched in the face during a fight at a grocery store 4 months ago. SFC Example denied any lasting pain resulting from the surgery and notes from his medical record indicate that he has fully recovered. He denied a history of head traumas and concussion.

Pain Assessment (*current pain*):

SFC Example denied current pain (0/10).

Mental Status Exam (*current*):

SFC Example arrived to his last appointment 15 minutes late and complaining that he overslept. He had dark circles under his eyes, was unshaven, and was dressed in his U.S. Army uniform of the day. He appeared his stated age, with multiple tattoos on his right arm. He walked without assistance and presented with some psychomotor agitation (leg tapping). He was awake, alert, and oriented to person, place, time, and situation. His speech was of normal rate, rhythm, prosody, and volume. He described his mood as "nervous" and his affect was mood congruent. His thoughts were logical, linear, and goal directed and focused on his current symptoms. There was no evidence of psychosis, and auditory, visual, olfactory, and tactile hallucinations were denied. Insight was fair. Judgment was fair and impulse control appeared intact during the session. Memory for past events appeared normal, and attention and concentration waned at times; however, he was responsive to redirection. Suicidal ideations, intentions, urges, or plans were consistently denied. Homicidal ideations, intentions, urges, or plans were also denied.

Suicidal/Homicidal Ideation Behavioral Review

SFC Example denied current suicidal or homicidal ideations, intentions, urges, or plans in our last session. During the initial evaluation, he also denied a history of suicidal or homicidal ideations, intentions, urges, or plans and described numerous deterrents to suicide, including a desire to see his children grow up, personal beliefs against suicide, and religious beliefs against suicide. He does not have a family history of suicide and does not have weapons at home. He was agreeable to following a clear safety plan should suicidal or homicidal ideations arise in the future.

Psychological Testing Results

SFC Example was administered a battery of psychological assessment measures on 23 August 2010: the Minnesota Multiphasic Personality Inventory–2-RF, the Millon Clinical Multiaxial Inventory, the Personality Assessment Inventory, and numerous self-report checklists. A full copy of these results is available in his electronic medical record.

Diagnosis

Axis I: Posttraumatic Stress Disorder

- ***Military Impairment*** (*clearly state how these symptoms impact the service member's occupational functioning and how current symptoms will likely impact the military mission; describe how the service member's symptoms impact ability to work in his or her MOS and whether impairment would be evident if he or she were moved to a new MOS*): SFC Example is unable to function fully in his current position as an MP. He will not be able to safely perform his role as an MP in a combat zone and has experienced continued difficulties with his duties in a garrison environment. He has trouble sleeping through the night, does not awake feeling rested, is easily distracted, has trouble focusing and concentrating when speaking to others and when writing reports, is often irritable, and experiences anxiety, which results in his leaving situations where more than three people are in attendance. He has been moved to an administrative position within his unit where he has fewer responsibilities and a more flexible schedule; however, he continues to have difficulties with interpersonal interactions and with writing. It is unlikely that another change in job responsibilities or change in MOS will be beneficial.

• *Social Impairment* (*clearly state how these symptoms impact the service member's family life, ability to attend school, ability to establish and maintain relationships*): SFC Example's family life has been greatly impacted by his current symptoms of PTSD. SFC Example noted that he has withdrawn from his wife, children, extended family, and friends. He stated that he loves his family very much and feels guilty that he has "cut off" others; however, he believes that he can no longer connect with those who were previously close with him. His interactions with his wife and children have improved while at home, but he continues to avoid social activities outside of the home, including his son's soccer games, the theater, and going out to a restaurant to eat. SFC Example enrolled in a course at the local community college, but dropped out because of the increased anxiety he felt around others in the classroom. He was able to successfully complete one online business course. Although his avoidant symptoms have been a target of treatment throughout the past year, he continues to struggle.

• *Treatment Plan:* It is recommended that SFC Example continue in weekly psychotherapy with a psychologist and continue to follow up for medication reviews on a monthly basis. His spouse has been given information regarding couple therapy and further resources for the family.

• *Barriers to Care:* SFC Example has avoided treatment in the past, and his ambivalence about attending psychotherapy was an impediment to treatment for the first month. His command has been flexible with his schedule and allowed him to attend all appointments as scheduled. When he transitions to a new provider in the VA system, his avoidance will likely need to be targeted.

Axis II: No Diagnosis on Axis II
Axis III: Noncontributory
Axis IV: Problems with Primary Support Group and Occupation
Axis V: Current Global Assessment of Functioning (GAF): 60
         GAF at intake: 50
         Highest in 12 months: 60

Administrative Recommendations:

Physical Evaluation Board

Recommendation for Medical Evaluation Board:

1. Is the service member considered fully competent to be discharged to his or her own custody?   YES
2. Are there past findings of incompetence or incapacitation?   NO
3. Is there pending disciplinary action, investigation, or administrative discharge pending?   NO
4. Is the service member considered fit to administer to his or her own financial and legal affairs?   YES

5. Is continued mental health treatment recommended during the processing of the board?   YES—see treatment plan

SIGNATURE OF WRITER

Specialty of Writer

Originating Department

CO-SIGNATURE

Specialty of Co-Signer

Department

CHAPTER 3

Assessment and Selection of High-Risk Operational Personnel

Identifying Essential Psychological Attributes

James J. Picano
Thomas J. Williams
Robert R. Roland

High-risk military personnel typically engage in critical and sensitive national security missions; employ nonroutine, nonstandard, or unconventional military tactics; deploy frequently and often for prolonged durations to denied or hostile environments in various cultural settings; operate fairly independently without much logistical or tactical support; and often encounter unknown and uncontrollable situational factors demanding ingenuity, expertise, initiative, and a high degree of common sense to avoid mission failure. Consequently, these personnel are often subjected to rigorous assessment and selection procedures in order to determine their suitability for high-risk military assignments.

The assessment and selection (A&S) of military personnel for high-risk jobs and special mission units is a central role of psychologists working in operational military settings (Staal & Stephenson, 2006; Williams, Picano, Roland, & Banks, 2006). Operational psychologists are often involved in either developing or providing direct input into A&S processes for individuals involved in high-demand and high-risk missions. Their involvement ranges from the identification, design, and development of A&S processes and procedures to program evaluation and validation of A&S decisions based on real-world operational outcomes.

Personnel who are especially well suited for high-risk operational occupations possess an identifiable set of core psychological attributes regardless of the specific mission or job they perform. Although these attributes may be essential to successful adaptation, they may not be sufficient for any one particular occupation because of additional unique mission requirements. However, such attributes represent the core of those required for success in high-risk operational positions, and their assessment is essential regardless of the position under consideration. In this chapter, we identify a number of these essential attributes from multiple sources: relevant published accounts of high-risk operational personnel; our experiences as operational psychologists within different operational assessment and selection programs; and the results of a survey of experts in the selection of special military populations conducted in the context of setting up a new A&S program for high-risk military personnel.

PSYCHOLOGICAL ASSESSMENT OF HIGH-RISK OPERATIONAL PERSONNEL

Personnel who must perform high-risk, nonroutine military duties under hazardous and demanding conditions almost always undergo stringent psychological A&S procedures. The goal of A&S is to evaluate the psychological fitness (Braun & Wiegand, 1991) of the applicants for unconventional military assignment. These high-risk operational personnel have in common special skills and abilities beyond those of their peers and pressure to perform "no-fail" missions under challenging or extreme environmental conditions (including combat). Common psychological A&S programs include those for military pilots (Turnbull, 1992; see also Hilton & Dolgin, 1991), military special operations forces (see, e.g., Stolrow, 1994), as well as personnel from other government agencies, such as astronauts (Santy, Holland, & Faulk, 1991). We differentiate these "special warriors" (Mountz, 1993) from other personnel whose positions demand reliability but with a lesser degree of environmental challenge, such as nuclear power plant operators, airline pilots, air traffic controllers, and most emergency services personnel (with the notable exceptions of police special operations personnel, bomb disposal personnel, and undercover agents). Personnel in these other "high-reliability" occupations (Flin, 2001) certainly have their own set of unique psychological demands. Other high-risk personnel who must work in isolated and/or confined environments (e.g., submariners, polar station inhabitants) probably occupy a borderland in our conceptualization, depending on how extreme and prolonged the environmental challenge (see Suedfeld & Steel, 2000, for a comprehensive discussion of issues related to these personnel).

Many military selection programs in the United States use the assessment center method for assessing and selecting high-risk operational personnel, the rich heritage of which dates back to World War II (Fiske, Hanfmann, MacKinnon, Miller, & Murray, 1948/1997; OSS Assessment Staff, 1948). Assessment centers comprise standardized evaluations of behavior by trained raters using multiple methods, including specially designed simulations with high job fidelity. Psychological evaluations occupy a central position in the assessment center method for high-risk operational personnel and constitute the most direct and distinguishing contribution of psychologists to these programs, although psychologists may play multiple key roles throughout the assessment center (Christian, Picano, Roland, & Williams, 2010).

Psychological evaluation in the selection of high-risk operational personnel typically comprises two stages: selecting out and selecting in (Suedfeld & Steel, 2000). In the selecting-out (or screening) phase, the assessment of psychological and emotional stability—that is, freedom from psychopathology and a minimal risk of developing psychological problems in the future—is of central concern. A&S screening procedures typically involve records reviews, psychological testing, and interviews. Some specialized high-risk military positions (e.g., sniper training) may depend entirely on a screening-out psychological selection process (e.g., screening out someone with high emotional instability using a personality inventory).

On the other hand, selecting in involves finding the best-suited candidates for the nature of the work. Put another way, select-in procedures are oriented to finding candidates with the complex skills and psychological attributes necessary for successful performance under unusually demanding conditions.

ESSENTIAL PSYCHOLOGICAL ATTRIBUTES FOR HIGH-RISK OPERATIONAL PERSONNEL

Psychological attributes necessary for successful performance in high-risk occupations are ideally identified a priori from a systematic job analysis. However, in our experience, attributes more often emerge from expert opinion or retrospectively from the empirical assessment of more general dispositions, qualities, or characteristics.

There is relatively little published in the psychological literature on the psychological attributes of successful high-risk operational personnel, because most organizations are understandably reluctant to expose the details of their A&S processes and procedures. For instance, many details for operational selection programs involving high-demand operational personnel are classified (a point made by Flin, 2001), and security concerns preclude the publication of data from such programs. Even when programs are not classified, the importance of maintaining the security of various A&S techniques and procedures results in reluctance among many psychologists to share the details of their efforts. This reluctance stems from both organizational and ethical considerations. First, psychologists involved in an A&S program have a legitimate ethical interest in preserving the integrity of the testing and assessment measures, consistent with both contractual and organizational interests (see, e.g., APA Ethics Code, 9.11, Maintaining Test Integrity; American Psychological Association, 2010). In most cases, the operational psychologists are consulting with an organization that has invested extensive resources into an A&S process and the psychologist, therefore, does not own the data. Measures and methods may lose their predictive value and utility as candidates gain information about the assessment process, either by word of mouth, access to scientific reports, or even repeated exposure (e.g., reapplying) to the assessment processes. In addition, psychologists who conduct specialized A&S are themselves operationally focused, and thus generally lack the time to engage in substantive research and rarely present formal data from their programs at scientific meetings. Whatever the reasons, there is a dearth of empirical literature identifying attributes for high-risk operational personnel. In addition, results that are available are rarely derived a priori through the use of job analyses or expert surveys. Most often, one encounters a scattering of studies of various personnel in high-risk occupations in which one group is contrasted with a reference sample from the general population (or a similar comparison group) on a number of personality and psychological characteristics in an attempt to establish a psychological "profile" for the personnel under study.

The first formal attempt in the U.S. military to identify and assess key psychological attributes for high-demand military operational personnel was the A&S program for the Office of Strategic Services (OSS) during World War II (Fiske et al., 1948/1997). Parenthetically, psychologists were involved in selection during World Wars I and II prior to the establishment of the OSS, but their efforts were primarily directed at the assessment of intelligence and other psychomotor skills (especially for military aeronautics; Resnick, 1997; see also Anastasi, 1988; Vane & Motta, 1984; Yoakum & Yerkes, 1920).

The OSS approach represented the first coherent effort in the United States to establish a structured method to assess qualities deemed necessary for successful performance of hazardous military duties. This ambitious project, begun toward the end of the war, comprised a set of processes and procedures designed to reveal significant aspects of personality functioning reflecting a recruit's potential to perform clandestine military operations, often deep behind enemy lines. It developed largely because prevailing selection methods (intelligence tests) proved ineffective in predicting success in the field among OSS operatives (Handler, 2001; OSS Assessment Staff, 1948). Led by Henry Murray, already prominent from his position as director of the Harvard Psychological Clinic, the OSS staff comprised some of the nation's foremost psychologists and psychiatrists of the time as well as others who went on to distinguished academic careers afterward (e.g., Donald Adams, Donald Fiske, Urie Bronfenbrenner, Kurt Lewin, O.H. Mowrer, Edward Tolman, Eugenia Hanfmann, and Morris Stein). The OSS A&S program was designed by these talented individuals in concert with military training specialists experienced in clandestine activities. However, they were almost certainly influenced by established selection programs in Germany and Great Britain (Handler, 2001).

As noted by the OSS staff (Fiske et al., 1948/1997; OSS Assessment Staff, 1948) and reinforced by Handler (2001), a number of factors made it difficult to identify specific attributes for assessment: There were no job analyses available; jobs varied widely; and often a candidate was later placed in a different position than that known to the staff at the time of assessment. As a result, the OSS staff decided that each candidate would be judged on a set of general dispositions, qualities, and abilities essential to the effective performance of the majority of assignments of OSS personnel overseas. In essence, these general qualifications became the core essential attributes of clandestine operations personnel, and were basic to the OSS assessment process regardless of the methods used to evaluate them. The seven general areas outlined by the OSS staff included motivation for assignment, energy and initiative, effective intelligence, emotional stability, social relations, leadership, and security. The OSS staff also evaluated additional special qualifications that were specific to one or two branches of the OSS, and added three of them to the list of general attributes: physical ability, observing and reporting, and propaganda skills (Fiske et al., 1948/1997; OSS Assessment Staff, 1948).

Kilcullen, Mael, Goodwin, and Zazanis (1999) identified individual attributes predicting effective on-the-job performance for U.S. Army Special Forces (SF) soldiers. Kilcullen et al. used a job analysis of SF positions conducted by Russell, Crafts, Tagliareni, McCloy, and Barkley (1994) as a basis for identifying attributes that were "best-bet" predictors of performance. In order to derive these, a group of psychologists and senior SF soldiers (subject matter experts) examined a wide array of attributes and identified 30 that were relevant to SF job performance. These critical individual attributes were broadly grouped into four categories: cognitive; communication; interpersonal, motivational, and character; and physical. *Cognitive* attributes included judgment and decision making, planning, adaptability, creativity, and specific cognitive skills (auditory, mechanical, spatial, math, and perceptual speed and accuracy). *Communication* attributes included reading and writing ability, language ability (learn new languages quickly), and communication abilities, verbal and nonverbal. *Interpersonal, motivational, and character* attributes included diplomacy, cultural adaptability, maturity (emotional stability), autonomy, team playership, dependability, initiative, perseverance, moral courage, motivational skills, and supervisory skills. Finally, *physical* attributes included swimming ability, flexibility and balance, strength, and endurance.

In attempting to assess which of the attributes were most predictive of successful performance among well-adapted SF soldiers, Kilcullen et al. (1999) used rationally developed bio-data scales that assessed similar though not exact constructs of the attributes they identified. Even in this relatively homogeneous sample, motivational attributes (cognitive flexibility, work motivation, achievement orientation) differentiated SF field performance.

Hartmann, Sunde, Kristensen, and Martinussen (2003) studied Norwegian naval special forces (NSF) candidates, searching for personality measures that predicted NSF training performance. They relied on both a job analysis and a description of the personal attributes required for success in NSF given by subject matter experts to select their measures and hypotheses. Of interest for our purposes are the attributes identified and reported in their article:

> The ideal marine aspirant was characterized as a highly gifted person, expressing above average emotional control, reality testing, and tolerance for stress. He has stamina, is able to quickly acquire theoretical knowledge and practical skills, can cope well with people, manages stress and ambiguity successfully, shows emotional stability, forms reasonable conclusions on the basis of sufficient evidence, and demonstrates goal-directed behavior based upon detached realistic judgments, and coherent cognition. (Hartmann et al., 2003, p. 88)

As part of an extended evaluation of a U.S. Air Force special duty assessment and selection program, Patterson, Brockway, and Greene (2004) described the critical attributes necessary for successful performance of high-risk operational aircrew duties. They identified the attributes in conjunction with a panel of experienced Air Force special duty personnel who primarily served in organizational leadership positions. Patterson et al. (2004) described 11 critical attributes for successful performance in Air Force special duty positions: emotional stability and stress tolerance; effective intelligence and problem-solving; motivation and commitment; integrity; attitudes toward and interactions with others; physical ability;

security; maturity and self-awareness; work ethic; flexibility; and positive impact of family. Of note, Patterson et al. (2004) found that assessment of an individual's overall suitability for assignment to special duty positions based upon a semistructured interview was correlated with later supervisor ratings for seven of the 11 attributes. Interestingly, supervisor ratings of attitudes and interactions with others, physical ability, work ethic, and flexibility (adaptability) were not related to the psychologists' recommendations, suggesting that certain attributes may have more predictive validity when assessed and/or observed over time.

Christian et al. (2010) described essential attributes for another sample of U.S. military elite: ground combat personnel undergoing A&S for unconventional military assignment. Attributes were derived using multiple methods in an extensive and extended job analysis involving interviews, focus groups, Q-sorts, and surveys with operational personnel as well as analysis of critical incidents of good/bad job performances. The essential attributes that they identified are remarkably similar to those reported by Patterson et al. (2004): adaptability; stress tolerance; physical ability; teamwork; integrity; initiative; effective intelligence; determination; dependability; and interpersonal skill.

Astronauts are an interesting group of high-risk operational personnel, comprising both military and civilian personnel, pilots and nonpilots, working within a quasi-military structure. There are two basic job classifications of astronauts: pilot and mission specialist. The skill requirements for these positions are quite different, and the mission profiles vary within the National Aeronautics and Space Administration. Not surprisingly, personnel wishing to become astronauts have quite different backgrounds and skills, and the subsequent performance demands are varied and multifaceted (Fogg & Rose, 1995). Thus, psychological assessment of the suitability of a candidate for astronautics demands an appraisal of general attributes that apply regardless of the specific position or mission profile.

In a review of astronaut selection criteria from projects Mercury through the space shuttle, Santy et al. (1991) found that qualities such as intelligence, drive, independence, adaptability, flexibility, motivation, emotional stability, and lack of impulsivity were necessary for success as an astronaut. Later work by Galarza and Holland (1999) identified 10 attribute areas that were required for success on both short- and long-duration space missions: family issues (ability to cope with long separations from family); performance under stressful conditions; group living skills (multicultural adaptability, humor); teamwork skills; self-regulation (emotional stability); motivation; judgment/decision making; conscientiousness (achievement, order, and integrity); communication skills (interpersonal, presentations, diplomacy); and leadership capability (decisive, flexible, motivate others).

Another nonmilitary group of high-risk operational personnel is under-cover law enforcement officers. These personnel are similar to the clandes-tine foreign operatives of the OSS in that they are required to misrepresent their identities and motives in performance of their duties (Girodo, 1997). The failure to do so effectively brings with it great risk to the mission and to one's life. Girodo (1997) conducted an analysis of attributes necessary for success as an undercover law enforcement agent. He found five categories that he concluded were "surprisingly similar to the dimensions of secret agent success identified by the OSS psychologists" (p. 247) approximately 60 years ago: nerve, daring, drive, and imagination; misrepresentation and tradecraft; good team interpersonal relations; adherence to rules and main-taining self-discipline; and stress resistance, mental health, and hardiness.

IDENTIFYING CORE ESSENTIAL ATTRIBUTES FOR HIGH-RISK OPERATIONAL PERSONNEL

In the aftermath of the September 11, 2001, terrorist attacks in the United States, two of us (JJP and RRR) served as consultants in the development of a specialized U.S. Department of Defense A&S program for military personnel possessing needed new capabilities in the Global War on Terror (GWOT). The positions carried with them a high need for security and behavioral reliability, multiple and extended separations from family, as well as performance of critical and sensitive missions under conditions of extreme threat.

In order to delineate core essential attributes, a list of more than 80 attributes, compiled from the literature as well as from materials accu-mulated in our experience with several special selection programs, were submitted to a panel of nine subject-matter experts for assessment. Our subject-matter experts had operational experience in one or more high-risk military operational organizations, and most were involved in the selec-tion and training of personnel for nonroutine and unconventional military positions. The panel members were asked to rate each of the attributes on a 5-point scale corresponding to how critical the attribute was for success-ful performance of high-risk military operations (5—absolutely essential, could not perform successfully without it; 1—unimportant to mission suc-cess). We considered an attribute as essential if it was rated as absolutely essential by at least five of the nine judges or if its average rating across all judges was greater than 4.0. We identified more than 40 essential individual attributes, conceptually grouped into seven broad categories comprising 20 different facets, as shown in Table 3.1 along with the overlap with attri-butes identified by others.

TABLE 3.1. Critical Attributes Identified by Subject-Matter Experts for Successful Performance of High-Demand Operational Jobs

Domain	Facet	Attribute	WWII clandestine operatives[a]	U.S. Army Special Forces soldiers[b]	U.S. Air Force special duty[c]	Norway naval special forces[d]	NASA astronauts[e]	Undercover law enforcement personnel[f]	High-risk military operational personnel[g]
Security	Operational security	Maintain operational security Avoid calling undue attention to oneself	X		X			X	X
Information processing	Observing and reporting	Report important information accurately and concisely Retain important information under pressure Extract important information under pressure Absorb new information quickly See beyond the surface appearance	X			X			X
Effective intelligence and reasoning	Planning	Plan and organize activities and resources to meet objectives Prioritize multiple critical tasks in a timely fashion	X	X					X
	Adaptability	Act promptly to changing demands; modify plans to fit situation	X	X	X	X	X	X	X
	Problem solving	Find novel ways to use resources at hand in solving problems—think outside the box Think creatively	X	X	X	X	X	X	
	Judgment	Assess risks, likely outcomes, and possible repercussions in problem-solving situations Carefully weight courses of action Be operationally patient—make the right decision	X	X	X	X	X		

58

Category	Trait	Description							
	Decisiveness	Make decisions in real time, under pressure, and meet operational deadlines			X			X	X
		Commit to a course of action							
	Communication	Listen effectively							
		Communicate well with others			X			X	X
Emotional stability	Composure	Demonstrate presence of mind, think and act promptly under stress			X	X	X	X	
		Be comfortable in high-pressure situations							
		Remain calm, composed, and in control of feelings and emotions under stress (e.g., fear, isolation, fatigue, detention)							
	Stress resilience	Be emotionally resilient, sturdy	X		X	X	X	X	X
		Tolerate difficulties and frustrations well							
		Be effective in an emergency or during periods of stress							
	Confidence	Be confident of abilities			X				
Initiative, motivation, and drive	Initiative	Be ambitious, motivated to advance and achieve	X		X	X	X	X	X
		Display initiative							
	Motivation	Be self-motivated and directed	X		X	X	X	X	
		Be self-sufficient and comfortable working alone							
		Be motivated by challenges							
	Perseverance	Persist, complete tasks despite boredom/distraction, hardship	X		X	X	X	X	
		Sustain a high level of effort over long periods of time despite hardships							

(cont.)

TABLE 3.1. (cont.)

Domain	Facet	Attribute	WWII clandestine operatives[a]	U.S. Army Special Forces soldiers[b]	U.S. Air Force special duty[c]	Norway naval special forces[d]	NASA astronauts[e]	Undercover law enforcement personnel[f]	High-risk military operational personnel[g]
Character	Self-discipline	Maintain self-discipline and self-control			X	X	X	X	X
	Dependability	Follow through on duties Be reliable		X	X	X	X		X
	Integrity	Own up to errors Accept responsibility for actions		X	X		X		X
	Moral courage	Do "the hard right thing"		X	X				
	Cooperation	Put group goals ahead of individual goals Share credit and accept blame	X	X	X	X	X	X	X
Physical ability	Fitness/stamina	Maintain physical readiness	X	X	X	X	X	X	X
			Add: Leadership ability; propaganda skills	*Add:* creativity; auditory, spatial, mechanical, math abilities; diplomacy, cultural adaptability; motivating others, supervising; swimming	*Add:* family stability; maturity and self-awareness		*Add:* leadership capability; family issues; teamwork skills	*Add:* nerve, daring; adherence to rules	

[a]Fiske et al. (1948/1997); [b]Kilcullen et al. (1999); [c]Patterson et al. (2004); [d]Hartmann et al. (2003); [e]Galarza and Holland (1999); [f]Girodo (1997); [g]Christian et al. (2010).

As is evident, there is considerable convergence regarding attributes essential for successful performance of high-risk operational positions. Most prominently, four attribute dimensions stand out as critical or essential across high-risk operational personnel over time (World War II to present day) and across cultures: stress resilience, adaptability, cooperation with others, and overall physical fitness and stamina.

Critical to successful performance of high-risk operational missions is psychological hardiness and stress tolerance. All of the accounts we reviewed emphasized some aspect of emotional stability, staying calm under pressure, effective performance under stress, and emotional control. In addition, adaptability—the ability to adapt to changing demands or circumstances—emerged across all of the samples. A third critical attribute area, cooperation, was captured by other terms such as teamwork ability or effective group interactions. It pertains to the degree to which the individuals are aware that they must work cooperatively with others and subordinate self-interest in order to accomplish goals. Finally, perhaps because high-risk operational occupations by definition involve extreme and unusual environmental and physical challenges, all of the samples stressed physical fitness and stamina.

To this listing we would add three other attribute areas that were identified by all but one of the samples: judgment, motivation, and initiative. Exercising good judgment and reasoning in decision making was described in various ways in most of the different accounts we reviewed, but certainly seems a critical part of effective functioning in high-demand operations. Likewise, nearly all of the descriptions emphasized the need for high intrinsic motivation, defined in terms of desire to perform a given mission, commitment to the work and organization, or patriotism. Initiative and self-sufficiency were also emphasized as important attributes. Notably, character or conscientiousness, described as, for example, such as integrity, moral courage, and dependability, emerged as a consistent predictor of on-the-job performance for modern-day selection programs in the United States (see, e.g., Barrick & Mount, 1991).

Two attribute areas identified in only two accounts were family stability and leadership, including supervising, and motivating others (Galarza & Holland, 1999; Kilcullen et al., 1999). Although it is tempting to see these areas as unique to the samples in which they were described, psychologists familiar with selecting high-risk operational personnel can easily appreciate their importance for success regardless of the specific mission. Especially in high-risk jobs involving repeated and extended deployments, the family's capacity to tolerate absences of the operational member directly impacts mission readiness and effectiveness. Family support programs are also important components of high-risk organizations. With respect to leadership, Flin (2001) asserts that "stress-resistance, decision making, and leadership skills are essential attributes" for high-reliability personnel (Flin, 2001, p. 254).

PERSONALITY CHARACTERISTICS OF HIGH-RISK OPERATIONAL PERSONNEL

Empirical studies of personality characteristics in high-risk operational personnel offer an additional way of identifying core attributes. The five-factor model (FFM) of personality (also known as the Big Five) has emerged as a useful framework for organizing and characterizing personality, especially with regard to predicting job performance (Barrick & Mount, 1991, 1993). It offers a comprehensive yet parsimonious approach that is replicable across different theoretical and assessment approaches (measures and sources), cultures, and languages. The FFM factors are (1) emotional stability, including stress tolerance, resilience, and freedom from negative emotionality; (2) extraversion, which comprises sociability, ambition, dominance, positive emotionality, and excitement seeking; (3) openness to experience or intellectance, which includes creativity, unconventionality, broad-mindedness, and receptiveness to inner life; (4) agreeableness, or an interpersonal stance of cooperation, trustfulness, compliance, and affability; and (5) conscientiousness, including dependability, achievement striving, organization, and planning.

Hogan and Lesser (1996) used the FFM as a way of framing the personality requirements for selecting personnel in hazardous occupations. On the basis of their review, they proposed emotional stability, conscientiousness, and openness to experience as important predictors of success in hazardous occupations.

A number of studies have contrasted various groups of high-risk operational personnel with normative samples on measures of personality in order to characterize the unique personality attributes of the sample. This method highlights the personality homogeneity of the personnel. The most developed literature involves military pilots.

Using the NEO Personality Inventory—Revised (NEO-PI-R; Costa & McCrae, 1992), a popular measure of the FFM, Callister, King, Retzlaff, and Marsh (1999) showed that U.S. Air Force (USAF) flight students were higher than the normative population in extraversion, and lower in agreeableness. They also scored higher than the normative sample on several facets of conscientiousness, such as achievement striving, dutifulness, and competence. Bartram (1995) found British student pilots to be higher than the normative population on FFM dimensions of emotional stability and extraversion.

Consistent findings across time and with different personality measures show that military pilots, regardless of gender, are more achievement oriented, outgoing, active, competitive, and dominant and less introspective, emotionally sensitive, and self-effacing than nonflying counterparts drawn from the general population (Ashman & Telfer, 1983; Callister et al., 1999, Fine & Hartmann, 1968; Picano, 1991; Retzlaff & Gibertini, 1987).

There also have been several personality studies of personnel who perform explosive ordnance disposal (EOD). Early studies using the 16PF (e.g., Cattell, 1964; Russell & Karol, 1994) to identify personality characteristics of successful bomb disposal operators found these personnel to have high levels of emotional control along with low levels of affiliation and to be more unconventional, and not bound by traditional thinking, than less experienced peers (Cooper, 1982). Using the Hogan Personality Inventory (HPI) with U.S. Navy EOD divers, Hogan and Hogan (1989) found these specialists to be more self-assured, well adjusted, agreeable, and adventuresome than referent groups from the general population.

Van Wijk and Waters (2001) used the 16PF to describe personality characteristics in South African Navy underwater sabotage device disposal (USDD) operators. According to their findings, USDD personnel were adventurous, assertive, self-assured, emotionally stable, and tough-minded. These personnel did not share the social distance found by Cooper (1982) among EOD personnel, a finding that Van Wijk and Waters (2001) attribute to the emphasis on teamwork in their sample and to differences in the larger population (divers) from which the USDD personnel were drawn.

As a whole, the findings suggest that personnel who perform explosive disposal share characteristics such as emotional stability, unconventional thinking, self-assurance, and adventure seeking. Sociability appears to vary by the sample studied.

In a study of U.S. NSF candidates, McDonald, Norton, and Hodgdon (1990) found that successful completers of demanding training differed from unsuccessful personnel on four dimensions of the HPI (which taps all of the dimensions of the FFM). Successful NSF candidates were more sociable (extraversion), emotionally stable, and likable (agreeableness) than unsuccessful candidates.

Contrasting successful and unsuccessful candidates for Norwegian NSF on dimensions of the FFM, Hartmann et al. (2003) found that both emotional stability and extraversion entered the logistic regression prediction equation. However, extraversion entered negatively, opposite that predicted and in contrast to the findings of McDonald et al. (1990).

Although somewhat variable, the personality findings with high-risk operational personnel do suggest some trends. When compared with the general population, personnel in high-risk operational positions are consistently higher in emotional stability and aspects of conscientiousness. Results for extraversion and agreeableness vary with the population under study. In general, high-risk populations tend to be higher than normative samples on facets of extraversion that tap boldness, dominance, and adventure seeking, with more variability on measures of gregariousness and sociability. Openness to experience does not figure prominently in findings, although successful performers in high-risk occupations tend not to be bound by traditional thinking. Darr (2011) provided empirical support for this narrative summary of findings on personality and military personnel in terms of work-related outcomes. In a meta-analysis of 20 independent military samples using the Self Description Inventory, based on the FFM of personality, Darr (2011) found that neuroticism (emotional stability) and conscientiousness—two of the Big Five factors—emerged as consistent predictors of work-related outcomes in military samples and in the range typically found in civilian occupations.

Although the broad dimensions of the FFM are helpful for examining general similarities and differences among high-risk personnel, much can be learned about the core as well as the unique personality attributes for different positions by looking at different facets of these broad domains. To illustrate this, we compare the patterns of normative differences on the NEO-PI-R for two samples: (1) USAF flight students (Callister et al., 1999) and (2) elite military personnel (mean age, 32 years) undergoing evaluation for suitability for high-stress, nonstandard positions (cf. Picano, Roland, Rollins, & Williams, 2006). All were extensively prescreened and passed medical, physical, occupational, and psychological standards. As Table 3.2 shows, candidates for high-demand positions differ from the general population in similar ways on a number of personality dimensions, suggesting core personality features or attributes for high-demand operational personnel. Descriptively, they appear resilient, dominant, assertive, and energetic. Reliable and responsible, they are competitive, with a strong drive for mastery and achievement. Tough-minded, they can be unsympathetic to the needs of others and manipulative when necessary. These characteristics are consistent with previous findings and expectations. Importantly, these two samples differ on a number of dimensions that might suggest personality attributes unique to their duties. For example, compared with the general population, flight students are more outgoing, gregarious, and receptive to inner emotional life, with more traditional values. Elite combat soldiers, relative to the general population, are lower in negative affectivity and more emotionally closed, methodical, and disciplined. It should be remembered that these findings pertain to candidates and not successful incumbents, although self-report FFM personality tests have not been robust predictors

TABLE 3.2. Differences from the General Population on the NEO-PI-R for Two Samples of High-Demand Operational Personnel

Domain	Male USAF flight students (n = 1,198)	Elite male U.S. soldiers (n = 340)
Neuroticism	Lower in Vulnerability	Lower in Vulnerability Anxiety Impulsiveness Depression Self-consciousness Anger
Extraversion	Higher in Excitement seeking Assertiveness Activity Gregariousness Positive emotions	Higher in Excitement seeking Assertiveness Activity
Openness to Experience	Higher in Actions Fantasy Feelings Ideas Lower in Values	Higher in Actions Lower in Fantasy Feelings Aesthetics
Agreeableness	Lower in Trust Straightforwardness Compliance Tender-mindedness Modesty	Higher in Trust Lower in Straightforwardness Compliance Tender-mindedness
Conscientiousness	Higher in Achievement striving Competence Dutifulness	Higher in Achievement striving Competence Dutifulness Self-discipline Deliberation

Note. Higher is greater than or equal to the 60th percentile for the normative sample. Lower is lower than or equal to the 40th percentile for the normative population.

of success in training for flight students (Martinussen, 1996) or for other high-risk operational military personnel (Hartmann & Grønnerød, 2009; Hartmann et al., 2003; Picano et al., 2002).

The FFM has helped make the dizzying array of personality attributes available for assessment more comprehensible by casting them within its nomological net, and has somewhat simplified the problem of developing an integrated formulation of personality, as recommended by the OSS staff. However, reliance on the FFM also raises the potential for oversimplification by ignoring other potentially useful formulations of personality (see, e.g., Block, 1995). For example, hardiness, a personality dimension related to psychological resilience, is not fully reflected in the Big Five dimensions (Bartone, Eid, Johnsen, Laberg, & Snook, 2009). Hardiness has been found to predict success in U.S. Army SF soldiers (Bartone, Roland, Picano, & Williams, 2008). Another personality construct not easily situated in the FFM is general self-efficacy. Derived from self-efficacy theory (Bandura, 1997), generalized self-efficacy reflects an enduring confidence in one's own abilities to meet situational demands. General self-efficacy was also shown to predict success in selection among U.S. Army SF candidates (Gruber, Kilcullen, & Iso-Ahola, 2009).

So-called projective personality measures, available to the staff of the OSS and long since abandoned by selection psychologists, appear to be again showing some promise for use in assessing high-risk operational personnel. Hartmann et al. (2003) studied Rorschach predictors of successful completion of NSF training among Norwegian candidates. Hartmann et al. (2003) focused on Rorschach variables thought to reflect psychological sturdiness under stress, reality testing, and deviant cognition. They found that Rorschach indices, but not self-report FFM scales, significantly predicted successful completion of NSF training.

Hartmann and Grønnerød (2009) tested an additional sample of Norwegian NSF candidates in an attempt to both replicate the initial study and extend Rorschach predictors using additional Rorschach indices tapping stress-related anxiety, self-criticism, and proneness to worry. In the initial study, Hartmann et al. (2003) administered the Rorschach under stress conditions (while the individual was undergoing training). Hartmann and Grønnerød (2009) varied their method so that participants were randomly assigned to one of two groups: one tested prior to training (i.e., calm test situation) and the second tested during the context of training (i.e., stressful test situation). This revised procedure allowed the investigators to test whether some Rorschach variables might have greater predictive validity under stress.

Results replicated those of the initial study: Selected Rorschach indices significantly predicted successful completion of NSF training, although the effect sizes were slightly lower than in the initial study. In addition, other

Rorschach indices also were significantly related to successful completion in the predicted direction. According to the Rorschach results, successful completion of NSF training was related to lower levels of inner tension and worry; more accurate perceptions of external reality; more logical and coherent ways of thinking; increased social adjustment; more accurate perceptions of others and more adequate interpersonal relationships; and higher levels of problem solving and general cognitive functioning. As in the Hartmann et al. (2003) study, FFM variables did not significantly predict successful completion of NSF training. Moreover, the Rorschach proved to be a better predictor of failing training (96%) than of passing training (23%). There were few significant differences in the Rorschach variables associated with the testing condition.

Picano et al. (2002) developed an index of responses to a sentence completion test (SCT) that reflected obvious attempts to avoid responding to the pull of the stems, which they termed "verbal defensiveness." In a sample of U.S. military personnel undergoing assessment for high-risk operational assignments, Picano et al. found that the number of defensive responses was higher among personnel who failed to complete a rigorous selection course.

In a second study involving another sample of elite military personnel, Picano, Roland, Williams, and Rollins (2006) found that candidates high in SCT verbal defensiveness were significantly less likely to complete a rigorous selection course for high-risk operational personnel, and were twice as likely as those low in verbal defensiveness to leave early in the course. In addition, candidates who were high in verbal defensiveness were rated lower by psychologists in psychological suitability for high-risk operational assignment after an extended interview.

CONCLUSION

Our purpose in this chapter was to highlight core psychological attributes among individuals who participate in high-demand, high-risk operational occupations. The picture that emerges from studies of personality as well as from reports using rationally developed a priori criteria is of an individual with exceptional stress tolerance, emotional stability, and physical fitness; a high degree of intrinsic motivation, initiative, and competitive drive; exceptional reliability and integrity; and sound judgment and reasoning under stress. Tough-minded and independent, such individuals may be more or less gregarious and interpersonally skilled. Although these core attributes may be helpful in the design of A&S programs for high-demand operational personnel, they are probably best considered necessary but insufficient for any one occupational group because of unique demands and functions.

Nevertheless, such core attributes can serve as the basis for establishing essential attributes for any high-demand operational position.

There is less convergence around the methods for assessing essential psychological attributes for high-demand personnel. Procedures range from the use only of psychological testing to select out candidates without the requisite emotional stability to the more complex and demanding assessment centers comprising structured interviews, psychological testing, and individual and group exercises to select in the best qualified applicants. In addition, psychological measures encompass a full range of cognitive and personality tests, including both self-report and performance personality measures.

Regardless of the nature of the program, there are some important considerations for assessment in specialized selection programs, all of which were identified by the OSS staff more than 60 years ago (OSS Assessment Staff, 1948). These include the principle of multiform procedures, defined as the use of many different kinds of evaluation techniques such as interviews and various tests; the use of lifelike tasks with operational fidelity that elicit essential attributes for the job as well an assessment of the candidate's potential for training; and the development of an integrated formulation of personality of the applicant (Fiske et al., 1948/1997; for a more detailed discussion, see Christian et al., 2010). Unfortunately, as Handler (2001) notes, these recommendations seem to have been forgotten with the emergence of the structured self-report personality test. In addition, following Campbell and Fiske (1959), each A&S process should consider and strive for a clear end state composed of a set of constructs for the types of traits or characteristics judged as important, along with a clear understanding of their interrelatedness, and use a variety of independent methods to then assess and predict success.

In this context, we urge the assessment of essential psychological attributes using tests and techniques that tap a wide array of personality characteristics, representing alternative models for conceptualizing personality, and the use of different measures and methods to assess similar constructs. It is only in consistent findings across different models and methods that an accurate portrait emerges of individuals who successfully engage in high-risk operational occupations.

FUTURE CONSIDERATIONS IN THE A&S OF HIGH-RISK OPERATIONAL PERSONNEL

Formal psychological A&S programs for high-risk military personnel are well established and have a long and distinguished history dating back in the United States to that developed by the OSS. There has been considerable growth in A&S programs over the past decade, with numerous specialized selection programs developed for the increased capabilities needed in the GWOT. We believe the future is equally bright. Continued expansion in the use of A&S programs brings with it new opportunities for operational psychologists. Still, challenges remain. For example, psychologists are often not involved in the initial stages of development of the program, and with urgent operational requirements, much of the initial groundwork such as job analyses and validation efforts is often neglected (Christian et al., 2010). To some extent, the attributes and personality characteristics we outline are useful starting points for assessment. Still, there is no shortcut to the development of a sound A&S program for high-risk operational personnel. Moving forward, operational psychologists should strive to insert themselves earlier in the development process.

We also note that, perhaps because of the increased use of psychological assessment in the selection of high-risk personnel, we are working with much better informed consumers of our services, who are increasingly asking tough methodological questions regarding predictive validity of measures and methods, demanding empirical support for psychological recommendations, and requesting the use of assessment methods and results in solving more strategic personnel issues. We expect this will continue to influence practice. For instance, personality tests have gained considerable respect in personnel selection in the past three decades owing to findings from meta-analytic studies (e.g., Barrick & Mount, 1991), and their use in military personnel selection is generally well accepted. However, other parts of the selection process, such as interviews, simulations and exercises, and other assessment techniques, have received less empirical attention in military selection programs. Operational psychologists are well advised to attend to issues of data and program validation and to systematically collect and analyze data in order to build the evidence basis for the methods and procedures they use and the operational selection decisions they recommend.

REFERENCES

American Psychological Association. (2010). *Ethical principles of psychologists and code of conduct.* Retrieved February 5, 2011, from *www.apa.org/ethics/ code/index.aspx.*

Anastasi, A. (1988). *Psychological testing* (6th ed.). New York: Macmillan.

Ashman, A., & Telfer, R. (1983). Personality profiles of pilots. *Aviation, Space, and Environmental Medicine, 54,* 940–943.

Bandura, A. (1997). *Self-efficacy: The exercise of control.* New York: Freeman.

Barrick, M. R., & Mount, M. K. (1991). The Big Five personality dimensions and job performance: A meta-analysis. *Personnel Psychology, 44,* 1–26.

Barrick, M. R., & Mount, M. K. (1993). Autonomy as a moderator of the relationship between the Big Five personality dimensions and job performance. *Journal of Applied Psychology, 78,* 111–118.

Bartone, P. T., Eid, J., Johnsen, B. H., Laberg, J. C., & Snook, S. A. (2009). Big Five personality factors, hardiness, and social judgment as predictors of leader performance. *Leadership and Organization Development Journal, 30*(6), 498–521.

Bartone, P. T., Roland, R. R., Picano, J. J., & Williams, T. J. (2008). Psychological hardiness predicts success in U.S. Army Special Forces candidates. *International Journal of Selection and Assessment, 16*(1), 78–81.

Bartram, D. (1995). The predictive validity of the EPI and 16PF for military flying training. *Journal of Occupational and Organizational Psychology, 68,* 219–236.

Block, J. (1995). Going beyond the five factors given: Rejoinder to Costa and McCrae (1995) and Goldberg and Saucier (1995). *Psychological Bulletin, 117*(2), 226–229.

Braun, P., & Wiegand, D. (1991). The assessment of complex skills and of personality characteristics in military services. In R. Gal & D. Mangelsdorff (Eds.), *Handbook of military psychology* (pp. 37–61). New York: Wiley.

Callister, J. D., King, R. E., Retzlaff, P. D., & Marsh, R. W. (1999). Revised NEO Personality Inventory profiles of male and female U.S. Air Force pilots. *Military Medicine, 164,* 885–890.

Campbell, D. T., & Fiske, D. W. (1959). Convergent and discriminant validation by the multitrait-multimethod matrix. *Psychological Bulletin, 56,* 81–105.

Cattell, R. B. (1964). *Handbook of 16 PF.* Savoy, IL: Institute of Personality and Ability Testing.

Christian, J. R., Picano, J. J., Roland, R. R., & Williams, T. J. (2010). Guiding principles for selecting high-risk operational personnel. In P. T. Bartone, B. H. Johnsen, J. Eid, J. M. Violanti, & J. C. Laberg (Eds.), *Enhancing human performance in security operations: International and law enforcement perspectives* (pp. 121–142). Springfield, IL: Charles C Thomas.

Cooper, C. (1982). Personality characteristics of successful bomb disposal experts. *Journal of Occupational Medicine, 24,* 653–655.

Costa, P. T., Jr., & McCrae, R. R. (1992). *Revised NEO Personality Inventory: Professional manual.* Odessa, FL: Psychological Assessment Resources.

Darr, W. (2011). Military personality research: A meta-analysis of the Self Description Inventory. *Military Psychology, 23,* 272–297.

Fine, P. M., & Hartman, B. O. (1968). *Psychiatric strengths and weaknesses of typical Air force pilots* (SAM-TR-68-121). San Antonio, TX: U.S. Air Force School of Aerospace Medicine, Brooks Air Force Base.

Fiske, D. W., Hanfmann, E., MacKinnon, D. W., Miller, J. G., & Murray, H. A. (1997). *Selection of personnel for clandestine operations: Assessment of men.* Laguna Hills, CA: Aegean Park Press. (Original work published 1948)

Flin, R. (2001). Selecting the right stuff: Personality and high-reliability occupations. In R. Hogan & B. R. Roberts (Eds.), *Personality psychology in the workplace* (pp. 253–275). Washington, DC: American Psychological Association.

Fogg, L. F., & Rose, R. M. (1995). Use of personal characteristics in the selection of astronauts. *Aviation, Space, and Environmental Medicine, 66*, 199–205.

Galarza, L., & Holland, A. (1999). *Critical astronaut proficiencies required for long-duration spaceflight* (SAE Technical Paper 1999-01-2097). Washington, DC: Society of Automotive Engineers.

Girodo, M. (1997). Undercover agent assessment centers: Crafting vice and virtue for importers. *Journal of Social Behavior and Personality, 11*(5), 237–260.

Gruber, K. A., Kilcullen, R. N., & Iso-Ahola, S. E. (2009). Effects of psychosocial resources on elite soldiers' completion of a demanding military selection program. *Military Psychology, 21*(4), 427–444.

Handler, L. (2001). Assessment of men: Personality assessment goes to war by the Office of Strategic Service Assessment Staff. *Journal of Personality Assessment, 76*(3), 558–578.

Hartmann, E., & Grønnerød, C. (2009). Rorschach variables and Big Five scales as predictors of military training completion: A replication study of the selection of candidates to the naval special forces in Norway. *Journal of Personality Assessment, 91*(3), 254–264.

Hartmann, E., Sunde, T., Kristensen, W., & Martinussen, M. (2003). Psychological measures as predictors of training performance. *Journal of Personality Assessment, 80*, 87–98.

Hilton, T. F., & Dolgin, D. L. (1991). Pilot selection in the military of the Free World. In R. Gal & A. David Mangelsdorff (Eds.), *Handbook of military psychology* (pp. 81–101). Oxford, UK: Wiley.

Hogan, J., & Lesser, M. (1996). Selection of personnel for hazardous performance. In J. Driskell & E. Salas (Eds.), *Stress and human performance* (pp. 195–222). Hillsdale, NJ: Erlbaum.

Hogan, R., & Hogan, J. (1989). Noncognitive predictors of performance during explosive ordnance training. *Military Psychology, 1*, 117–133.

Kilcullen, R. N., Mael, F. A., Goodwin, G. F., & Zazanis, M. M. (1999). Predicting U.S. Army Special Forces field performance. *Human Performance in Extreme Environments, 4*, 53–63.

Martinussen, M. (1996). Psychological measures as predictors of pilot performance. *Internal Journal of Aviation Psychology, 6*, 1–20.

McDonald, D. G., Norton, J. P., & Hodgdon, J. A. (1990). Training success in U.S. Navy Special Forces. *Aviation, Space, and Environmental Medicine, 61*, 548–554.

Mountz, T. (1993). Special warriors, special families and special concerns. In F. W. Kaslow (Ed.), *The military family in peace and war* (pp. 121–129). New York: Springer.

OSS Assessment Staff. (1948). *Assessment of men.* New York: Rinehart.

Patterson, J. C., Brockway, J., & Greene, C. (2004). *Evaluation of an Air Force special duty assessment and selection program* (Contract F41624-00-6/1001/0001). San Antonio, TX: Conceptual MindWorks.

Picano, J. J. (1991). Personality types among experienced military pilots. *Aviation, Space, and Environmental Medicine, 62*, 517–520.

Picano, J. J., Roland, R. R., Rollins, K. D., & Williams, T. J. (2002). Development and validation of a Sentence Completion Test measure of defensive responding in military personnel Assessed for nonroutine missions. *Military Psychology,* *14,* 279–298.

Picano, J. J., Roland, R. R., Williams, T. J., & Rollins, K. D. (2006). Sentence Completion Test Verbal defensiveness as a predictor of success in military personnel. *Military Psychology, 18*(3), 207–218.

Resnick, R. J. (1997). A brief history of psychology–expanded. *American Psychologist, 52,* 463–468.

Retzlaff, P. D., & Gibertini, M. (1987). Air Force pilot personality: Hard data on the right stuff. *Multivariate, Behavioral Research, 22,* 383–389.

Russell, M., & Karol, D. (1994). *16PF fifth edition: Administrator manual* (2nd ed.). Savoy, IL: Institute for Personality and Ability Testing.

Russell, T. L., Crafts, J. L., Tagliareni, F. A., McCloy, R. A., & Barkley, P. (1994). *Job analysis of Special Forces jobs* (ARI Research Note 96-76). Alexandria, VA: U.S. Army Research Institute for the Behavioral and Social Sciences.

Santy, P. A., Holland, A. W., & Faulk, D. M. (1991). Psychiatric diagnoses in a group of astronaut applicants. *Aviation, Space, and Environmental Medicine, 62,* 969–973.

Staal, M. A., & Stephenson, J. A. (2006). Operational psychology: An emerging subdiscipline. *Military Psychology, 18*(4), 269–282.

Stolrow, J. P. (1994). The assessment and selection of Special Forces qualification course candidates with the MMPI. *Dissertation Abstracts International, 55*(6), 2413B.

Suedfeld, P., & Steel, G. D. (2000). The environmental psychology of capsule habitats. *Annual Review of Psychology, 51,* 227–253.

Turnbull, G. (1992). A review of pilot selection. *Aviation, Space, and Environmental Medicine, 63,* 825–830.

Van Wijk, C., & Waters, A. H. (2001). Psychological attributes of South African Navy underwater sabotage device disposal operators. *Military Medicine, 166,* 1069–1073.

Vane, J. R., & Motta, R. W. (1984). Group intelligence tests. In G. Goldstein & M. Hersen (Eds.), *Handbook of psychological assessment* (pp. 100–116). New York: Pergamon.

Williams, T. J., Picano, J. J., Roland, R. R., & Banks, L. M. (2006). Introduction to operational psychology. In C. H. Kennedy & E. A. Zillmer (Eds.), *Military psychology: Clinical and operational applications* (pp. 193–214). New York: Guilford Press.

Yoakum, C. S., & Yerkes, R. M. (1920). *Army mental tests.* New York: Henry Holt.

CHAPTER 4

Assessment and Management of Acute Combat Stress on the Battlefield

Bret A. Moore
Shawn T. Mason
Bruce E. Crow

The concept of stress is one that is very familiar to the service member. From the first days of recruit training, leaders spend countless hours covering the topic. They distinguish between the different types of stress. They present graphs explaining the "perfect," or optimal, balance of stress with extremes of inactivity (i.e., too little stress) and overload (i.e., too much stress). And when appropriate they purposefully induce high levels of stress during training in order to simulate battlefield conditions and test performance (Franken & O'Neil, 1994; Harris, Hancock, & Harris, 2005; Salas, Priest, Wilson, & Burke, 2006; see also Chapter 12, this volume).

Although at times seen as excessive by the individual service member, the military's seemingly obsessive penchant for stress awareness and education and realistic training is quite appropriate. Gleaned from decades of studying the effects of both acute and prolonged periods of stress, military leaders have recognized that stress has a far-reaching influence on the battlefield (Jones, 1995a; Sladen, 1943; see also Chapter 1, this volume). Stress can decrease the performance of, and even disable, the individual service member and overwhelm the entire unit. It can dampen morale, create an environment for poor decision making, and even lead to refusal of orders. In short, it can negatively impact the overall military mission. However, at times the opposite is overlooked or neglected: Stress has many positive influences. It can initiate a cascade of neurochemicals that can help focus the mind, prepare the body for a difficult task, and promote a general sense of well-being (Contrada & Baum, 2010).

In this chapter, we address the important issues of evaluating and managing acute combat stress on the battlefield. After brief reviews of the history of battlefield stress and the impact of acute stress on the service member during combat, we provide a detailed review of stress assessment and the provision of psychoeducational, psychological, and pharmacological interventions.

HISTORY OF BATTLEFIELD STRESS

A detailed account of the history of battlefield stress is beyond the scope of this chapter (see Figley & Nash, 2007, and Jones, 1995b, for more comprehensive reviews as well as Chapter 1, this volume). Here we provide a brief review of the history of the terminology used and progress made in understanding battlefield stress over the centuries.

Acknowledgment of the wide-reaching impact of the psychological injuries of war can be traced back to early antiquity. However, it was not until the mid-18th century that an attempt was made to apply a diagnostic label to this phenomenon: "nostalgia." Originally called "Swiss disease" after it appeared in Swiss villagers who were involuntarily placed in rogue armies, military leaders began to recognize that an unexplained collection of physical and psychological symptoms prevented their men from fighting (Moore & Reger, 2007). Jones (1995a) provided an excerpt from Rosen (1975) in his account of Leopold Auenbruger's 18th-century description of this phenomenon. Auenbruger wrote:

> When young men who are still growing are forced to enter military service and thus lose all hope of returning safe and sound to their beloved homeland, they become sad, taciturn, listless, solitary, musing, full of sighs and moans. Finally, they cease to pay attention and become indifferent to everything which the maintenance of life requires of them. (Rosen, 1975, p. 344)

In 1871, J. M. Da Costa, an Army physician during the U.S. Civil War, wrote about a condition known as *irritable heart*. The condition was characterized by what we now describe as classic panic symptoms (e.g., racing heart, nausea, sweating, chest pain). Da Costa (1871) also noticed that many of the soldiers improved just by removing them from the forward lines and allowing them to rest, hence the first documentation of the success of one basic combat stress management principle used today.

The terms *shell-shock* and *battle fatigue* have also been used to describe stress on the battlefield and are still used in current vernacular. These terms are precursors to today's formal diagnostic criteria of post-traumatic stress disorder (PTSD; American Psychiatric Association, 2000) which was added to the *Diagnostic and Statistical Manual of Mental Disorders* (DSM) in 1980. However, PTSD represents a longer-term, ongoing condition (e.g., lasting 30 days or more) and only addresses the immediate responses of *fear, helplessness, or horror* to stressors (DSM Criterion A). The current clinical diagnoses addressing responses to stress in the shorter period after an event (e.g., < 30 days) are acute stress reaction (ASR; World Health Organization, 1992) and acute stress disorder (ASD; American Psychiatric Association, 2000). However, for the purposes of this chapter and the specific and immediate window of time being addressed, the generally accepted nonclinical term is combat stress (CS) or combat and operational stress (COS).

At this point, it should be noted that the focus of this chapter is not to sift through the various definitions and diagnoses associated with acute stress that occurs on the battlefield. To do so would complicate the ultimate intent of the chapter, which is to help the wide range of providers better evaluate and treat service members in the deployed setting. Therefore, we use the broad concept of acute combat stress except when assessment and intervention strategies are uniquely germane to a particular concept (e.g., reviewing evidence-based strategies for ASD). The reader is referred to Isserlin, Zerach, and Solomon (2008) for an intriguing and informative review of how ASR, ASD, and combat stress response fit together within the larger context of acute stress theory and practice.

EFFECTS OF ACUTE COMBAT STRESS ON THE SERVICE MEMBER

Acute combat stress, as defined in this chapter, is the short-term activation of the stress response on the battlefield, which immediately sends physical and psychological clues to the person that a threat is imminent and can have residual effects of various degrees for weeks. It occurs in service members who have suffered a serious psychological event during combat operations, such as being in a vehicle when hit with an improvised explosive device (IED), coming under small-arms fire, having to perform emergency first aid on the severely wounded, or witnessing the injury or death of a fellow service member in battle. In popular terms, it is referred to as the fight-or-flight system, which is governed by the sympathetic and parasympathetic divisions of the autonomic nervous system (Robertson, 2004). By definition, it is intense in nature and short in duration and can be reactivated by various stimuli (see Barlow, 2004, for a comprehensive review of anxiety and panic).

The impact of acute combat stress on service members varies considerably (Bonanno, 2005; Kelly & Vogt, 2009). Some individuals can become incapacitated and unable to function, which can have grossly negative consequences if this it occurs during enemy contact. For others, the shock to the system can propel them to perform selfless and heroic acts as if overtaken by an unknown force. Most service members fall somewhere in the middle of these two reactions, and the stress reaction may persist for days or weeks (Grossman & Christensen, 2007). Regardless of the individual differences in reacting to acute stress, common symptoms and reactions may be seen, both positive and negative.

Adaptive Acute Stress Effects during Combat

Activation of the stress response on the battlefield can be a highly protective event. Physiologically, several important things happen, which translate to adaptive responses on the battlefield. The most salient are presented next.

Catecholamine Surge

Norepinephrine, epinephrine, and dopamine, the most abundant catecholamines in the nervous system, facilitate immediate physical reactions associated with a preparation for violent muscular action. This surge accelerates the heart, which pumps blood at a greater velocity and ensures that all the vital organs are provided for so that the body can defend itself or retreat (Goldstein, Eisenhofer, & McCarty, 1998). In combat, this immediate surge of catecholamines can provide a greater level of strength, excitement, and aggression, all of which are needed when confronting an enemy threat. It is notable, however, that epinephrine and norepinephrine have also been components of the reexperiencing symptoms associated with ASD and PTSD (McNeil & Morgan, 2010), indicating a trade-off at times in the response to life-threatening and traumatic stimuli.

Liberation of Energy

Once the acute stress response is activated, the body releases stored glucose and fat for the purpose of supporting increased energy (Scanlon & Sanders, 2006). With increased fuel available to the muscles, the individual is able to react with more force and agility. This energy release, in combination with increased blood flow and catecholamine release, allows for adaptive maneuvers on the battlefield, such as sprinting short distances, scaling walls, or carrying/dragging heavy loads for short distances.

Faster Reflexes

During acute stress, the speed of the person's reflexes, both innate and learned, is increased (Goldstein et al., 1998). Increased reaction time can be the most critical factor when it comes to protecting oneself or others from a threat on the battlefield. This is part of the rationale of overlearning in the military. In an attempt to override any instinct to freeze during an attack, defensive and aggressive tactics are continuously rehearsed during training so that the more adaptive learned instincts will be chosen, albeit unconsciously.

Memory and Learning

Stress hormones play an important role in memory functioning (Lupien et al., 2002), and acute stress promotes associative learning and classical conditioning (Joëls, Pug, Wiegert, Oitzl, & Krugers, 2006; Shors, Weiss, & Thompson, 1992). Therefore, it has been proposed that acute stress can facilitate more effective decision making and aid in memory formation. If true, this could prove invaluable for service members during periods of acute stress associated with combat exposure. However, this is not a uniform phenomenon, and it is important to note that while some memory and learning processes may be enhanced, acute stress and chronic stress have their drawbacks on the process as well. Operational demand-related cognitive decline, the "decrements in cognitive performance or decision making resulting from the manifold pressures or acute stressors characteristic of extreme environments" (McNeil & Morgan, 2010, p. 363), is described as a normal and expected process in many military environments.

Less Adaptive Acute Stress Effects during Combat

As indicated earlier, the stress response can be a double-edged sword for the service member on the battlefield. The same processes that support adaptive behavior during stressful situations are also responsible for less adaptive ones.

Panic

Probably the most well-known battlefield reaction to acute stress is panic, or "freezing," commonly played out in television dramas as an overwhelmed service member under intense combat strain who becomes immobilized in his foxhole or behind the remnants of a battle-scarred building in an urban war zone. Although this certainly happens, the frequency of this type of reaction is actually quite low and varies widely in severity. For example, a Marine Corporal who had been shot and was still engaged in the firefight noted that another Marine, a Lance Corporal, during the same firefight screamed "I've been shot" and sat down and stopped firing. The Corporal yelled at him, "We're all shot! Just fire back!" which was all the Lance Corporal needed to get back in the battle. The other extreme of the response can result in nonfunction. For example, immediately after their vehicle hit an IED, a Marine was convinced that his Sergeant, who was unharmed, had been killed. The Marine became catatonic and nonresponsive and had to be medically evacuated from the battlefield. It is important to note that, with immediate intervention, the Marine's psychological condition cleared within 3 hours and he returned to his unit in a full-duty status 48 hours later. (More on interventions is presented later).

Tunnel Vision and Auditory Exclusion

Two sensory events than can happen during periods of acute stress are tunnel vision and auditory exclusion (Bremner, 2005; LeDoux, 1996). As its name implies, tunnel vision is the narrowing of one's peripheral vision. It is caused by blood leaving the head and being redistributed to other areas of the body, which are critical for defense. Also related to blood flow, auditory exclusion, sometimes referred to as tunnel hearing, involves a temporary filtering of irrelevant external noise. In theory, tunnel vision and auditory exclusion could be viewed as adaptive (e.g., allow for greater focus on threat); however, the ability to identify additional threats via peripheral vision and hear verbal commands clearly is critical on the battlefield.

ASSESSMENT OF ACUTE COMBAT STRESS ON THE BATTLEFIELD

Clinicians in practice on the battlefield primarily specialize in rapid assessment and disposition of patients under difficult conditions (Linnerooth, Mrdjenovich, & Moore, 2011). As much as they try to categorize "typical" reactions and homogenize assessment and intervention strategies, individual variability and highly fluid situations can make rapid assessment difficult. In general, for practical assessment purposes, acute battlefield stress can be viewed in two ways: immediate stress (present time) and postimmediate stress (within a few hours to a few weeks).

Immediate Stress Reaction

A number of terms are used to describe the immediate responses to a major stressor, among them *psychological shock, acute crisis reaction*, and *peritraumatic stress response*. However, these terms have been used inconsistently and have implications that either do not apply to the context or do not readily account for the range of responses observed on the battlefield. Thus, we use the term *immediate stress reaction* to describe the array of stress reactions that occur during combat.

Immediate stress reaction is a useful means of conceptualizing the truly acute psychological and physiological consequences of trauma on the battlefield, particularly with regard to battlefield psychological triage. When assessing a service member in such a situation, the corpsman/medic must assess two things: orientation and functionality. In other words, the field medical asset must perform a brief mental status examination. Regarding orientation, the clinician asks questions such as "What is your name?", "Do you know where you are?", and "What is your serial/social security number?" If the service member is oriented at the most basic level, it is then important to increase the complexity of the questions: for example, "What just happened?" "What should you do next?" It is important that that the clinician only assess a potentially severe reaction but also, as a normal course of the evaluation, orient the service member and provide information as to what happened. The medic/corpsman will have information regarding any other wounded, and often this is the service member's primary concern (i.e., "Is everyone okay?" "Is my best friend okay?"). The provision of accurate information in this stage can be critical to the outcome of the event for the service member.

Regarding functionality, it is the clinician's responsibility to ensure that the service member is able to continue with his or her mission safely and, if not, to consider medical evacuation from the battlefield. The service member should be checked for deficiencies in gait, tremulousness in hands, irregularities in breathing patterns (e.g., hyperventilation), and so on. The service member's level of activity should also be evaluated. A slow and lethargic or overly excitable and impulsive presentation can put the service member, as well as those around him or her, at risk of harm. It is important to note that service members will, as a normal course, exhibit hyperarousal, possibly pressured speech, and other reactions following a life-threatening event. These do not typically result in the need for battlefield evacuation. Not uncommonly, hyperarousal—combined with the need to talk— often results in the service member spontaneously recounting the entire event, including the most traumatic parts. This can be capitalized on in the immediate and postimmediate reaction phases but must be carefully managed.

Finally, it is imperative that the service member's state of mind be assessed. Does the service feel he or she can continue with the mission safely? Is his or her next choice of action logical (e.g., providing perimeter security while an injured service member is being evacuated from the "hot zone")? Is the service member overcome with fear?

It is important to understand that the ultimate goal is to keep the service member and the other members of the unit safe. Differential diagnoses, processing of the event, and quality of life are of little relevance in the immediate phases of acute stress on the battlefield.

Post-Immediate Stress

Post-immediate stress is a way to understand the effects of combat stress within the first hours to weeks following an intense exposure on the battlefield and while the service member is still in the combat zone. When assessing the service member during this period, it is important to be aware of differential diagnoses, risk to self or others, mission readiness, and the need for follow-up evaluation. This stage begins at the time of arrival to a higher echelon of combat zone care or once the service member/unit is out of immediate harm's way.

Differential Diagnoses

After some degree of stability has been attained, it is important to determine whether the service member's symptoms are typical and expected or are indicative of a potentially more serious problem, such as a chronic mental health disorder exacerbated by the combat experience (e.g., major depressive disorder or preexisting PTSD), an acute psychotic or acute stress disorder, or the effects of a physical injury (e.g., blast concussion). Many people equate combat stress and ASD. However, these are different entities. ASD is a diagnosable clinical disorder and is characterized by the development of severe anxiety, dissociation, and other symptoms within 1 month after exposure to an extreme traumatic stressor. Often, individuals with ASD show decreased emotional responsiveness, increased apathy, fatigue, and many other affective, cognitive, and physical symptoms. Although CS/COS, ASD, and PTSD have considerable symptom overlap (Isserlin et al., 2008), the dissociative nature of ASD and the timeline of symptoms are the primary defining characteristics. The DSM includes a review of diagnostic criteria for ASD (American Psychiatric Association, 2000).

It is also important to be aware that because of the relatively high rate of preexisting PTSD and acute concussion in service members (Tanielian & Jaycox, 2008) as well as the overlap of various symptoms (Kennedy et al., 2007; Vasterling, Verfaellie, & Sullivan, 2009), diagnostic accuracy can be difficult. Therefore, close attention to symptom presentation and history is crucial. (See Chapter 8 of this volume for more information on blast concussion.)

In addition to mental health and medical disorders, the presentation of any given service member in a war zone is compounded by environmental and physiological stressors (U.S. Department of the Army, 1994; see Table 4.1).

Once it has been determined that there are no other causes for the symptoms or symptoms have been parsed out from other diagnoses or conditions (e.g., blast concussion, dehydration), in general, reactions in both the immediate and post-immediate reaction phases are placed under the umbrella of CS/COS. This refers to any stress that occurs during the course of combat-related duties, whether as a result of enemy action or other sources, and is not initially considered pathological.

CS/COS has been described as what happens when a person experiences a normal reaction to what would be considered an abnormal experience. The service member may manifest many different stress symptoms within four specific areas (Moore & Reger, 2007): physical (e.g., fatigue/exhaustion, numbness and/or tingling in extremities, nausea/vomiting,

TABLE 4.1. Physical and Mental Stressors in the Combat Zone

Physical stressors	Mental stressors
Environmental	Cognitive
Heat, cold, or wetness	Information: too much or too little
Vibration, noise, blast	Sensory overload versus deprivation
Hypoxia, fumes, poisons, chemicals	Ambiguity, uncertainty, isolation
Directed energy weapons/devices	Time pressure versus waiting
Ionizing radiation	Unpredictability
Infectious agents/diseases	Rules of engagement, difficult judgments
Skin irritants or corrosives	Organizational dynamics
Physical work	Hard choices versus no choices
Bright light, darkness, haze, and obscuration	Recognition of impaired functioning
Difficult or arduous terrain	
Physiological	Emotional
Sleep debt	Fear and anxiety-producing threats
Dehydration	Grief-producing losses
Malnutrition, poor hygiene	Resentment, anger, and rage
Muscular and aerobic fatigue	Boredom-producing inactivity
Impaired immune system	Conflicting motives
Overuse or underuse of muscles, organ systems	Spiritual confrontation or temptation causing loss of faith
Illness or injury	Interpersonal feelings

Note. From U.S. Department of the Army (1994).

insomnia, psychomotor agitation); cognitive (e.g., difficulties in concentration, memory loss, nightmares, flashbacks, depersonalization); emotional (e.g., fear and hopelessness, mood lability, anger); and behavioral (e.g., misconduct, carelessness, impulsivity).

It is important to note that there is an expectancy that with time and basic intervention, the symptoms present in both the immediate and post-immediate phases will remit and the service member will continue with his or her duties. In extreme cases, however, the service member may fail to improve and may require more extensive treatment or medical evacuation from the combat theater. However, regarding the latter, this assessment should only be made once the service member has had a period of stabilization and continued evaluation. Unnecessary evacuation from the combat theater for a psychological injury can potentially have lasting effects on the service member's morale, confidence, and overall psychological health (Jones, 1995a).

The accepted nomenclature for CS/COS intervention is based on the principles of BICEPS: brevity, immediacy, centrality, expectancy, proximity, and simplicity. Brevity refers to the importance of brief and targeted treatment; immediacy stresses the positive benefits of intervening early; centrality ensures that the service member maintains communication and connection with his or her unit peers and superiors as a means to stay connected to the mission; expectancy acknowledges the transient nature of the symptoms; proximity allows the service member to stay close to his or her unit during recovery; and simplicity stresses the importance of keeping focused and pragmatic goals, such as returning the service member back to his or her unit or minimizing the use of medication. In sum, BICEPS recognizes the importance of focusing on existing strengths, refrains from placing the service member in the "sick" role, and views reconstruction, reorientation, and reintegration as the main objectives in recovery (U.S. Department of the Army, 2009).

Risk

Every mental health provider, civilian or military, must possess the core competencies of suicide and homicide risk assessment and management (Moore, Hopewell, & Grossman, 2009; Rudd, Cukrowicz, & Bryan, 2008). On the battlefield, these competencies will be tested.

The first days and weeks after a stress reaction can be emotionally charged and confusing for the service member. Therefore, it is imperative that the battlefield clinician be cognizant of the service member's psychiatric history, level of connection with others, presence of guilt and/or remorse, and relationships with leadership and peers among other possible factors that could potentially contribute to suicidal ideation. If the service member does become suicidal, swift and decisive action should be taken (see American Psychiatric Association, 2003; Rudd, 2009).

In addition to assessing suicidal behavior, it is also important to assess homicidal ideation. Although it is known that severe combat exposure can increase physical aggression postdeployment (Kilgore et al., 2008) and increased hostility and anger are associated with posttraumatic stress symptoms in returning service members (Elbogen et al., 2010), little is known about aggression and hostility in the days following a severe stress episode. However, in our experience, thoughts of hurting local innocent civilians, particularly if the service member or his or her fellow troops were attacked, are not uncommon. Consequently, precautions should be taken. For example, in some of the combat hospitals there is no segregation of locals from injured service members in the emergency rooms and/or on the ward. In this scenario, it may be very difficult for a service member to revert immediately to a position of not feeling threatened when surrounded by local male civilians who dress identically to the individuals responsible for his or her hospitalization. The reader is referred to Moore et al. (2009) for further information on the assessment and management of violence in the service member.

Return to Duty

Although responsibilities are vast, a general guideline is that during a time of war the battlefield clinicians' job often comes down to determining "fit for duty" or "not fit for duty" (Linnerooth, Mrdjenovich, & Moore, 2011). Can the senior noncommissioned officer, grieving for a service member killed in action, return to the battlefield? Can the newly minted lieutenant overcome with fear continue to lead his men after narrowly escaping an ambush? Will the combat medic/corpsman be able to provide care on the battlefield after watching his best friend die, unable to save him? Unfortunately, there are no clear guidelines for clinicians with regard to such decision making. Therefore, they must rely on their clinical training, experience, and knowledge of the service member's occupational specialty and the overall mission.

Follow-Up

Following the service member closely during the first few weeks is important. Manifestation of some symptoms can be delayed, whereas others that were relatively mild in the beginning can worsen. Although the clinician will unlikely have any useful baseline data except for the mental status exam, more formal data collection at this point can be helpful if the service member experiences a subsequent traumatic episode or decompensates at a later time in the deployment. It is also important to note that most providers now have access to the Theater Data Management System, and clinical notes from prior deployments are available in the combat zone.

MANAGEMENT OF COMBAT STRESS
ON THE BATTLEFIELD

As detailed previously, the primary goal when dealing with an immediate stress reaction is to ensure the service member's safety. The following sections provide recommendations for the first few hours to weeks after the stress reaction (during the post-immediate stress period).

Psychoeducation

The use of psychoeducation in the military to prevent and treat psychiatric problems has a long and prominent history. It is provided to service members in all branches of the military before, during, and after deployment and comes in various forms such as tip cards, slide shows, formal and informal briefings, leadership training, and videos. Furthermore, it is a primary component of the CS/COS model of early and nonpathological focused intervention (U.S. Department of the Army, 1994), the Battlemind training program (WRAIR Land Combat Study Team, 2006), the Operational Stress Control & Readiness program (Hoyt, 2006), the U.K. Trauma Risk Management program (e.g., Royal Air Force, 2009), and disaster response (see Chapter 7, this volume), as well as one aspect of psychological debriefing (PD; for a review, see Rose, Bisson, Churchill, & Wessely, 2002).

Wessely and colleagues (2008) identified five primary assumptions that support the foundation of psychoeducation. First, it is believed that if people are educated about what symptoms they may experience subsequent to a trauma, the symptoms will be less disturbing to them. Second, people are less distressed by their symptoms when they receive reassurance that what they are experiencing is normal and that many people experience some difficulties following traumatic experiences—in short, that they are experiencing a normal response to an abnormal event. Third, people may be propelled to ask for and receive help because of the knowledge gleaned from the educational intervention. Fourth, psychoeducation may actually provide more adaptive corrective information that challenges maladaptive views of oneself or the event. Finally, psychoeducation increases self-efficacy and empowers people to take ownership of their recovery and draws on their inner resiliency.

Psychoeducation during the immediate aftermath of an extreme stressor on the battlefield promotes a sense of safety, calmness, and cohesion (if provided in a group format) and instills hope. These are all principles outlined by Hobfoll et al. (2007) as necessary in the early stages of disaster intervention. The provision of psychoeducation can be easily applied in an individual or group setting. However, it is important to note that providing psychoeducation in a group format is not the same as conducting a PD. Clinicians should be flexible and not prescriptive in the provision of services during the early aftermath of trauma (Litz, 2008). In sum, psychoeducation that focuses on typical reactions to stress, the natural tendency to recover, and resources for help if symptoms persist appears to be the most prudent method for minimizing the early effects of acute stress.

For example, a Marine was medically evacuated to a combat hospital for shrapnel injuries after a rocket attack. During his acute evaluation, he exhibited pressured speech. After admission to the open bay ward, he exhibited hyperstartle every time a door or drawer was closed, relived the experience as if watching a movie of it repeatedly, and exhibited open hostility toward an injured local male who was on the same ward. These reactions were considered common, and brief intervention focusing heavily on psychoeducation was implemented. The Marine was provided psychoeducation regarding the normalcy and origin of his hyperstartle (and that it would be present to some degree until after redeployment), education about how to address the reexperiencing symptoms so that he could sleep, and information that the local male was not a terrorist and had also been wounded in the same terrorist attack. His psychoeducation was administered jointly by a psychologist and a psychiatric technician, who also arranged for command and peer visitation and the use of a satellite phone to call home.

Cognitive Therapy

The primary strategy of cognitive therapy (CT) with trauma victims is to provide them the opportunity to identify, critically examine, and change the way they view the traumatic event and the meanings and implications of the trauma as related to self and others (Litz & Bryant, 2009).

Unfortunately, there is little evidence to support using CT strategies in the first days and weeks after a stress reaction, certainly none with service members on the battlefield. What the literature does show, however, is that CT is effective in reducing posttraumatic stress symptoms within the first several months of exposure (Ehlers et al., 2003; Echeburúa, de Corral, Sarasua, & Zubizarreta, 1996).

Freeman and Moore (2009) discuss how, in general, service members are ideal candidates for cognitive-behavioral therapy (CBT). CBT is active, directive, goal oriented, time limited, and structured, all which are consistent with military culture. Furthermore, it can be approached from a single-session perspective. There is a beginning, middle, and end to each session. Based on the same principles of CBT, particularly the latter, it is reasonable to assume that CT would be a useful and effective approach in alleviating the acute combat stress symptoms in service members during the first few days and weeks. Most likely the clinician will have limited contact with the service member, which means that any contact within a clinical context must be maximized. Considering that many early interventions are "one-shot" events, a single structured CT session that assists the service member in making sense of the event and that directly challenges maladaptive thoughts may prove beneficial. Possible CT interventions are provided in Table 4.2.

Prolonged Exposure Therapy

Prolonged exposure (PE) is a CBT-based treatment that is gaining much attention in military clinical and research circles. PE includes four primary components: (1) imaginal exposure, (2) *in vivo* exposure, (3) psychoeducation related to common reactions to trauma, and (4) breathing retraining (Peterson, Foa, & Riggs, 2011). The typical PE treatment protocol is 10 to 12 individual sessions, each 90 -minutes in length; however, there can be considerable flexibility in the actual number used. The sessions can be conducted once or twice weekly, which is an added benefit considering potential time constraints working with service members in a combat zone.

As with CT and psychoeducation, the number of studies on the use of PE during the early stages of acute stress is limited. To our knowledge, only three case studies in the literature report using PE with combat-related posttraumatic symptoms. Two (Nacasch et al., 2007, 2011) were conducted

TABLE 4.2. Cognitive Therapy Interventions during Acute Stress

Questioning the evidence	"How do you know your friend would still be alive if you had reacted faster?"
Reattribution	"It wasn't your fault. Horrible things happen in war."
Examining options	"What other things can you do besides focus on your friend's death?"
Decatastrophizing	"What is the worst thing that could happen if you talked with someone about how you're feeling?"
Turning adversity to advantage	"How can this make you stronger?"
Direct disputation	"I disagree that you are powerless and have no control over your situation. You've overcome difficult obstacles in the past."

with veterans with combat-related PTSD and the third was conducted with active-duty military personnel in Iraq who met criteria for ASD (Cigrang, Peterson, & Shobitz, 2005). The results of all three studies showed significant improvement in symptoms.

The Cigrang et al. (2005) case study is informative in that it provided evidence of a modified four-session PE format that was more intensive in nature. Prior to initiating PE therapy, the three military personnel who received the treatment were at risk of being medically evacuated from the combat theater because of their symptoms. After treatment, they were able to remain in theater and continue with their mission.

It is reasonable to assume that a modified form of PE, similar to the one just mentioned, may be a viable intervention choice for service members suffering from posttraumatic stress symptoms within weeks, if not days, of exposure. However, because of the lack of data supporting the use of PE in this manner, caution should be taken, and service members should not be pushed to emotionally engage in traumatic material unless they are ready. Furthermore, this modified use of PE in this situation should be limited to clinicians with significant experience with the treatment approach.

Pharmacotherapy

The use of psychoactive medication with service members is a highly controversial topic in the military today. Much of the controversy stems from a proposed correlation between the increase in psychiatric medication use by service members and the increasing suicide rate in the military. Granted, there are risks with the use of psychiatric medications in deployed settings; however, the lack of use when indicated likely incurs more problems.

Generally, the literature does not support the use of medications in the immediate and post-immediate periods of stress. However, in certain situations, pharmacotherapy can be useful. Specifically, in extreme cases of hyperarousal or panic, benzodiazepines (e.g., lorazepam) and certain beta blockers (e.g., propranolol) can reduce these symptoms. Results from a small study of victims of terrorism support this approach (Jiménez, Romero, Diéguez, & Aliño, 2007). It should be noted, however, that research has shown that benzodiazepines can hinder CT interventions for a variety of disorders, including anxiety disorders (Sammons & Levant, 1999; Sammons & Schmidt, 2001). Therefore, if at all possible, benzodiazepines should not be the first-line choice for intervention during an ASR.

Sleep medications (e.g., zolpidem, trazodone) can be effective in restoring both quantity and quality of sleep. However, it should be noted that people taking these medications should be able to dedicate a sufficient amount of time (6–8 hours) to sleep, as a "hangover" effect may be present upon waking. Thus, for service members who are likely to be roused in the night for a mission, these medications may not be the most prudent choice (Moore & Krakow, 2009).

FINAL THOUGHTS

A major responsibility of any behavioral health clinician who works with service members in the deployed setting is the assessment and management of acute stress. The military clinician should have a firm understanding of the different types of stressors that service members encounter during combat operations and which interventions are most appropriate to help deal with those stressors. The good news is that proper assessment and management are well within the knowledge area and skill set of most trained behavioral health clinicians. With careful thought, reassurance, and focus on the best psychological interests of the service member, acute stress on the battlefield can be managed and psychological health protected.

REFERENCES

American Psychiatric Association. (2000). *Diagnostic and statistical manual of mental disorders* (4th ed., text rev.). Washington, DC: Author.

American Psychiatric Association. (2003). *Practice guideline for the assessment and treatment of patients with suicidal behaviors.* Arlington, VA: Author.

Barlow, D. H. (2004). *Anxiety and its disorders: The nature and treatment of anxiety and panic* (2nd ed.). New York: Guilford Press.

Bonanno, G. A. (2005). Resilience in the face of potential trauma. *Current Directions in Psychological Science, 14*, 135–138.

Bremner, J. (2005). Effects of traumatic stress on brain structure and function: Relevance to early responses to trauma. *Journal of Trauma and Dissociation, 6*, 51–68.

Cigrang, J. A., Peterson, A. L., & Schobitz, R. P. (2005). Three American troops in Iraq: Evaluation of a brief exposure therapy treatment for the secondary prevention of combat-related PTSD. *Pragmatic Case Studies in Psychotherapy, 1*, 1–25.

Contrada, R., & Baum, A. (2010). *The handbook of stress science: Biology, psychology and health.* New York: Springer.

Da Costa, J. M. (1871). On irritable heart; a clinical study of a form of functional cardiac disorder and its consequences. *American Journal of the Medical Sciences, 61*, 17–52.

Echeburúa, E., de Corral, P., Sarasua, B., & Zubizarreta, I. (1996). Treatment of acute posttraumatic stress disorder in rape victims: An experimental study. *Journal of Anxiety Disorders, 10*, 185–199.

Ehlers, A., Clark, D. M., Hackmann, A., McManus, F., Fennell, M., Herbert, C., et al. (2003). A randomized controlled trial of cognitive therapy, a self-help booklet, and repeated assessments as early interventions for posttraumatic stress disorder. *Archives of General Psychiatry, 60,* 1024–1032.

Elbogen, E. B., Wagner, H. R., Fuller, S. R., Calhoun, P. S., Kinneer, P. M., Mid-Atlantic Mental Illness Research, Education, and Clinical Center Workgroup, et al. (2010). Correlates of anger and hostility in Iraq and Afghanistan war veterans. *American Journal of Psychiatry, 167*(9), 1051–1058.

Figley, C., & Nash, W. (2007). *Combat stress injury: Theory, research, and management.* New York: Routledge/Taylor & Francis Group.

Franken, J., & O'Neil, H., Jr. (1994). Stress induced anxiety of individuals and teams in a simulator environment. In H. F. O'Neil, Jr., & P. M. Drillings (Eds.), *Motivation: Theory and research* (pp. 201–218). Hillsdale, NJ: Erlbaum.

Freeman, A., & Moore, B. A. (2009). Theoretical base for treatment of military personnel. In S. M. Freeman, B. A. Moore, & A. Freeman (Eds.), *Living and surviving in harm's way: A psychological treatment handbook for pre- and post-deployment of military personnel* (pp. 171–192). New York: Routledge/Taylor & Francis Group.

Goldstein, D. S., Eisenhofer, G., & McCarty, R. (1998). *Catecholamines: Bridging basic science with clinical medicine.* San Diego, CA: Academic Press.

Grossman, D., & Christensen, L.W. (2007). *On combat: The psychology and physiology of deadly conflict in war and in peace* (2nd ed.). Millstadt, IL: PPCT Research.

Harris, W., Hancock, P., & Harris, S. (2005). Information processing changes following extended stress. *Military Psychology, 17,* 115–128.

Hobfoll, S., Watson, P., Bell, C., Bryant, R., Brymer, M., Friedman, M., et al. (2007). Five essential elements of immediate and mid-term mass trauma intervention: Empirical evidence. *Psychiatry: Interpersonal and Biological Processes, 70,* 283–315.

Hoyt, G. B. (2006). Integrated mental health within operational units: Opportunities and challenges. *Military Psychology, 18,* 309–320.

Isserlin, L., Zerach, G., & Solomon, Z. (2008). Acute stress response: A review and synthesis of ASD, ASR, and CSR. *American Journal of Orthopsychiatry, 78,* 423–429.

Jiménez, J., Romero, C., Diéguez, N., & Aliño, J. (2007). Pharmacological treatment of acute stress disorder with propranolol and hypnotics. *Actas Españolas de Psiquiatría, 35*(6), 351–358.

Joëls, M., Pu, Z., Wiegert, O., Oitzl, M. S., & Krugers, H. J. (2006). Learning under stress: How does it work? *Trends in Cognitive Sciences, 10,* 152–158.

Jones, F. D. (1995a). Psychiatrics lessons of war. In F. D. Jones, L. R. Sparacino, V. L. Wilcox, & J. M. Rothberg (Eds.), *Textbook of military medicine* (pp. 1–33). Falls Church, VA: Office of the Surgeon General, U.S. Department of the Army.

Jones, F. D. (1995b). Traditional warfare combat stress casualties. In F. D. Jones, L. R. Sparacino, V. L. Wilcox, J. M. Rothberg, & J. W. Stokes (Eds.), *War psychiatry* (pp. 35–61). Washington, DC: Borden Institute.

Kelly, M., & Vogt, D. (2009). Military stress: Effects of acute, chronic, and traumatic stress on mental and physical health. In S. M. Freeman, B. A. Moore,

& A. Freeman (Eds.), *Living and surviving in harm's way: A psychological treatment handbook for pre- and post-deployment of military personnel* (pp. 85–106). New York: Routledge/Taylor & Francis Group.

Kennedy, J. E., Jaffee, M. S., Leskin, G. A., Stokes, J. W., Leal, F. O., & Fitzpatrick, P. J. (2007). Posttraumatic stress disorder and posttraumatic stress disorder-like symptoms and mild traumatic brain injury. *Journal of Rehabilitation Research and Development, 44*, 895–920.

Kilgore, W. D., Cotting, D. I., Thomas, J. L., Cox, A. L., McGurk, D., Vo, A. H., et al. (2008). Post-combat invincibility: Violent combat experiences are associated with increased risk-taking propensity following deployment. *Journal of Psychiatric Research, 42*, 1112–1121.

Le Doux, J. E. (1996). *The emotional brain.* New York: Simon Schuster.

Linnerooth, P. J., Mrdjenovich, A. J., & Moore, B. A. (2011). Professional burnout in clinical military psychologists working with service members: Challenges and recommendations, before, during, and after deployment. *Professional Psychology: Research and Practice, 42*(1), 87–93.

Litz, B. (2008). Early intervention for trauma: Where are we and where do we need to go?: A commentary. *Journal of Traumatic Stress, 21*, 503–506.

Litz, B., & Bryant, R. (2009). Early cognitive-behavioral interventions for adults. In E. B. Foa, T. M. Keane, & M. J. Friedman (Eds.), *Effective treatments for PTSD: Practice guidelines from the International Society for Traumatic Stress Studies* (2nd ed., pp. 117–135). New York: Guilford Press.

Lupien, S. J., Wilkinson, C. W., Brière, S., Ménard, C., Ng Ying Kin, N. M., & Nair, N. P. (2002). The modulatory effects of corticosteroids on cognition: Studies in young human populations. *Psychoneuroendocrinology, 27*, 401–416.

McNeil, J. A., & Morgan, C. A. (2010). Cognition and decision making in extreme environments. In C. H. Kennedy & J. L. Moore (Eds.), *Military neuropsychology* (pp. 361–382). New York: Springer.

Moore, B. A., Hopewell, C. A., & Grossman, D. (2009). Violence and the warrior. In S. M. Freeman, B. A. Moore, & A. Freeman (Eds.), *Living and surviving in harm's way: A psychological treatment handbook for pre and postdeployment of military personnel* (pp. 307–327). New York: Routledge.

Moore, B. A., & Krakow, B. (2009). Characteristics, effects, and treatment of sleep disorders in service members. In S. M. Freeman, B. A. Moore, & A. Freeman (Eds.), *Living and surviving in harm's way: A psychological treatment handbook for pre- and post-deployment of military personnel* (pp. 281–306). New York: Routledge/Taylor & Francis Group.

Moore, B. A., & Reger, G. M. (2007). Historical and contemporary perspectives of combat stress and the Army Combat Stress Control Team. In C. R. Figley & W. P. Nash (Eds.), *Combat stress injury: Theory, research, and management* (pp. 161–182). New York: Routledge/Taylor & Francis Group.

Nacasch, N., Foa, E. B., Fostick, L., Polliack, M., Dinstein, Y., Tzur, D., et al. (2007). Prolonged exposure therapy for chronic combat-related PTSD: A case report of five veterans. *CNS Spectrums, 12*, 690–695.

Nacasch, N., Foa, E. B., Huppert, J. D., Tzur, D., Fostick, L., Dinstein, Y., et al.

(2011). Prolonged exposure therapy for combat- and terror-related posttraumatic stress disorder: A randomized control comparison with treatment as usual. *Journal of Clinical Psychiatry, 72,* 1174–1180.

Peterson, A. L., Foa, E. B., & Riggs, D. S. (2011). Prolonged exposure therapy. In B. A. Moore & W. E. Penk (Eds.), *Treating PTSD in military personnel: A clinical handbook* (pp. 42–58). New York: Guilford Press.

Robertson, D. (2004). *Primer on the autonomic nervous system* (2nd ed.). San Diego, CA: Academic Press.

Rose, S. C., Bisson, J., Churchill, R., & Wessely, S. (2002). Psychological debriefing for preventing post traumatic stress disorder (PTSD). *Cochrane Database of Systematic Reviews, 2,* DC000560.

Rosen, G. (1975). Nostalgia: A forgotten psychological disorder. *Psychological Medicine, 5,* 340–354.

Royal Air Force. (2009). *Stress handbook: TRiM.* London: Air Media Centre.

Rudd, M. (2009). Depression and suicide: A diathesis–stress model for understanding and treatment. In S. M. Freeman, B. A. Moore, & A. Freeman (Eds.), *Living and surviving in harm's way: A psychological treatment handbook for pre- and post-deployment of military personnel* (pp. 239–258). New York: Routledge/Taylor & Francis Group.

Rudd, M., Cukrowicz, K., & Bryan, C. (2008). Core competencies in suicide risk assessment and management: Implications for supervision. *Training and Education in Professional Psychology, 2,* 219–228.

Salas, E., Priest, H. A., Wilson, K., & Burke, C. S. (2006). Scenario-based training: Improving military mission performance and adaptability. In A. B. Adler, C. A. Castro, & T. W. Bitt (Eds.), *Military life: The psychology of serving in peace and combat: Volume 2. Operational stress* (pp. 32–53). Westport, CT: Praeger Security International.

Sammons, M., & Levant, R. (1999). *Combined psychosocial and pharmacological treatments.* New York: Plenum.

Sammons, M., & Schmidt, N. (2001). *Combined treatment for mental disorders: A guide to psychological and pharmacological interventions.* Washington, DC: American Psychological Association.

Scanlon, V. C., & Sanders, T. (2006). *Essentials of anatomy and physiology.* Philadelphia: Davis.

Shors, T. J., Weiss, C., & Thompson, R. F. (1992). Stress-induced classification of classical conditioning. *Science, 257,* 537–539.

Sladen, F. (1943). *Psychiatry and the war: A survey of the significance of psychiatry and its relation to disturbances in human behavior to help provide for the present war effort and for post-war needs.* Oxford, UK: C. C. Thomas.

Tanielian, T., & Jaycox, L. H. (Eds.). (2008). *Invisible wounds of war: Psychological and cognitive injuries, their consequences, and services to assist recovery.* Santa Monica, CA: RAND Center for Military Health Policy Research.

U.S. Department of the Army. (1994). *FM 22-51, leaders' manual for combat stress control.* Washington, DC: Author.

U.S. Department of the Army. (2009). *FM 6-22.5, combat and operational stress control manual for leaders and soldiers.* Washington, DC: Author.

Vasterling, J., Verfaellie, M., & Sullivan, K. (2009). Mild traumatic brain injury and posttraumatic stress disorder in returning veterans: Perspectives from cognitive neuroscience. *Clinical Psychology Review, 29,* 674–684.

Wessely, S., Bryant, R., Greenberg, N., Earnshaw, M., Sharpley, J., & Hughes, J. (2008). Does psychoeducation help prevent posttraumatic psychological distress? *Psychiatry: Interpersonal and Biological Processes, 71,* 287–302.

World Health Organization. (1992). *International classification of diseases* (10th rev.). Geneva, Switzerland: Author.

WRAIR Land Combat Study Team. (2006). *Battlemind training.* Walter Reed Army Institute of Research. Retrieved from *www.battlemind.army.mil.*

CHAPTER 5

Posttraumatic Stress Disorder, Depression, and Other Psychological Sequelae of Military Deployment

Greg M. Reger
Nancy A. Skopp

More than 2 million military service members have deployed in support of Operation Enduring Freedom (OEF) and Operation Iraqi Freedom (OIF) since the attacks of September 11, 2001. These deployments increase the risk of combat exposure and often impose a number of psychosocial stressors, resulting in a growing number of behavioral health problems among previously deployed military personnel. Posttraumatic stress disorder (PTSD), depression, and substance abuse are frequently acknowledged as common problems, but there are a range of additional psychological sequelae as well. After a brief discussion of the stressors common to the deployment experience, we review the psychological challenges facing single service members, common difficulties associated with postdeployment family life, and the psychosocial challenges of the postdeployment transition period. We then review relevant literature on the treatment of deployment-related PTSD, depression, and substance abuse.

Military deployments change the warrior. These changes can manifest in numerous ways, perhaps as unique as each individual who deploys. It is also true that there are common postdeployment difficulties that many warriors experience. In general, military personnel adjust well and effectively transition to new missions, duty stations, or civilian roles. Some, however, face considerable and broad-ranging difficulties affecting many aspects of their lives, including problems on the job, in their relationships, and in society. Some service members face adjustment to visible or invisible wounds or losses. Still others may experience a combination of difficulties and personal growth as a result of their deployments (Pietrzak et al., 2010). The discussion that follows seeks to emphasize some of the most commonly observed psychosocial and behavioral health challenges.

THE DEPLOYMENT EXPERIENCE

Common postdeployment experiences can be better comprehended through an understanding of the context and environment in which deployment occurs. Stressors during combat and other military operations are typically conceptualized within four categories (U.S. Department of the Army, 1996). First, *environmental stressors* can include the temperature and weather conditions of the area of operations. Excessive heat and cold, sandstorms, extended precipitation, and unusual or difficult terrain can all exact their toll. Service members can face environment-based health threats, such as vectors or other infectious agents. A second category of challenges includes *physiological stressors,* such as the commonplace challenge of maintaining a high level of performance under significant sleep deprivation. Sleep debt can be due to insomnia or simply limited sleep opportunities and is known to reduce efficiency on the battlefield (Wesensten & Balkin, 2010). Maintaining adequate hydration and nutrition also can be challenging in austere environments with searing heat and high operational tempos. Exhaustion can result from the combination of long work hours, poor sleep, and heavy labor performed in cumbersome personal protective equipment. The confluence of these factors can negatively impact service members' physical conditions, putting them at increased risk of illness or injury.

A number of *emotional stressors* also arise, and relationship problems and homefront worries are common. Issues range from financial concerns, anxiety about partner fidelity, and family health issues to child behavioral problems. Deployments are rife with significant events that will challenge the psyche of warriors. In recent conflicts in both Iraq and Afghanistan, deaths of fellow service members, having to kill the enemy, frequent firefights, having to perform emergency first aid on friends, improvised explosive device (IED) and rocket/mortar attacks, and significant physical injuries have been the norm for ground personnel. Finally, common *cognitive stressors* include the challenge of life-and-death decision making in accordance with the rules of engagement in the context of extreme physical and psychological stressors (for more on cognition and decision making in extreme environments, see McNeil & Morgan, 2010). Some service members have access to limited information, and this can be difficult, particularly when it impacts them individually (e.g., length of deployment, possibility of deployment extension, timing of 2-week R & R). All of these stressors occur within a context in which service members have limited access to typical coping approaches and resources. Service members are separated from a large portion of their normal support network, consisting of spouses, families and nonmilitary friends, faith communities, and typical recreation. It is self-evident that military service members execute their duties under challenging circumstances, often with life-and-death consequences.

Given the stressful context associated with deployment, one might assume that the homecoming would be a consistent time of great joy. Although this is the case for many, in some instances the initial happiness of the homecoming can give way to a number of postdeployment difficulties. Alternatively, the homecoming may be stressful from the outset, perhaps even dreaded. Given the range of experiences, we cannot assume that any given service member "must be so glad to be home!"

UNIQUE CHALLENGES
OF THE SINGLE SERVICE MEMBER

"My first day home I watched everyone joyfully reuniting with spouses and partners and I stood alone just wanting to get out of there. As a single soldier, I went back to an empty barracks room after the ceremony. It was so quiet, and I felt like a loser. During the deployment, we lived in a small tent and talked to each other day or night. It sounds crazy, but I wanted to be back in Afghanistan."

—A PREVIOUSLY DEPLOYED SOLDIER

Studies of civilian populations and the relationship between marital status and mental health disorders generally suggest that divorced individuals are at greater odds of psychiatric problems than married/cohabitating or single individuals. For example, a study of the lifetime risk of mental health disorders among a nationally representative sample of 9,282 Americans (Kessler, Berglund, Demler, Jin, & Merikangas, 2005) found that *previously married* individuals had 80% higher odds of anxiety disorders and 90% higher odds of mood disorders relative to married/cohabitating participants. Previously married participants were 3.9 times more likely than married/cohabitating individuals to have a substance use disorder.

Interestingly, there were no significant differences in the odds of any categories of mental health disorders between never-married and married/cohabitating individuals.

Longitudinal data from the National Survey of Families and Households included 10,005 individuals who were surveyed in 1987–1988 and again in 1992–1993 (Kim & McKenry, 2002). The study found that individuals who transitioned from single/noncohabitating to married status reported a decrease in depressive symptoms, whereas married individuals who divorced or separated reported higher depressive symptoms. Interestingly, those who persisted as single (never married/non-cohabitating) reported higher levels of depressive symptoms at the second survey than those who were continuously married, although not as high as married individuals who divorced/separated or those who were continuously divorced/separated.

There is limited research on the impact of military deployments on single service members. What evidence there is may suggest that single military personnel perceive fewer negative consequences from deployment (Newby, McCarroll, et al., 2005) and experience less stress (Hammelman, 1995). However, a comparison study of a random sample of U.S. troops deployed in support of Operations Desert Shield and Desert Storm and same-era non-deployed troops (Fiedler et al., 2006) found that service members who were single during the war had 83% higher odds of having drug or alcohol dependence. There was no difference in the odds of having an anxiety disorder.

Regarding veterans of OIF and OEF, a large study of more than 100,000 veterans seen at U.S. Department of Veterans Affairs healthcare facilities found small differences in rates of PTSD diagnoses according to marital status. Divorced and separated/widowed veterans were 20% and 21% more likely, respectively, to receive a diagnosis of PTSD relative to veterans who were married or those who had never married (Seal, Bertenthal, Nuber, Sem, & Marmar, 2007). Consistent with this research, a study of more than 4,000 active-duty soldiers included marital status in the analyses of those previously deployed in support of OIF/OEF (Lapierre, Schwegler, & LaBauve, 2007). The authors found that, among those deployed to Iraq, separated and divorced service members reported significantly higher PTSD symptoms and depression relative to married soldiers. However, among soldiers previously deployed to Afghanistan, being single was unexpectedly associated with decreased PTSD symptoms relative to those who were married.

In fairness, it is likely not the status of being single that is singularly important but rather the presence or absence of positively perceived intimate others who can provide support during challenges (Holt-Lundsted, Birmingham, & Jones, 2008). Similarly, the body of research just reviewed suggests that it may be relevant if someone is single and never married or currently single because they divorced. Regardless, single service members do face unique challenges as they redeploy from combat. As the prior quote illustrates, from the moment that single service members arrive back home, their experience may be unique relative to those with partners. Military welcoming home ceremonies can leave some single service members standing alone, feeling awkward, and can transform a joyous occasion into disappointment.

Similar challenges can persist after the ceremony. While others go out to celebrate with their partners and families, single service members may be left to celebrate alone. One soldier observed that he had "dreamt of my favorite restaurant all year and when I got home, I ended up going there alone." Some military personnel are offered half-day work schedules for the first 2 weeks following redeployment. This may be a wonderful time to reconnect with family and friends for some. For others, it is downtime without clear purpose.

Single service members with children face the transition of children back into their day-to-day custody. These children may have grown accustomed to the homes and routines of their grandparents or other caregivers during the deployment. Particularly when children are young, it can be challenging for redeployed service members to redevelop their mutual bond and attachment with their own child.

In general then, some single military personnel may face less immediately available social support, whereas others may experience a less complicated deployment and redeployment experience. It can be problematic when a single service member is struggling postdeployment and has limited social support. The detection of a service member in need of help could be delayed if the individual lives off post/base and is not meaningfully engaged with other unit members.

POSTDEPLOYMENT READJUSTMENT TO FAMILY LIFE

Family separations associated with operational deployments have been associated with high levels of stress and may present a number of challenges for both deployed service members and their families (Mabe, 2009). Deployment may engender increased parenting stress in the nondeployed partner as well as unpleasant emotions such as numbness, shock, loneliness emotional distance, and anger (see Palmer, 2008, for a review). In addition, children of deployed parents may experience adjustment problems, including depression, anxiety, aggression, and academic difficulties (Jensen & Shaw, 1996; Kelley et al., 2001; Schwab et al., 1995).

Although deployment separations are associated with increased levels of family stress, postdeployment reunions present their own set of challenges. The postdeployment reunion, although typically joyous, may also be marked by anxiety and a number of readjustment difficulties (Moore & Kennedy, 2011), including the service member feeling like an outsider, communication issues, disagreements about parenting practices, and decreased relationship intimacy (see Palmer, 2008).

Unfortunately, relatively scant research has focused on family issues postdeployment from OIF/OEF. Goff, Crow, Reisbig, and Hamilton (2007) found trauma symptoms as well as sexual and sleep problems related to lower relationship satisfaction in recently redeployed OIF/OEF male soldiers and their female partners. Lapp and colleagues (2010) conducted a qualitative analysis of problems reported by spouses of National Guard and Reserve members following OIF/OEF deployment. They reported that couples struggled with attaining equilibrium or "new normal" adjustment, and there appeared to be a persistent sense among nondeployed partners that their spouses, whom they had known well, were changed in significant ways following deployment. For example, one spouse of a deployed service member described the postdeployment reunion as a "mixed bag" in which "you get used to living without that person, and then when they come back they are a different person" (Lapp et al., 2010, p. 53). Other spouses expressed a sense that their postdeployed spouses were reluctant to share their experiences, and they also reported experiencing frustration over not being able to understand, as articulated in the following description: "There's no way for me to understand what he went through and the things he saw or did or anything like that. And, I want to. I want to be there for him, but I don't know how" (Lapp et al., 2010, pp. 53–54). With regard to help seeking, some spouses of deployed service members expressed reluctance to access support for fear of rumors and a preference for relating their difficulties to someone who could understand their problems through similar personal experiences.

Karney and Crown (2007) examined marital dissolution trends at the military population level from 1996–2005 and reported that deployment length was positively associated with marital dissolution only among enlisted members and officers of the active Air Force. In fact, among enlisted members of the other branches of service and officers in the Navy and the Marines Corps, deployment length was inversely associated with marital dissolution. These results were also found to hold for enlisted members and officers of the Army, officers in the Navy Reserve, enlisted members of the Air Force Reserve, and all ranks of the Army and Air National Guard. Karney and Crown (2007) concluded that several factors may account for the negligible association found between deployment length and marital dissolution. For example, it may be that exposure to combat and traumatic experiences, rather than deployment per se, relate to marital dissolution; it is also possible that for some service members deployment can lead to personal fulfillment and career growth. However, the authors also reported that the rate of both military marriage and marital dissolution have been gradually increasing since 2000. To help explain this finding, they put forth a *selection hypothesis* that posits that the military tends to recruit the most vulnerable individuals (in terms of age, opportunities for career advancement in the civilian arena) and unwittingly offers incentives for marriage. Moreover, with the prospect of impending deployment, some military personnel may initiate marriages that they would not have otherwise initiated. These younger couples then may face financial stress as well as separation from their families. Collectively, these findings suggest that postdeployed service members who are younger and junior enlisted may be at increased risk for marital problems following deployment.

Although a number of studies support the notion that deployment affects children adversely (Jensen, Martin, & Watanabe, 1996; Kelley et al., 2001; Rosen, Teitelbaum, & Westhuis, 1993), other research indicates that children appear to be relatively resilient to parental deployment (see Mabe, 2009, for a review). A consistent preoccupation of many children of deployed parents appears to be the deployed parents' safety; thus, children whose parents are injured during deployment may be at more risk for difficulties than those whose parents do not sustain combat injuries (Mabe, 2009). Some children, however, may remain resilient to maladaptive psychological outcomes despite (or because of) exposure to deployment-related adversities (Luthar, Cicchetti, & Becker, 2000). Moreover, a comprehensive understanding of effects of deployment on child adjustment requires consideration of sources of influence at multiple levels. These include child characteristics (e.g., age, gender, temperament, problem-solving skills, intelligence, premorbid psychological functioning), the nature of deployment (e.g., deployment length, combat exposure, death risk, parental injury, forms of communication available during deployment, public support of the mission), family circumstances (e.g., two parents deployed, gender of deployed parent, psychological health of parents, marital status), and the availability of community support (Mabe, 2009). For example, younger or older children may be more or less affected by parental deployment as a function of developmental factors such as reasoning capacity and/or coping style. However, the influence of such individual factors in relation to adjustment to parental deployment may be further modified by contextual and family-level factors (e.g., multiple deployments, combat injuries, parental psychopathology).

There has been speculation that intimate partner violence may increase following deployment because of increased stress associated with readjustment that is placed on poorly functioning families (Newby, Ursano, et al.,

2005). However, the literature on this topic is sparse and equivocal. Newby, Ursano, and colleagues (2005) examined postdeployed intimate partner violence among wives of soldiers deployed to Bosnia for 6 months. Results indicated that deployment was not significantly associated with increases in postdeployment reports of intimate partner violence reported anonymously by wives. However, younger wives and those who experienced predeployment intimate partner abuse were more likely to report abuse at postdeployment. This finding is consistent with McCarroll et al. (2003), who also did not find deployment per se to be associated with increased intimate partner violence. Other research, however, suggests modest increases in intimate partner violence following deployment (e.g., Gimbel & Booth, 1994; Orcutt, King, & King, 2003). PTSD-related aggression may also increase the risk for intimate partner violence. Sherman, Sautter, Jackson, Lyons, and Han (2006) studied 179 couples seeking relationship therapy at a Veterans Affairs medical center. Based on their survey of the combined veteran and spouse self-reports, 81% of veterans diagnosed with depression or PTSD reported that they had perpetrated minor violence (e.g., threw something) or severe violence (e.g., kicked, bit, or hit with a fist) against intimate partners in the past year.

Impact on the Family of PTSD in the Postdeployed Service Member

PTSD in the returning service member (discussed in greater detail shortly) is among the strongest predictors of postdeployment relationship and family problems. Research on PTSD in service members spanning several decades and military conflicts beginning with World War II indicate that PTSD is associated with a 62% increase in failed marriages (Ruger, Wilson, & Waddoups, 2002). Emotional numbing associated with PTSD appears to be an especially strong predictor of intimate relationship problems (Riggs, Byrne, Weathers, & Litz, 1998). Withdrawal and anger are additional consequences of PTSD that exact a toll on intimate relationships and the family unit as a whole.

POSTDEPLOYMENT TRANSITIONS

Whether single or married, postdeployment transitions are a common challenge. This point in time often requires consequential decisions about a number of issues. First, service members face occupational decision points. During or shortly after deployment, enlisted personnel often have fulfilled their obligated period of service and are faced with the decision of whether or not to reenlist. This decision can be a complex one. Positive deployment experiences may cause some personnel to consider extending service; difficult deployments may cause hesitation. Enticing monetary bonuses for some occupational specialties can make reenlistment opportunities particularly appealing. Those considering exiting the service may wonder what civilian employment will hold; since "The military is all I've ever known."

For those choosing to reenlist, additional decision points include whether to use their reenlistment to acquire a new military occupational specialty (MOS), or job. Some consider this change because of an interest in jobs with better promotion potential. Others might be interested in a job with training relevant to future interests in the civilian job market. Some desire to move out of combat arms roles to reduce the risk of future combat exposure. Whatever the reason, those choosing to use reenlistment to pursue a new job typically require retraining, which may involve months spent at a different installation and a new duty station to follow. Another opportunity is to use reenlistment to acquire a desired new duty station. Although this may indeed be a desired change, a relocation following deployment is a significant change and a transition that may well still be stressful.

Of course, not all service members who have fulfilled their service obligation choose to reenlist. Some decide to leave the military and transition to civilian jobs. It can be challenging for some to translate their military skills and training (e.g., infantry) into experience relevant to a civilian job search. Additionally, an adverse economic climate on the home front can make a civilian job search difficult.

Other service members face postdeployment transitions involving new family adjustments. Children born during the deployment can bring great joy to returning fathers. However, infants often add significant stress to family life, requiring significant changes in day-to-day life. Others return to significant marital problems that developed during deployment and face the difficult road of reunion and reconciliation. Still others who have made the decision to divorce during deployment must deal with the aftermath of this decision upon their return home, which can add considerable stress to the postdeployment transition (Moore & Kennedy, 2011).

PTSD FOLLOWING DEPLOYMENT

Postdeployment difficulties in the current historical context must be considered in tandem with the potential for problems with posttraumatic stress. PTSD is an anxiety disorder that some people develop in response to traumatic events. Following the event, based on DSM criteria, symptoms will last at least 1 month (American Psychiatric Association, 2000) and include reexperiencing of the traumatic event in the form of upsetting, intrusive thoughts; nightmares; a sense of reliving the event as if it were recurring;

and psychological and physiological distress when confronted with cues or reminders of the traumatic event. Affected individuals can experience avoidance of stimuli related to the event and numbing symptoms, including avoidance of trauma-related thoughts, feelings, and conversations; avoidance of places, people, or other circumstances that are reminders of the trauma; poor recollection of important parts of the event; decreased interest in meaningful activities; interpersonal detachment; difficulties experiencing emotions; and a sense of a foreshortened future. Symptoms can also include anxiety and arousal, including sleep problems; irritability or anger; problems concentrating; hypervigilance; and an increased startle response.

PTSD Rates among Military Personnel Deployed to Iraq and Afghanistan

A number of studies have attempted to determine the rates of PTSD among those who have deployed to Iraq and Afghanistan. There has been some variance in rates reported depending on the tool used for detection, the point in history when data were collected, the research method used, and the population studied. For example, the first study of veterans of OIF/OEF (Hoge et al., 2004) included a cross-sectional sample of soldiers and Marines from combat brigades assessed 3 to 4 months after deployment to Iraq or Afghanistan. The PTSD Checklist (Weathers, Huska, & Keane, 1991) was used to determine the presence of PTSD, and two scoring methods were used. First, participants were categorized as positive for PTSD if they reported at least moderate symptoms in a pattern that was consistent with DSM-IV criteria (i.e., at least one reexperiencing symptom, three avoidance symptoms, and two arousal symptoms). A second more conservative scoring approach was also used, which required the same pattern of symptoms just described with the additional criterion of a total score of at least 50. Rates of PTSD among Army personnel previously deployed to Iraq were 18% and 12.9% for the broad and strict definitions of PTSD, respectively. Similarly, rates of PTSD among Marines previously deployed to Iraq were 19.9% and 12.2%, respectively. Given that data for this study were collected during 2003, prior to increased combat operations in Afghanistan, it is not surprising that rates of PTSD were lower for personnel previously deployed in support of OEF. Rates of PTSD among soldiers previously deployed to Afghanistan were 11.5% and 6.2% for the broad and strict definitions, respectively.

Another study reported on all soldiers and Marines who completed a routine postdeployment health assessment in May 2003–April 2004 within 2 weeks of returning from deployment to Iraq or Afghanistan (Hoge, Auchterlonie, & Milliken, 2006). As part of this assessment, military personnel completed a four-item screen for PTSD, which was developed for primary care settings (PC-PTSD; Prins et al., 2003). Any person who endorsed two of four items was deemed at risk of PTSD. According to this study, the rates of personnel at risk of PTSD were 9.8% and 4.7% of personnel previously deployed to Iraq and Afghanistan, respectively.

Because of concerns that screenings completed within 2 weeks of redeployment (a term denoting return from deployment) underestimated the rates of behavioral health problems, the U.S. Department of Defense launched a second assessment that was conducted 3–6 months postdeployment. A longitudinal study using PC-PTSD compared rates of behavioral health problems for Army soldiers at both assessment time points collected between June 2005 and December 2006 (Milliken, Auchterlonie, & Hoge, 2007). At the first assessment immediately postdeployment, 11.8% of active duty soldiers were at risk of PTSD. Three to 6 months postdeployment, this rate increased to 16.7%.

One of the limitations of these studies is the cross-sectional nature of the research and the absence of predeployment data. A notable exception to this body of literature is Smith et al.'s (2008) prospective study of a large, representative cohort of military personnel with a longitudinal research design. Using results from the PTSD Checklist, the investigators reported the new cases of PTSD detected during a follow-up survey of previously deployed personnel surveyed in June 2004 to February 2006. On the basis of DSM-IV symptomatic criteria for PTSD and a minimum total score of 50, 4.3% of the cohort reported new-onset PTSD.

PTSD has been associated with other difficulties as well. As noted previously, PTSD puts individuals at greater risk of marital problems. In addition, it has been found to be a predictor of increased antisocial behavior among Vietnam War veterans (Resnick, Foy, Donajoe, & Miller, 1989). Similar findings were reported in a recent study of more than 1,500 Marines who had deployed in support of combat (Booth-Kewley, Larson, Highfill-McRoy, Garland, & Gaskin, 2010). The authors found that those who screened positive for PTSD were more than six times as likely to have engaged in antisocial behavior as those who did not. The second-order effects of these types of behaviors (e.g., physical altercations, disobedience to orders, conflicts with law enforcement, increased disciplinary action) undoubtedly result in increased stress, interpersonal problems, and occupational difficulties. A snowball effect of functional difficulties can occur that both reflect and exacerbate mental health difficulties.

Treatment of PTSD

Research has identified several effective psychotherapeutic treatments for PTSD. A range of clinical practice guidelines (CPGs; Institute of Medicine, 2008; American Psychiatric Association, 2004; Foa, Keane, Friedman,

& Cohen, 2009; U.S. Department of Veterans Affairs & Department of Defense, 2010) recommend exposure therapy; cognitive therapies, including cognitive processing therapy (CPT; Resick, Monson, & Chard, 2007); eye movement desensitization therapy (EMDR; Shapiro, 2001); and other cognitive-behavioral therapies such as stress inoculation therapy (SIT; Kilpatrick, Veronen, & Resick, 1982; Meichenbaum, 1974).

Exposure therapy was historically delivered according to Mowrer's (1960) two-factor theory about the acquisition and maintenance of PTSD. However, this theory did not adequately account for all of the symptoms observed in those with PTSD (Foa, Steketee, & Rothbaum, 1989; Foa & Hearst-Ikeda, 1996). In order to better explain the full clinical presentation, emotional processing theory was proposed (Foa & Kozak, 1986). According to this theory, PTSD is the continuation of a pathological fear structure made up of associations between stimuli from the event, responses (e.g., physiological responses), and the meaning of the event to the individual. When components of the fear structure are encountered by individuals with PTSD, they frequently use cognitive and behavioral avoidance to avoid the resulting distress. However, this avoidance also prevents the learning of new, corrective information that would modify the fear structure and result in decreased anxiety. Exposure therapies aim to activate the fear structure through intentionally confronting aspects of it in order to facilitate the new learning required for recovery.

Prolonged exposure (PE; Foa, Hembree, & Rothbaum, 2007) is one of the best researched exposure therapy protocols. Aspects of the PE protocol have been studied in the treatment of female assault survivors (Resick, Nishith, Weaver, Astin, & Feuer, 2002; Foa et al., 1999, 2005), female veterans (Schnurr et al., 2007), and mixed-trauma groups (Marks, Lovell, Noshirvani, Livanou, & Thrasher, 1998), among others. Although dozens of randomized clinical trials for exposure therapy have been completed, none had large enough samples of military personnel to allow separate analyses of its efficacy with active-duty service members.

CPT (Resick et al., 2007) is a manualized cognitive therapy for patients with PTSD, which is based on social-cognitive theory. CPT addresses cognitions within the social context and aims to address the common emotions beyond just fear. It seeks to address a range of common trauma-related affective responses, including anger, horror, guilt, sadness, and humiliation. In CPT, existing cognitive schemas are thought to interact with the trauma event in one of two pathological ways: assimilation and *overaccommodation*. In assimilation, the patient has interpreted new information in a manner consistent with their prior beliefs (e.g., "Since good things happen to good people, I must be getting what I deserve"). Second, overaccommodation occurs when the trauma survivor alters his or her beliefs in an extreme way to feel safe ("I can't ever go to a crowded public place again"). Therapists work toward accommodation, that is, incorporating the true elements of the trauma into balanced beliefs. The therapist helps the patient to identify and challenge problematic thoughts and beliefs, with particular attention paid to repetitive cognitive patterns, or "stuck points"—feelings and beliefs from the traumatic event that are inconsistent with prior beliefs.

A number of randomized clinical trials that have examined the efficacy of CPT demonstrate consistent benefit to many patients. One noteworthy, well-designed study compared the efficacy of CPT, PE, and wait-list control in the treatment of female rape survivors (Resick et al., 2002). There were no statistical differences between PE and CPT on PTSD, but both showed large improvement compared with the wait-list control group. Additional studies of military personnel are needed, but based on existing research CPT is recommended for the treatment of active-duty military personnel and veterans with PTSD (U.S. Department of Veterans Affairs & Department of Defense, 2010).

EMDR (Shapiro, 2001) is based on adaptive information processing and involves accessing information networks related to the trauma memory, stimulating the information-processing system, and adaptively resolving the information. The treatment involves dual-attention tasks to help the patient process the trauma. The external stimulus usually requires lateral eye movements, although other external stimuli have also been used (Shapiro, 1995). For example, the patient may be asked to look at flashing lights presented from left to right while being encouraged to recall memories and feelings associated with the traumatic event. EMDR proposes that the protocol reduces distress and increases belief in appropriate positive cognitions.

EMDR is an eight-phase treatment for PTSD, including history gathering, client preparation (e.g., rapport building and introducing bilateral stimulation), systematic assessment of trauma-relevant targets, desensitization and reprocessing the identified memory network, installation of alternative positive cognitive networks, body scan (i.e., reprocessing physical manifestations of the memory), closure (bringing the session to an end), and reevaluation (follow-up from the previous EMDR session). A number of studies have found generally positive treatment outcomes for EMDR among, for example, sexual assault survivors (Rothbaum, Astin, & Mosteller, 2005), combat veterans (Carlson, Chemtob, Rusnak, Hedlund, & Muraoka, 1998), and mixed-trauma groups (Devilly & Spence, 1999; Marcus, Marquis, & Sakai, 1997). However, dismantling studies have found limited evidence that the eye movements contribute to the efficacy of the treatment (Hembree & Foa, 2003).

Finally, in SIT the therapist provides a variety of coping skills to the patient that are useful in managing anxiety. Trained skills often include cognitive restructuring, self-talk, muscle relaxation, breathing retraining, and role playing. SIT may also include graduated *in vivo* exposure. The goal of this type of therapy is to increase stress management skills and decrease avoidance and anxious responses related to the trauma-related memories, thoughts and feelings. Studies have found SIT to be effective in the treatment of rape and assault victims (Foa, Rothbaum, Riggs, & Murdock, 1991; Foa et al., 1999) and mixed-trauma survivors (Lee, Gavriel, Drummond, Richards, & Greenwald, 2002).

DEPRESSION AMONG PREVIOUSLY DEPLOYED MILITARY PERSONNEL

Disorders involving depression are typically mood disorders in which a change from baseline functioning occurs as a result of subjectively depressed mood or decreased interest in most activities, with the presence of some combination of additional depressive symptoms (American Psychiatric Association, 2000). Sleep disturbance, guilt or feelings of worthlessness, low energy, decreased appetite or overeating, decreased concentration, feelings of hopelessness, and thoughts of death or suicide may accompany the mood disturbance. Suicidality can be of particular concern among individuals with depression, and careful assessment of risk is indicated (for an in-depth discussion of suicide and military personnel, see Chapter 9, this volume).

Depression Rates

As with studies of military personnel and PTSD, results of research on the prevalence of depression after military deployments have varied, likely because of differences in the amount of combat exposure and variation in screening measures and research designs. Population-based research of deployed military personnel found that 70.3 per 10,000 military personnel reported depression (Riddle, Sandersa, Jones, & Webb, 2008). Rates among personnel returning from deployment have generally been higher. Results from a cross-sectional study of infantry units (Hoge et al., 2004) found that 15.2% of soldiers and 14.7% of Marines met broad screening criteria for depression after deployment to Iraq. When strict screening criteria were used, these rates decreased to 7.9 and 7.1%, respectively. A longitudinal study of more than 88,000 soldiers previously deployed to Iraq found that rates of depression increased from the initial weeks after deployment (4.7%) to six months postdeployment (10.3%). Rates of depression were slightly higher 6 months postdeployment among Reserve component soldiers (13%). Similarly, a large study of active-duty and National

Guard infantry brigade combat teams (Thomas et al., 2010) found that rates of positive depression screens were similar 3 and 12 months postdeployment for active-component soldiers (16.0% and 15.7%, respectively) but increased, from 11.5 to 15.9%, for National Guard soldiers.

Treatment of Depression

There are several effective psychotherapies for the treatment of depression, among them cognitive-behavioral therapy (CBT) and interpersonal therapy (IPT). A number of meta-analytic reviews have generally found similar outcomes for the efficacy of both (de Mello, de Jesus Mari, Bacaltchuk, Verdeli, & Neugebauer, 2005; Jacobson et al., 1996; Luty et al., 2007). Accordingly, patient preference should be considered in the selection of an evidence-based treatment approach.

CBT is one of the best researched treatments for depression. CBT utilizes a combination of behavioral interventions and cognitive techniques to identify and modify maladaptive thoughts, life rules, and core beliefs. There are a number of different treatment CBT protocols available to treat depression (e.g., Beck, 1976; Beck, 2011), and meta-analytic reviews of the body of scientific literature clearly establish the efficacy of these treatments (e.g., Ekers, Richards, & Gilbody, 2008; Imel, Malterer, McKay, & Wampold, 2008).

One CBT treatment, behavioral activation, views depression as a reduction in opportunities for positive reinforcement. Depressed individuals engage in pleasant activities less often and, accordingly, experience less positive reinforcement (MacPhillamy & Lewinsohn, 1974). In behavioral activation, patients track their mood and activities to increase awareness. Activities are then rescheduled to reduce avoidance and increase positive reinforcement (Lewinsohn, Sullivan, & Grosscap, 1980). A number of studies support the efficacy of behavioral activation to treat depression (for reviews, see Cuijpers, van Straten, & Warmerdam, 2007; Mazzucchelli, Kane, & Rees, 2009).

IPT (Klerman, Weissman, Rounsaville, & Chevron, 1984; Weissman, Markowitz, & Klerman, 2000) focuses on current interpersonal problems and events that are related to the depressive symptoms. It is a time-limited protocol (often 12–16 sessions) that aims to resolve here-and-now interpersonal problems in order to improve depressive symptoms (Markowitz, Svartberg, & Swartz, 1998). Depressive symptoms are conceptualized within environmental situations (e.g., interpersonal role transitions or role disputes), and patients explore actions they can take to impact their situation and, as a result, decrease depression.

Dozens of randomized controlled trials have studied IPT in the treatment of adolescents (e.g., Mufson et al., 2004), adults (e.g., Markowitz,

Kocsis, Bleiberg, Christos, & Sacks, 2005), older adults (e.g., Van Schaik et al., 2006), and patients whose depression was associated with specific medical conditions (e.g., Markowitz et al., 1998). Previous meta-analytic reviews have determined that IPT is an effective treatment for depression (Cuijpers et al., 2011; de Mello et al., 2005). Limited research exists, however, evaluating the effectiveness of IPT with veterans and active-duty service members. One pilot study used a group format of IPT to treat nine Vietnam War veterans with PTSD, depression, and interpersonal problems (Ray & Webster, 2010). Participants reported meaningful reductions in depression, interpersonal problems, and PTSD symptoms at posttreatment relative to the pretreatment baseline. IPT is a recommended treatment in the CPG for management of major depressive disorder issued by the U.S. Department of Veterans Affairs and Department of Defense (2009).

Substance Abuse among Postdeployed Service Members

Substance abuse is a significant health problem in the U.S. military, accounting for upward of 16,997 criminal offenses reported for the Army in 2009 (U.S. Department of the Army, 2010; see also Chapter 10, this volume). Alcohol abuse, in particular, appears to be a significant postdeployment problem, estimated to affect 20 to 25% of service members. Hoge et al. (2004) conducted a population-based study of soldiers and Marines deployed in support of OIF/OEF and found that one in four service members reported difficulty controlling alcohol use postdeployment. Rona and colleagues (2007) reported a similar rate (i.e., 20%) of alcohol abuse among U.K. soldiers following deployment in support of OIF. More recently, Wilk et al. (2010) revealed that 25% of soldiers deployed to Iraq screened positive for alcohol misuse at 3–4 months postdeployment.

Less is known about abuse of controlled substances among service members. Data indicate that illegal drug use is more common among civilians compared to military personnel (see Freeman & Hurst, 2009, for a discussion). Illicit drug use also declined steeply from 1980 to 1998 and has remained low, whereas alcohol abuse increased sharply from 1998 to 2002 and has remained high (Bray & Hourani, 2007). This lower rate of illicit drug use compared with alcohol use may be attributable to greater acceptance of alcohol use within the military culture, random drug testing, and serious disciplinary repercussions of illegal drug use, including military separation (i.e., the zero-tolerance policy). Other reports, however, indicate that use of illicit substances among service personnel is on the rise. The U.S. Army Health Promotion, Risk Reduction, and Suicide Prevention report (2010) indicates that recent lapses in drug surveillance have resulted in undetected illicit drug use among some 40,000 soldiers. In addition, an estimated 106,000 soldiers are prescribed pharmaceutical drugs to assuage pain and psychiatric symptoms, which suggests an obvious potential for misuse.

Service members at greatest risk for postdeployment substance abuse problems appear to be younger than 25, junior enlisted, and unmarried (Wilk et al., 2010; Williams et al., 2010). Additional risk factors for postdeployment substance abuse include combat exposure and mental health problems such as major depressive disorder and PTSD (Wilk et al., 2010). Service members with predeployment substance misuse problems are also likely to be at increased risk for substance misuse postdeployment.

Postdeployment Psychosocial Stressors and Substance Abuse

A large body of research documents the strong link between emotional distress and problematic substance use, with high rates of comorbity reported for substance abuse disorders and mood and anxiety disorders (e.g., Hasin, Stinson, Ogburn, & Grant, 2007; Kessler et al., 1996; Schneier et al., 2010). Theory and data suggest that substance misuse may serve as a coping mechanism to allay mood disturbances, anxiety, work and relationship problems, and social isolation (Byrne, Jones, & Williams, 2004; Duncan, 1974; Schneier et al., 2010; Tomlinson, Tate, Anderson, McCarthy, & Brown, 2006). Such problems may be prominent among some service members during the reintegration period following an operational deployment. Return from deployment may engender a number of psychosocial stressors such as readjustment to family life, disrupted intimate relationships, feelings of isolation, future plans, work-related problems, and boredom. Redeploying service members may experience depressive and anxiety symptoms in relation to such stressors and use substances to relieve unpleasant emotions and social circumstances associated with their return.

Links between Combat Exposure and Postdeployment Substance Abuse

Combat exposure appears to be an especially salient risk factor for postdeployment substance abuse. The vast majority of ground troops deployed in support of OIF/OEF are exposed to high levels of combat trauma, such as ambush, IED attacks, firefights, exposure to the gravely wounded as well as the dead, and artillery fire (see Bernhardt, 2009, for a review). Exposure to such trauma is strongly associated with alcohol misuse. For example, Rona and colleagues (2007) reported that almost 20% of military personnel deployed for 9–12 months reported severe alcohol problems, which were, in part, associated with exposure to combat trauma. There is also evidence that specific appraisals surrounding combat exposure are associated with heavy drinking. For example, the thought that combat-related death is imminent appears to relate to problematic alcohol consumption (Browne et al., 2008; Hooper et al., 2008). In a similar vein, Wilk and colleagues (2010) reported that exposure to combat atrocities as well as situations characterized by threat of death or injury to self were significantly associated with hazardous alcohol consumption. The link between traumatic combat experiences, such as witnessing atrocities, and heavy drinking may be mediated by unresolved guilt and other negative emotions surrounding the event (Wilk et al., 2010). Moreover, emotional responses to combat trauma are complex and may involve feelings of grief, sorrow, anguish, shame, and guilt (Conoscenti, Vine, Papa, & Litz, 2009).

Although combat exposure has been shown to relate to alcohol abuse independently of the effects of PTSD symptoms (Wilk et al., 2010), PTSD is a clear predictor of postdeployment substance abuse (Nunnick et al., 2010; Ouimette, Read, Wade, & Tirone, 2010; Sharkansky, Brief, Peirce, Meehan, & Mannix, 1999; Stewart, 1996). Postdeployed service personnel suffering from PTSD may attempt to cope with unpleasant trauma symptoms with alcohol or other substances. For example, Sharkansky et al. (1999) found that conflict with others, physical discomfort, and unpleasant emotions triggered substance use among veterans diagnosed with PTSD. Service members may use alcohol and other substances to ameliorate problems with combat trauma-induced nightmares. A recent study indicated that insomnia and nightmares mediated the association between combat stress and PTSD, underscoring the importance of addressing sleep disturbances in returning service members exposed to combat stress (Picchioni et al., 2010). An additional consideration is that female service members dually diagnosed with substance abuse and PTSD may be a particularly vulnerable group. Research conducted with female veterans indicated that the dually diagnosed veterans experienced more severe and enduring problems than female veterans solely diagnosed with PTSD (Najavits, Weiss, & Shaw, 1999; Nunnick et al., 2010).

In sum, deployment to a war zone may give rise to unique problems that are linked with postdeployment substance abuse. Younger, single, junior enlisted service members appear to be at elevated risk for postdeployment substance misuse, and female service members dually diagnosed with PTSD and substance abuse represent a particularly vulnerable subgroup. Risk factors for postdeployment substance misuse include predeployment history of substance misuse, psychosocial stressors associated with redeployment, combat trauma, PTSD, and other mental health problems. The research findings reviewed here suggest the need for clinicians working with postdeployed service members to consider the following issues:

- Predeployment problems with substance misuse.
- Specific types of combat experiences, and combat exposure, in general, that may increase the propensity toward alcohol misuse.
- Potential misuse of prescription drugs to cope with redeployment stress and mental health symptoms.
- Importance of assessing PTSD at the symptom level to facilitate the management of substance misuse and relapse.
- Awareness of social circumstances and redeployment stressors associated with substance abuse.
- Focus on the development of specific skills to cope with unpleasant emotions and circumstances that may trigger substance use.
- Use of interventions that target mood tolerance and emotional regulation, relationship building, and communication skills.
- Treatment of trauma symptoms and other mental health problems after substance misuse has been successfully treated may reduce potential for relapse.

For further discussion of substance use problems, military personnel, relationship of PTSD to substance abuse, and treatment options, see Chapter 10, this volume.

ASSESSMENT OF POSTDEPLOYMENT READJUSTMENT

Given the potential for significant readjustment problems following deployment and possible enduring effects, thorough assessment across multiple domains of functioning and psychological well-being is indicated to inform treatment planning. This is true when working with either individual service members or military families following deployment. Assessment should cover domains such as interpersonal, family, relationship, and work functioning; current stressors; risks; strengths; barriers to treatment; military history; and current psychological symptoms. Meichenbaum (2009) provides a case conceptualization model designed specifically for soldiers returning from deployment. It is also prudent to assess children of parents who present for postdeployment adjustment difficulties, across multiple domains of functioning, including psychological health, family relationships, and interpersonal and academic functioning. The parent–child relationship is a key area of assessment, because the effects of combat deployment on child psychosocial and academic functioning may be mediated by parental stress and psychopathology (Palmer, 2008).

Stigma is widely acknowledged as a barrier to service members getting the assessment and treatment they need. Following a peacekeeping mission in Bosnia, 61% of 708 U.S. military service members indicated that admission of a psychological problem would negatively impact their career. Similar results have been reported among previously deployed personnel supporting OIF/OEF. Only 38–45% of service members self-reporting symptoms that met screening criteria for a mental health problem indicated an interest in treatment (Hoge et al., 2004). A number of innovative solutions are attempting to increase access to resources for service members who are hesitant to seek face-to-face care inside the military medical system. For example, *www.afterdeployment.org* is a resource designed by the U.S. Department of Defense to help service members and their families manage the challenges that are often faced following a deployment. This website contains information and self-guided solutions for dealing with common postdeployment problems, such as stress, anger, depression, and relationship issues. Although it is not designed as a substitute for treatment when professional help is indicated, this tool may provide self-assessment and self-care solutions to those who have not yet identified their need for help or whose difficulties are preclinical in nature. For those seeking face-to-face counseling, active-duty service members, National Guard, Reserves members, and their families can access *militaryonesource.com* for 12 no-cost counseling sessions to address issues that are not medically diagnosable (e.g., improving home or work relationships, grief and loss, postdeployment transitions).

CONCLUSION

Service members and their families make significant sacrifices during military deployments, and their sacrifices often do not cease at the redeployment ceremony. Instead, challenges can persist, ranging from normative adjustment problems to clinical conditions that warrant treatment. These persisting difficulties can be experienced by the service member, their spouse, other loved ones, and their children. Significant work is under way to ensure that help is available to those who need it, whether through innovative web-based self-care or nonstigmatizing face-to-face care. Furthermore, previous research suggests that effective treatments are available for many deployment-related problems. However, significant questions remain. There is limited clinical research of the efficacy of evidence-based psychological treatments for active-duty military personnel. Many questions also remain about the relationship between military deployments and future mental health. In particular, limited information is known about the long-term mental health implications of deployments to Iraq and Afghanistan. Longitudinal studies of representative samples are needed to address these and related questions.

REFERENCES

American Psychiatric Association. (2000). *Diagnostic and statistical manual of mental disorders* (4th ed., text rev.). Washington, DC: Author.

American Psychiatric Association. (2004). *Practice guideline for the treatment of patients with acute stress disorder and posttraumatic stress disorder*. Washington, DC: Author.

Beck, A. T. (1976). *Cognitive therapy and the emotional disorders*. New York: New American Library.

Beck, J. S. (2011). *Cognitive behavior therapy: Basics and beyond* (2nd ed.). New York: Guilford Press.

Bernhardt, A., (2009). Rising to the challenge of treating OEF/OIF veterans with co-occurring PTSD and substance abuse. *Smith College Studies in Social Work, 79*, 344–367.

Booth-Kewley, S., Larson, G. E., Highfill-McRoy, R. M., Garland, C. F., & Gaskin, T. A. (2010). Factors associated with antisocial behavior in combat veterans. *Aggressive Behavior, 36*, 330–337.

Bray, R. M., & Hourani, L. L. (2007). Substance use trends among active duty military personnel: Findings from the United States Department of Defense Health Related Behavior Surveys, 1980–2005. *Addiction, 102*, 1092–1101.

Browne, T. E., Iversen, A., Hull, L., Workman, L., Barker, C., Horn, O., et al. (2008). How do experiences in Iraq affect alcohol use amongst male UK armed forces personnel? *Occupational and Environmental Medicine, 65*, 628–633.

Byrne, P., Jones, S., & Williams, R. (2004). The association between cannabis and alcohol use and the development of mental disorder. *Current Opinion in Psychiatry, 17*, 255–261.

Carlson, J. G., Chemtob, C. M., Rusnak, K., Hedlund, N. L., & Muraoka, M. Y. (1998). Eye movement desensitization and reprocessing (EMDR) treatment for combat-related posttraumatic stress disorder. *Journal of Traumatic Stress, 11*, 3–24.

Conoscenti, L. M., Vine, V., Papa, A., & Litz, B. T. (2009). Scanning for danger: Readjustment to the noncombat environment. In S. M. Freeman, B. A. Moore, & A. Freeman (Eds.), *Living and surviving in harm's way* (pp. 123–146). New York: Routledge/Taylor & Francis Group.

Cuijpers, P., Geraedts, A. S., van Oppen, P., Andersson, G., Markowitz, J. C., & van Straten, A. (2011). Interpersonal psychotherapy for depression: A meta-analysis. *American Journal of Psychiatry, 168*, 581–592.

Cuijpers, P., van Straten, A., & Warmerdam, L. (2007). Behavioral activation treatments of depression: A meta-analysis. *Clinical Psychology Review, 27*, 318–326.

de Mello, M. F., de Jesus Mari, J., Bacaltchuk, J., Verdeli, H., & Neugebauer, R. (2005). A systematic review of research findings on the efficacy of interpersonal therapy for depressive disorders. *European Archives of Psychiatry and Clinical Neuroscience, 255*, 75–82.

Devilly, G. J., & Spence, S. H. (1999). The relative efficacy and treatment distress of EMDR and a cognitive-behavior trauma treatment protocol in the amelioration of posttraumatic stress disorder. *Journal of Anxiety Disorders, 13,* 131–157.

Duncan, D. F. (1974). Drug abuse as a coping mechanism. *American Journal of Psychiatry, 131,* 724.

Ekers, D., Richards, D., & Gilbody, S. (2008). A meta-analysis of randomized trials of behavioural treatment of depression. *Psychological Medicine, 38,* 611–623.

Fiedler, N., Ozakinci, G., Hallman, W., Wartenberg, D., Brewer, N. T., Barrett, D. H., et al. (2006). Military deployment to the Gulf War as a risk factor for psychiatric illness among US troops. *British Journal of Psychiatry, 188,* 453–459.

Foa, E. B., Dancu, C. V., Hembree, E. A., Jaycox, L. H., Meadows, E. A., & Street, G. P. (1999). The efficacy of exposure therapy, stress inoculation training, and their combination in ameliorating PTSD for female victims of assault. *Journal of Consulting and Clinical Psychology, 67,* 194–200.

Foa, E. B., & Hearst-Ikeda, D. (1996). Emotional dissociation in response to trauma: An information-processing approach. In L. K. Michelson & W. J. Ray (Eds.), *Handbook of dissociation: Theoretical and clinical perspectives* (pp. 207–222). New York: Plenum Press.

Foa, E. B., Hembree, E. A., Cahill, S. P., Rauch, S. A., Riggs, D. S., Feeny, N. C., et al. (2005). Randomized trial of prolonged exposure for PTSD with and without cognitive restructuring: Outcome at academic and community clinics. *Journal of Consulting and Clinical Psychology, 73,* 953–964.

Foa, E. B., Hembree, E. A., & Rothbaum, B. O. (2007). *Prolonged exposure therapy for PTSD: Emotional processing of traumatic experiences, therapist guide.* New York: Oxford University Press.

Foa, E. B., Keane, T. M., Friedman, M. J., & Cohen, J. A. (2009). *Effective treatments for PTSD: Practice guidelines from the International Society for Traumatic Stress Studies.* New York: Guilford Press.

Foa, E. B., & Kozak, M. J. (1986). Emotional processing of fear: Exposure to corrective information. *Psychological Bulletin, 99*(1), 20–35.

Foa, E. B., Rothbaum, B. O., Riggs, D. S., & Murdock, T. B. (1991). Treatment of posttraumatic stress disorder in rape victims: A comparison between cognitive-behavioral procedures and counseling. *Journal of Consulting and Clinical Psychology, 59,* 715–723.

Foa, E. B., Steketee, G., & Rothbaum, B. O. (1989). Behavioral/cognitive conceptualizations of posttraumatic stress disorder. *Behavior Therapy, 20,* 155–176.

Freeman, S. M., & Hurst, M. R. (2009). Substance use, misuse, and abuse: Impaired problem solving and coping. In S. M Freeman, B. A. Moore, & A. Freeman (Eds.), *Living and surviving in harm's way* (pp. 259–280). New York: Routledge./Taylor & Francis Group.

Gimbel, C., & Booth, A. (1994). Why does military combat experience adversely affect marital relations? *Journal of Marriage and the Family, 56,* 691–703.

Goff, B. S. N., Crow, J. R., Reisbig, A. M. J., & Hamilton, S. (2007). The impact of individual trauma symptoms of deployed soldiers on relationship satisfaction. *Journal of Family Psychology, 21,* 344–353.

Hammelman, T. L. (1995). The Persian Gulf conflict: The impact of stressors as perceived by Army reservists. *Health and Social Work, 20,* 140–145.

Hasin, D. S., Stinson, F. S., Ogburn, E., & Grant, B. F. (2007). Prevalence, correlates, disability, and comorbidity of DSM-IV alcohol abuse and dependence in the United States: Results form the National Epidemiologic Survey on Alcohol and Related Conditions. *Archives of General Psychiatry, 64,* 830–842.

Hembree, E. A., & Foa, E. B. (2003). Interventions for trauma-related emotional disturbances in adult victims of crime. *Journal of Traumatic Stress, 16,* 187–199.

Hoge, C. W., Auchterlonie, J. L., & Milliken, C. S. (2006). Mental health problems, use of mental health services, and attrition from military service after returning from deployment to Iraq or Afghanistan. *Journal of the American Medical Association, 295*(9), 1023–1032.

Hoge, C. W., Castro, C. A., Messer, S. C., McGurk, D., Cotting, D. I., & Koffman, R. L. (2004). Combat duty in Iraq and Afghanistan, mental health problems, and barriers to care. *New England Journal of Medicine, 351,* 13–22.

Holt-Lundsted, J., Birmingham, W., & Jones, B. Q. (2008). Is there something unique about marriage? The relative impact of marital status, relationship quality, and network social support on ambulatory blood pressure and mental health. *Journal of Behavioral Medicine, 35,* 239–244.

Hooper, R., Rona, R. J., Jones, M., Fear, N. T., Hull, L., & Wessely, S. (2008). Cigarette and alcohol use in the UK armed forces, and their association with combat exposures: A prospective study. *Addictive Behavior, 33,* 1067–1071.

Imel, Z. E., Malterer, M. B., McKay, K. M., & Wampold, B. E. (2008). A meta-analysis of psychotherapy and medication in unipolar depression and dysthymia. *Journal of Affective Disorders, 110,* 197–206.

Institute of Medicine. (2008). *Treatment of posttraumatic stress disorder: An assessment of the evidence.* Washington, DC: National Academies Press.

Jacobson, N. S., Dobson, K. S., Truax, P. A., Addis, M. E., Koerner, K., Gollan, J. K., et al. (1996). A component analysis of cognitive-behavioral treatment of depression. *Journal of Consulting and Clinical Psychology, 64,* 295–304.

Jensen, P., Martin, D., & Watanabe, H. (1996). Children's response to parental separation during Operation Desert Storm. *Journal of the American Academy of Child and Adolescent Psychiatry, 35,* 433–441.

Jensen, P., & Shaw, J. A. (1996). The effects of war and parental deployment upon children and adolescents. In R. J. Ursano & A. E. Norwood (Eds.), *Emotional aftermath of the Persian Gulf War: Veterans, families, communities, and nations.* Washington, DC: American Psychiatric Press.

Karney, B. R., & Crown, J. S. (2007). *Families under stress: An assessment of data, theory, and research on marriage and divorce in the military.* Santa Monica, CA: RAND National Defense Research Institute.

Kelley, M., Hock, E., Smith, K., Jarvis, M., Bonney, J., & Gaffney, M. (2001). Internalizing and externalizing behavior of children with enlisted Navy mothers experiencing military-induced separation. *Journal of the American Academy of Child and Adolescent Psychiatry, 40,* 464–471.

Kessler, R. C., Berglund, P., Demler, O., Jin, R., & Merikangas, K. R. (2005). Lifetime prevalence and age-of-onset distributions of DSM-IV disorders in the National Comorbidity Survey replication. *Archives of General Psychiatry, 62,* 593–603.

Kessler, R. C., Nelson, C. B., McGonagle, K. A., Edlund, M. J., Frank, R. G., & Leaf, P. J. (1996). The epidemiology of co-occurring addictive and mental disorders: Implications for prevention and service utilization. *American Journal of Orthopsychiatry, 66,* 17–31.

Kilpatrick, D. G., Veronen, L. J., & Resick, P. A. (1982). Psychological sequelae to rape: Assessment and treatment strategies. In D. M. Dolays & R. L. Meredith (Eds.), *Behavioral medicine: Assessment and treatment strategies* (pp. 473–497). New York: Plenum Press.

Kim, H. K., & McKenry, P. C. (2002). The relationship between marriage and psychological well-being: A longitudinal analysis. *Journal of Family Issues, 23,* 885–911.

Klerman, G., Weissman, M., Rounsaville, B., & Chevron, E. (1984). *Interpersonal psychotherapy of depression.* New York: Basic Books.

Lapierre, C. B., Schwegler, A. F., & LaBauve, B. J. (2007). Posttraumatic stress and depression symptoms in soldiers returning from combat operations in Iraq and Afghanistan. *Journal of Traumatic Stress, 20,* 933–943.

Lapp, C. A., Taft, L. B., Tollefson, T., Hoepner, A., Moore, K., & Divyak, K. (2010). Stress and coping on the home front: Guard and Reserve spouse searching for a new normal. *Journal of Family Nursing, 16,* 45–67.

Lee, C., Gavriel, H., Drummond, P., Richards, J., & Greenwald, R. (2002). Treatment of PTSD: Stress inoculation training with prolonged exposure compared to EMDR. *Journal of Clinical Psychology, 58,* 1071–1089.

Lewinsohn, P. M., Sullivan, J. M., & Grosscap, S. J. (1980). Changing reinforcing events: An approach to the treatment of depression. *Psychotherapy: Theory, Research, and Practice, 17,* 322–334.

Luthar, S. S., Cicchetti, D., & Becker, B. (2000). The construct of resilience: A critical evaluation and guidelines for future work. *Child Development, 71,* 543–562.

Luty, S. E., Carter, J. D., McKenzie, J. M., Rae, A. M., Frampton, C. M. A., Mulder, R. T., et al. (2007). Randomised controlled trial of interpersonal psychotherapy and cognitive-behavioural therapy for depression. *British Journal of Psychiatry, 190,* 496–502.

Mabe, P. A. (2009). War and children coping with parental deployment. In S. M. Freeman, B. A. Moore, & A. Freeman (Eds.), *Living and surviving in harm's way* (pp. 349–370). New York: Routledge/Taylor & Francis Group.

MacPhillamy, D. J., & Lewinsohn, P. M. (1974). Depression as a function of levels of desired and obtained pleasure. *Journal of Abnormal Psychology, 83,* 651–657.

Marcus, S. V., Marquis, P., & Sakai, C. (1997). Controlled study of treatment of PTSD using EMDR in an HMO setting. *Psychotherapy: Therapy, Research, Practice, Training, 34,* 307–315.

Markowitz, J. C., Kocsis, J. H., Bleiberg, K. L., Christos, P. J., & Sacks, M. (2005). A comparative trial of psychotherapy and pharmacotherapy for 'pure' dysthymic patients. *Journal of Affective Disorders, 89,* 167–175.

Markowitz, J. C., Kocsis, J. H., Fishman, B., Spielman, L. A., Jacobsberg, L. B.,

Frances, A. J., et al. (1998). Treatment of depressive symptoms in human immunodeficiency virus-positive patients. *Archives of General Psychiatry, 55,* 452–457.

Markowitz, J. C., Svartberg, M., & Swartz, H. A. (1998). Is IPT time-limited psychodynamic psychotherapy? *Journal of Psychotherapy Practice and Research, 7,* 185–195.

Marks, I., Lovell, K., Noshirvani, H., Livanou, M., & Thrasher, S. (1998). Treatment of posttraumatic stress disorder by exposure and/or cognitive restructuring: A controlled study. *Archives of General Psychiatry, 55,* 317–325.

Mazzucchelli, T., Kane, R., & Rees, C. (2009). Behavioral activation treatments for depression in adults: A meta-analysis and review. *Clinical Psychology: Science and Practice, 16,* 383–411.

McCarroll, J. E., Ursano, R. J., Newby, J. H., Lui, X., Fullerton, C. S., Norwood, A. E., et al. (2003). Domestic violence and deployment in US Army soldiers. *Journal of Nervous and Mental Disease, 191,* 3–9.

McNeil, J. A., & Morgan, C. A. (2010). Cognition and decision making in extreme environments. In C. H. Kennedy & E. A. Zillmer (Eds.), *Military neuropsychology* (pp. 361–382). New York: Springer.

Meichenbaum, D. (1974). Self-instructional methods. In F. H. Kanfer & A. P. Goldstein (Eds.), *Helping people change* (pp. 357–391). New York: Pergamon Press.

Meichenbaum, D. (2009). Core psychotherapeutic tasks with returning soldiers: A case conceptualization approach. In S. M. Freeman, B. A. Moore, & A. Freeman (Eds.), *Living and surviving in harm's way* (PP. 193–210). New York: Routledge/Taylor & Francis Group.

Milliken, C. S., Auchterlonie, J. L., & Hoge, C. W. (2007). Longitudinal assessment of mental health problems among active and Reserve component soldiers returning from the Iraq War. *Journal of the American Medical Association, 298*(18), 2141–2148.

Moore, B. A., & Kennedy, C. H. (2011). *Wheels down: Adjusting to life after deployment.* Washington, DC: American Psychological Association.

Mowrer, O. H. (1960). *Learning theory and behavior.* New York: Wiley.

Mufson, L. H., Dorta, K. P., Wickramaratne, P., Nomura, Y., Olfson, M., & Weissman, M. M. (2004). A randomized effectiveness trial of interpersonal psychotherapy for depressed adolescents. *Archives of General Psychiatry, 61,* 577–584.

Najavits, L. M., Weiss, R. D., & Shaw, S. R. (1999). A clinical profile for women with posttraumatic stress disorder and substance dependence. *Psychology of Addictive Behaviors, 13,* 98–104.

Newby, J. H., McCarroll, J. E., Ursano, R. J., Fan, Z., Shigemura, J., & Tucker-Harris, Y. (2005). Positive and negative consequences of a military deployment. *Military Medicine, 170,* 815–819.

Newby, J. H., Ursano, R. J., McCarroll, J. E., Lui, X., Fullerton, C. S., & Norwood, A. E. (2005). Postdeployment domestic violence by US Army soldiers. *Military Medicine, 170,* 642–647.

Nunnick, S. E., Goldwaser, G., Heppner, P. S., Pittman, J. O. E., Nievergelt, C. M., & Baker, D. G. (2010). Female veterans of the OEF/OIF conflict:

Concordance of PTSD symptoms and substance misuse. *Addictive Behaviors, 35,* 655–659.

Orcutt, H. K., King, L. A., & King, D. W. (2003). Male-perpetrated violence among Vietnam veteran couples: Relationships with veteran's early life characteristics, trauma history, and PTSD symptomatology. *Journal of Traumatic Stress, 16,* 381–390.

Ouimette, P., Read, J. P., Wade, M., & Tirone, V. (2010). Modeling associations between posttraumatic stress symptoms and substance use. *Addictive Behavior, 35,* 64–67.

Palmer, C. (2008). A theory of risk and resilience factors in military families. *Military Psychology, 20,* 205–217.

Picchioni, D., Cabrera, O. A., McGurk, D., Thomas, J. L., Castro, C. A., Balkin, T. J., et al. (2010). Sleep symptoms as a partial mediator between combat stressors and other mental health symptoms in Iraq War veterans. *Military Psychology, 22,* 340–355.

Pietrzak, R. H., Goldstein, M. B., Malley, J. C., Rivers, A. J., Johnson, D. C., Morgan, C. A., et al. (2010). Posttraumatic growth in veterans of Operations Enduring Freedom and Iraqi Freedom. *Journal of Affective Disorders, 126,* 230–235.

Prins, A., Ouimette, P., Kimerling, R., Cameron, R. P., Hugelshofer, D. S., Shaw-Hegwer, J., et al. (2003). The Primary Care PTSD Screen (PC-PTSD): Development and operating characteristics. *Primary Care Psychiatry, 9,* 9–14.

Ray, R., & Webster, R. (2010). Group interpersonal therapy for veterans with posttraumatic stress disorder: A pilot study. *International Journal of Group Psychotherapy, 60,* 131–140.

Resick, P. A., Monson, C. M., & Chard, K. M. (2007). *Cognitive processing therapy: Veteran/military version.* Washington, DC: Department of Veterans Affairs.

Resick, P. A., Nishith, P., Weaver, T. L., Astin, M. C., & Feuer, C. A. (2002). A comparison of cognitive-processing therapy with prolonged exposure and a waiting condition for the treatment of chronic posttraumatic stress disorder in female rape victims. *Journal of Consulting and Clinical Psychology, 70*(4), 867–879.

Resnick, H. S., Foy, D. W., Donahoe, C. P., & Miller, E. N. (1989). Antisocial behavior and post-traumatic stress disorder in Vietnam veterans. *Journal of Clinical Psychology, 45,* 860–866.

Riddle, M. S., Sandersa, J. W., Jones, J. J., & Webb, S. C. (2008). Self-reported combat stress indicators among troops deployed to Iraq and Afghanistan: An epidemiological study. *Comprehensive Psychiatry, 49,* 340–345.

Riggs, D. S., Byrne, C. A., Weathers, F. W., & Litz, B. T. (1998). The quality of the intimate relationships of male Vietnam veterans: Problems associated with posttraumatic stress disorder. *Journal of Traumatic Stress, 11,* 87–101.

Rona, R. J., Fear, N. T., Hull, L., Greenberg, N., Earnshaw, M., Hotopf, M., et al. (2007). Mental health consequences of overstretch in the UK armed forces: First phase of a cohort study. *British Journal of Medicine, 335,* 603.

Rosen, L. N., Teitelbaum, J. M., & Westhuis, D. J. (1993). Children's reactions to the Desert Storm deployment: Initial findings from a survey of Army families. *Military Medicine, 158,* 465–469.

Rothbaum, B. O., Astin, M. C., & Marsteller, F. (2005). Prolonged exposure versus eye movement desensitization and reprocessing (EMDR) for PTSD rape victims. *Journal of Traumatic Stress, 18,* 607–616.

Ruger, W., Wilson, S. E., & Waddoups, S. L. (2002). Warfare and welfare: Military service, combat, and marital dissolution. *Armed Forces and Society, 29,* 85–107.

Schneier, F. R., Foose, T. E., Hasin, D. S., Heimberg, R. G., Liu, S. M., & Grant, B. F. (2010). Social anxiety disorder and alcohol use disorder co-morbidity in the National Epidemiologic Survey on alcohol and related conditions. *Psychological Medicine, 40,* 977–988.

Schnurr, P. P., Friedman, M. J., Engell, C. C., Foa, E. B., Shea, M. T., Chow, B. K., et al. (2007). Cognitive behavioral therapy for posttraumatic stress disorder in women: A randomized controlled trial. *Journal of the American Medical Association, 297,* 820–830.

Schwab, J., Ice., J., Stephenson, J., Raymer, K., Houser, K., Graziano, L., et al. (1995). War and the family. *Stress Medicine, 11,* 131–137.

Seal, K. H., Bertenthal, D., Nuber, C. R., Sen, S., & Marmar, C. (2007). Bringing the war back home: Mental health disorders among 103,788 US veterans returning from Iraq and Afghanistan seen at Department of Veterans Affairs facilities. *Archives of Internal Medicine, 167,* 476–482.

Shapiro, F. (1995). *Eye movement desensitization and reprocessing (EMDR): Basic principles, protocols, and procedures.* New York: Guilford Press.

Shapiro, F. (2001). *Eye movement desensitization and reprocessing: Basic principles, protocols, and procedures* (2nd ed.). New York: Guilford Press.

Sharkansky, E. J., Brief, D. J., Peirce, J. M., Meehan, J. C., & Mannix, L. M. (1999). Substance abuse patients with posttraumatic stress disorder (PTSD): Identifying specific triggers of substance use and their associations with PTSD symptoms. *Psychology of Addictive Behaviors, 13,* 89–97.

Sherman, M. D., Sautter, F., Jackson, M. H., Lyons, J. A., & Han, X. (2006). Domestic violence in veterans with posttraumatic stress disorder who seek couples therapy. *Journal of Marital Family Therapy, 32,* 479–490.

Smith, T. C., Ryan, M. A. K., Wingard, D. L., Slymen, D. J., Sallis, J. F., & Kritz-Silverstein, D. (2008). New onset and persistent symptoms of post-traumatic stress disorder self reported after deployment and combat exposures: Prospective population based US military cohort study. *British Medical Journal, 336,* 366–371.

Stewart, S. H. (1996). Alcohol abuse in individuals exposed to trauma: A critical review. *Psychological Bulletin, 120,* 83–112.

Thomas, J. L., Wilk, J. E., Riviere, L. A., McGurk, D., Castro, C. A., & Hoge, C. W. (2010). Prevalence of mental health problems and functional impairment among active component and National Guard soldiers 3 and 12 months following combat in Iraq. *Archives of General Psychiatry, 67,* 614–623.

Tomlinson, K. L., Tate, S. R., Anderson, K. G., McCarthy, D. M., & Brown, S. A. (2006). An examination of self-medication and rebound effects: Psychiatric symptomatology before and after drug relapse. *Addictive Behaviors, 31,* 461–474.

U.S. Department of the Army. (1996). *Combat operational stress control.* Washington, DC: Author.

U.S. Department of the Army. (2010). *Health promotion risk reduction, and suicide prevention.* Washington, DC: Author.

U.S. Department of Veterans Affairs & Department of Defense. (2009). *VA/DoD clinical practice guideline for management of major depressive disorder (MDD).* Washington, DC: Author.

U.S. Department of Veterans Affairs & Department of Defense. (2010). *VA/DoD clinical practice guideline for the management of post-traumatic stress.* Washington, DC: Author.

Van Schaik, A., van Marwijk, H., Ader, H., van Dyck, R., de Haan, M., Penninx, B., et al. (2006). Interpersonal psychotherapy for elderly patients in primary care. *American Journal of Geriatric Psychiatry, 14,* 777–786.

Weathers, F. W., Huska, J., & Keane, T. M. (1991). *The PTSD Checklist Military Version (PCL-M).* Boston: National Center for PTSD.

Weissman, M. M., Markowitz, J. C., & Klerman, G. L. (2000). *Comprehensive guide to interpersonal psychotherapy.* New York: Basic Books.

Wesensten, N. J., & Balkin, T. J. (2010). Cognitive sequelae of sustained operations. In C. H. Kennedy & J. L. Moore (Eds.), *Military neuropsychology* (pp. 297–320). New York: Springer.

Wilk, J. E., Bliese, P. D., Kim, P. Y., Thomas, J. L., McGurk, D., & Hoge, C. W. (2010). Relationship of combat experiences to alcohol misuse among US soldiers returning from the Iraq War. *Drug and Alcohol Dependence, 108,* 115–121.

Williams, J., Jones, S. B., Pemberton, M. R., Bray, R. M., Brown, J. M., & Vandermaas-Peeler, R. (2010). Measurement invariance of alcohol use motivations in junior military personnel at risk for depression or anxiety. *Addictive Behaviors, 35,* 444–451.

CHAPTER 6

Clinical Health Psychology and Behavioral Medicine in Military Healthcare Settings

Alan L. Peterson
Ann S. Hryshko-Mullen
Donald D. McGeary

This chapter reviews the specialty area of behavioral medicine and clinical health psychology in military healthcare. We begin with the definition of various terms used to describe this area. Next, the recommended education and training for individuals interested in working in this specialty are evaluated. The chapter examines the spectrum of applications of behavioral medicine and clinical health psychology, including disease management and health interventions. Finally, we provide a brief review of individual and group evidence-based interventions for common behavioral risk factors and medical conditions treated in military behavioral medicine and clinical health psychology settings.

DEFINITIONS OF CLINICAL HEALTH PSYCHOLOGY AND BEHAVIORAL MEDICINE

A number of terms have been used to describe this specialty area, including "behavioral medicine" (Schwartz & Weiss, 1978), "medical psychology" (Prokop & Bradley, 1981), "psychosomatic medicine" (Lipowski, Lipsitt,

& Whybrow, 1977; Weddington & Blindt, 1983), "behavioral health" (Matarazzo, 1980), "behavioral health psychology" (Matarazzo, Weiss, Herd, Miller, & Weiss, 1984), "health psychology" (Goldberg, Carlson, & Paige-Dobson, 1994; Millon, 1982; Stone et al., 1987), and "clinical health psychology" (Belar & Deardorff, 2009).

As a multidisciplinary profession, "behavioral medicine" probably best describes this specialty area. The Society of Behavioral Medicine (SBM) was established in 1978 with 60 charter members who were originally part of the Association for Behavioral and Cognitive Therapies (ABCT; previously called the Association for Advancement of Behavior Therapy). The fact that SBM was spawned from ABCT is a testament to the strong behavioral and scientific underpinnings in this professional organization. The emergence of behavioral medicine was due in part to the success of the fields of behavior modification, applied behavioral analysis, and behavior therapy (Blanchard, 1982). SBM includes psychologists, psychiatrists, social workers, nurses, dentists, and physicians from a number of nonpsychiatric specialties such as internal medicine. SBM now has more than 2,000 members, the largest proportion of which comprises psychologists (Society of Behavioral Medicine, 2012).

There are some limitations of the term "behavioral medicine" as it relates to the discipline of psychology. By definition, individuals who work in the field of behavioral medicine collaborate closely with medical and dental colleagues. However, the term "medicine" is a bit of a misnomer, because it relates to departments (e.g., academic departments of psychology) or clinics that are staffed exclusively by psychologists. Therefore, "behavioral medicine" in this context can be misconstrued to mean that psychologists are practicing medicine. In the Army, "behavioral medicine" has been used somewhat synonymously with "mental health."

The best term to describe this specialty, that is, the clinical practice of psychologists in healthcare settings, is "clinical health psychology." The term was initially archived by the American Psychological Association (APA) in 1997 and is defined as follows:

> Clinical Health Psychology applies scientific knowledge of the interrelationships among behavioral, emotional, cognitive, social and biological components in health and disease to the promotion and maintenance of health; the prevention, treatment and rehabilitation of illness and disability; and the improvement of the health care system. The distinct focus of Clinical Health Psychology (also known as behavioral medicine, medical psychology and psychosomatic medicine) is at the juncture of physical and emotional illness, understanding and treating the overlapping challenges. (American Psychological; Association, 2012)

Behavioral medicine and clinical health psychology have been the fastest growing specialties in psychology over the past 25 years. Clinical health psychology is currently the most popular specialty in postdoctoral training. Of the 126 postdoctoral fellowship programs listed in the Association of Psychology Postdoctoral and Internship Centers guide (2010), 66 programs (52%) provide training in clinical health psychology, compared with 52 (41%) for neuropsychology, one of the other popular fellowship programs.

Another testament to the growth of this specialty is the number of psychologists who work at medical schools. In 1953, 255 psychologists were employed by American medical schools. By 1993 that number had grown to more than 3,500. Similarly, the average number of psychologists employed by each medical school grew from 2 in the 1950s to 28 in the 1990s (Sheridan, 1999).

The specific names of clinics and clinical services in military healthcare that offer this type of clinical assessment and treatment have varied over the past two decades, to include the terms "behavioral medicine clinic" and "behavioral health psychology service." Currently, the term "clinical health psychology" best describes the practice of this specialty in most military and civilian healthcare settings.

CLINICAL PROBLEMS ADDRESSED BY BEHAVIORAL MEDICINE AND CLINICAL HEALTH PSYCHOLOGY

Clinical health psychologists at major medical centers in the military provide nonpharmacological, nonsurgical interventions for conditions in which behavioral factors play a primary or secondary role. Common areas of emphasis include chronic pain, insomnia, obesity, tobacco dependence, diabetes, hypertension, gastrointestinal disorders, chronic obstructive pulmonary disease, cancer, and behavioral cardiology. Patients are usually treated outside of the usual mental health clinic population to help avoid the mental health stigma and to differentiate clearly between the treatment of medical and mental health conditions. Clinical health psychologists usually provide treatment primarily for diagnosed medical conditions or behavioral factors that affect health (e.g., smoking). Patients referred by physicians to clinical health psychologists often believe that this means that their physicians think their problem is "not real" or "all in their head." Therefore, it is often helpful to reassure patients early in the evaluation that it is presumed that they are being evaluated for a true medical or dental condition and that if it were believed that they had a primary mental health condition, then they would have been referred to the mental health clinic instead. This is one reason why many clinical health psychology clinics are established as separate and independent clinics from mental health clinics. In most cases, patients referred to a clinical health psychology service are seen for evaluation only when referred by a physician, dentist, or other healthcare provider. In most cases, patients should be medically cleared by the referring provider before the initiation of behavioral treatment to ensure that there is no underlying physical cause that has not yet been adequately evaluated or treated (e.g., a headache caused by a brain tumor).

Clinical health psychologists evaluate and treat a wide variety of health-related conditions. Belar and Deardorff (2009) outlined a variety of healthcare services provided by clinical health psychologists such as:

1. Assessment for medical procedures such as organ transplants, bone marrow transplants, or bariatric surgery.
2. Anxiety reduction for medical and dental treatments.
3. Pain management interventions.
4. Interventions to control symptoms (e.g., vomiting associated with chemotherapy).
5. Support groups for patients with chronic medical conditions.
6. Rehabilitation interventions after traumatic injury or stroke.
7. Interventions targeting leading health risk behaviors such as smoking, obesity, and physical inactivity.
8. Consultations regarding medical staff working relationships and communication.
9. Development of worksite health promotion programs.
10. Neuropsychological assessment after head injury.

Many military clinical or counseling psychologists have experience and training in the assessment and treatment of a number of these conditions. However, fellowship training in clinical health psychology is recommended for individuals whose primary clinical practice consists of the evaluation and treatment of patients with these conditions. Fellowship-trained clinical health psychologists often serve as the chief of a clinical health psychology service or clinic at a major military medical center and are often the final tertiary referral source for many of these patients. In these settings, clinical health psychologists are often the only specialty-trained provider for assessment and treatment for all of the different conditions outlined by Belar and Deardorff (2009). Military psychologists who are generalists as well as those who are specialists must be sure they have adequate education and training to be able to practice within their scope of care (APA, 2002).

RECOMMENDED EDUCATION AND TRAINING

Formal training in clinical health psychology occurs at the doctoral, internship, and postdoctoral levels (Sheridan et al., 1988; Stone et al., 1987). Within the last 5 years, there have been numerous influences advancing the education and training of clinical health psychologists. Consistent with the movement in professional psychology training, there has been an emphasis on identifying competencies required of clinical health psychologists and appropriate levels of training for these competencies. In March 2007, a working group of clinical health psychology educators and trainers held an executive summit in Tempe, Arizona ("Tempe Summit") to identify the foundational and functional competencies expected of a well-trained, entry-level clinical health psychologist based on the Rodolfa et al. (2005) cube model of competency development (France et al., 2008). Another outcome of the Tempe Summit was the reactivation of the health psychology training council that had been inactive since the mid-1990s; this newly renamed Council of Clinical Health Psychology Training Programs held its inaugural meeting in January 2008 in San Antonio, Texas. Further developments in the training guidelines and recommendations for clinical health psychology were described in a series of articles published in *Training and Education in Professional Psychology* in 2009, identifying "best practices" and addressing training at the doctoral training program, predoctoral internship, and postdoctoral levels and beyond to recognize lifelong competency development (Masters, France, & Thorn, 2009; Larkin, 2009; Kerns, Berry, Frantsve, & Linton, 2009). Another significant development in the elucidation of education and training guidelines in clinical health psychology was the Riverfront Conference held in February 2010 (Suls, 2010). During this APA Division 38-sponsored meeting, participants explored what 21st-century clinical health psychology training should look like in basic and clinical science/practice; this was the first time this question was formally addressed since the Arden House Conference in 1983.

Many graduate programs in clinical and counseling psychology have specialty tracks in clinical health psychology or behavioral medicine. Individuals in these programs take specialty coursework and complete at least one clinical practicum in a healthcare setting. Similarly, many psychology internship programs have either a primary emphasis or a major rotation in clinical health psychology or behavioral medicine. Postdoctoral fellowships in clinical health psychology are usually 1 or 2 years long. The specific focus of each fellowship varies, depending on the program. Most programs include supervised training in the following areas: (1) assessment and management of chronic disease and illness, (2) maintenance of health through prevention efforts, (3) evaluation of intervention effectiveness, (4) development of interdisciplinary collaboration with other healthcare providers, (5) skills necessary to develop disease management teams, (6) use of population health assessment and treatment strategies, and (7) development of skills necessary to complete applied clinical research.

Most civilian fellowship programs have a targeted focus in one or two specific areas of behavioral medicine such as pain management or weight management. The military-sponsored fellowships at Wilford Hall

Ambulatory Surgical Center in San Antonio, Texas, and Tripler Army Medical Center in Hawaii are much broader and prepare graduates to serve as the chief of clinical health psychology at a military medical center (James, Folen, Porter, & Kellar, 1999). These programs prepare clinical health psychologists to handle almost any type of behavioral medicine referral. The military fellowship programs do allow for a specific emphasis in an area of interest of the postdoctoral fellow along with the more broad-based clinical health psychology training.

The number of APA-accredited postdoctoral fellowship programs has increased significantly since 1999, when the APA first offered to evaluate specialty accreditation applications. There are currently six APA-accredited postdoctoral residency training programs in clinical health psychology. The clinical health psychology program at Wilford Hall Ambulatory Surgical Center was the first postdoctoral fellowship program in the country to apply to the APA as a specialty program. The Army also sponsors a postdoctoral fellowship in clinical health psychology at Tripler Army Medical Center. Both the Air Force and Army fellowships in clinical health psychology are accredited by the APA; the Air Force program is accredited as a specialty practice program, whereas the Army program is accredited as a traditional practice program. In addition, the Air Force program is accredited as a Behavioral Sleep Medicine program by the American Academy of Sleep Medicine. The Navy utilizes the Army program to train clinical health psychologists.

The capstone of education and training in clinical health psychology is to become board certified by the American Board of Professional Psychology (ABPP). Graduates of the fellowship programs at Wilford Hall and Tripler have been very successful in obtaining an ABPP in clinical health psychology. Military psychologists currently receive board certification pay of $6,000 per year for obtaining a diplomate in one of the ABPP specialties.

EVIDENCE-BASED TREATMENT APPROACHES

Numerous excellent textbooks provide comprehensive reviews of behavioral medicine and clinical health psychology (Baum, Revenson, & Singer, 2001; Belar & Deardorff, 2009; Boll, Johnson, Perry, & Rozensky, 2002; Frank, Baum, & Wallander, 2004; Frank & Elliott, 2000; Llewelyn & Kennedy, 2003; Nicassio & Smith, 1995; Raczynski & Leviton, 2004). Therefore, detailed information on epidemiology, assessment, and empirically supported treatment for each of these conditions is not reviewed in this chapter. The *Journal of Consulting and Clinical Psychology* has published a special issue devoted to behavioral medicine and clinical health psychology every decade since 1982 (Blanchard, 1982, 1992; Smith, Kendall, & Keefe, 2002). This special issue provides one of the best reviews of the literature on the assessment and treatment of individual patients that are most commonly seen in a behavioral medicine or clinical health psychology service.

There are a variety of behavioral medicine and clinical health psychology treatments with specific relevance to military healthcare settings, including tobacco cessation, weight management, pain management, insomnia management, diabetes management, temporomandibular disorders management, cardiac rehabilitation, and pulmonary rehabilitation. Formal, manualized treatment programs for all of these areas are available from me (A. S. H.-M.) through the Clinical Health Psychology Service at Wilford Hall, including both provider and patient manuals for most of these areas. Four of these areas—tobacco cessation, weight management, chronic pain management, and insomnia management—are of significant importance to military clinical health psychologists and are subsequently addressed here in depth.

Tobacco Cessation

Tobacco cessation is the most important target of behavioral medicine interventions for psychologists in both military and civilian settings (Niaura & Abrams, 2002; Peterson, Vander Weg, & Jaén, 2011; Wetter et al., 1998). Tobacco use is the leading cause of preventable death in the United States (Centers for Disease Control and Prevention, 1997), and more than 400,000 Americans die each year from smoking-related causes (Mokdad, Marks, Stroup, & Gerberding, 2004). About 48 million Americans smoke (Centers for Disease Control and Prevention, 2000), and it can be expected that between one-third and one-half will die from smoking-related causes (Mokdad et al., 2004).

Smoking is also the single most important health risk for the U.S. military. More Americans will die this year from smoking-related illnesses than have died in the past 100 years in military combat. Additional healthcare and decreased productivity costs related to smoking in the U.S. military have been estimated at $930 million per year (Robbins, Chao, Coil, & Fonseca, 2000). Service members who smoke are significantly more likely to be prematurely discharged from active duty than nonsmokers, resulting in an approximate annual cost of more than $130 million in excess training costs across all service branches (Klesges, Haddock, Chang, Talcott, & Lando, 2001). Smoking affects personnel readiness through lower levels of physical fitness, increased risk for injuries, and more sick days (Altarac et al., 2000; Lincoln, Smith, Amoroso, & Bell, 2003). Although smoking by active-duty U.S. military personnel steadily declined for almost 2 decades (1980–1998), there has been a significant increase in smoking from 1998 to

2002 (Bray et al., 2003). We have no scientific data identifying the cause of this increase, but one theory posits that it may be related to the increase in stress on military members related to deployments and other work-related demands since September 11, 2001. The current prevalence of smoking in the military (any smoking in the past 12 months) is as follows: Army, 35.6%; Navy, 36.0%; Marine Corps, 38.7%; Air Force, 27.0%. Service comparisons in the prevalence of any smokeless tobacco use in the past 12 months is as follows: Army, 14.0%; Navy, 9.0%; Marine Corps, 20.4%; Air Force, 8.8% (Bray et al., 2003).

Almost every U.S. military installation offers programs for tobacco cessation. The specific details of each program differ, depending on the location and available resources, but most include some combination of a behaviorally based program combined with nicotine replacement therapy (NRT) such as patches and gum (Fiore, Smith, Jorenby, & Baker, 1994; Hatsukami et al., 2000) and bupropion hydrochloride (Zyban; Hurt et al., 1997). Current research indicates that the combination of those three components (behavioral counseling, NRT, and bupropion) results in the greatest quit rates (Fiore et al., 2008; Jorenby et al., 1999). Most programs result in quit rates of about 25–35%, as seen by 7-day point prevalence measures at 1-year follow-up (Fiore et al., 2008). Many military cessation programs have advertised themselves as having extremely high quit rates (e.g., >75%). However, on closer scrutiny, these high rates are usually an artifact of the mode of measurement (e.g., not including all who start a program—only those who can be contacted at follow-up or reflecting poor measurement of tobacco use status). The only recent published study of tobacco cessation in a military setting found a 27% abstinence rate through the Tripler Tobacco Cessation Program (Faue, Folen, James, & Needels, 1997).

It is recommended that tobacco cessation programs be based on currently available scientific evidence and practice guidelines (Abrams et al., 2003; Fiore et al., 2008; Niaura & Abrams, 2002; Wetter et al., 1998). *Nicotine and Tobacco Dependence* (Peterson et al., 2011) can be used as a guide for tobacco cessation facilitators. It is based in part on the eight-session Wilford Hall Tobacco Cessation Program. In the program, bupropion is started during week 2 for those who are medically eligible, and the quit date is usually at the start of week 3. The newest tobacco cessation medication, varenicline (Chantix), can also be used as an alternative to NRT and bupropion. Weeks 4–8 focus on overcoming urges, relapse prevention, limiting weight gain (Talcott et al., 1995; Peterson, 1999; Peterson & Helton, 2000; Russ, Fonseca, Peterson, Blackman, & Robbins, 2001), stress management, relaxation training, and assertive communication. The program is designed for cigarette smoking as well as smokeless tobacco cessation (Cigrang, Severson, & Peterson, 2002; Peterson et al., 2007; Severson et al., 2009).

Four to 8 weeks of NRT, involving the nicotine patch or nicotine gum, are available as part of the program for those participants who are medically qualified (Fiore et al., 1994). NRT begins at the third session, which is the established quit date for the program, although some programs use it longer. However, nicotine patch treatment of 4–8 weeks has been shown to be as efficacious as longer treatment periods (Fiore et al., 1994). Therefore, we use 6 weeks of nicotine patches, gum, or both for our program. When both nicotine patches and nicotine gum are used, the patches are the primary form of NRT, with a few pieces of gum (usually fewer than six per day) to help with additional cravings. Bupropion is also available for 8 weeks, beginning the second week of the program. It is recommended that participants take bupropion for at least a week prior to their quit date. In most military tobacco cessation programs, the medications are bundled with the program, meaning that individuals must participate in the program and attend weekly sessions to obtain the medications. Research indicates that these medications do not work well unless combined with a comprehensive behavioral treatment program. However, there is evidence that less intensive programs can also be somewhat effective if delivered by a primary care provider (Fiore et al., 2008) or behavioral health consultant (Hunter & Peterson, 2001; James, Folen, Porter, et al., 1999).

A tobacco cessation program can be administered by a number of types of clinicians. Programs offered by a clinician (e.g., psychologist, physician, dentist, health educator, nurse) increases the smoking cessation rates relative to interventions in which there is no provider (Fiore et al., 2008). There is no evidence that cessation rates are increased if the program is administered by a former tobacco user as opposed to a clinician who has never used tobacco regularly. In the U.S. Air Force, psychologists receive training in tobacco cessation during their residency program and are the primary providers in these programs at most Air Force bases. In the Navy, individuals working or volunteering in health and wellness departments (e.g., dieticians, personal trainers, former tobacco users), psychologists, and substance abuse counselors are the primary facilitators of tobacco cessation courses, with augmentation by a family practice physician or physician's assistant, who provides prescriptions and assists enrollees in choosing their most optimal quit method.

One unique aspect of tobacco cessation in the military is related to tobacco use policies. Over the years, all four of the military services have banned tobacco use during basic training (Woodruff, Conway, & Edwards, 2000). Several studies have evaluated the impact of this ban as well as whether cessation rates can be improved with the addition of cessation and prevention programs. Most research has indicated that the policy banning tobacco use has a significant impact in helping some individuals remain abstinent after basic training (Klesges, Haddock, Lando, & Talcott, 1999;

Woodruff et al., 2000). However, the impact of the additional interventions has yielded much more modest effects (Conway et al., 2004). Additional research is needed to further evaluate population-based interventions and policy.

Weight Management

Obesity is second only to tobacco use in the risk for morbidity and mortality in the United States (Mokdad et al., 2004). According to national surveys that track weight trends, rates of overweight and obesity have increased steadily among adults over the past 40 years. For example, according to data from the National Health and Nutrition Examination Survey (NHANES), obesity [body mass index (BMI) > 30] prevalence has increased from 13.4% in 1960–1962 to 30.9% in 1999–2000 (Flegal, Carroll, Ogden, & Johnson, 2002). Not surprisingly, the prevalence of overweight (BMI > 25) has demonstrated similar patterns. For example, among adults surveyed in NHANES, the number of individuals who are overweight has increased from 45% in 1960–1962 to 64% in 1999–2000 (Fried, Prager, MacKay, & Xia, 2003). Similarly, the annual Behavioral Risk Factor Surveillance System Survey, using a random telephone survey of self-reported weight and height, has documented similar trends among adults. Overweight and obesity combined climbed from 44.7% in 1990 to 59.1% in 2002 (Centers for Disease Control and Prevention, 2004).

Despite an emphasis on fitness and readiness, the U.S. military has also had substantial increases in overweight and obese personnel. For example, Bray et al. (2003) report that the number of individuals who were overweight in 1995 amounted to 49.0%, increasing to 57.2% by 2002. A more recent report based on the National Health and Nutrition Examination Survey revealed that up to 33% of all American males and 53% of American females ages 17 to 24 years were overweight for armed forces enlistment between 2001 and 2004 (Yamane, 2007). The author notes that the increasing obesity rate among individuals eligible for enlistment in the military will result in a recruitment strain for the services in the future. Hsu, Nevin, Tobler, and Rubertone (2007) found that the rate of overweight among 18-year-old applicants for U.S. military enlistment rose from 23% in 1993 to 27% in 2006, and the rate of applicant obesity rose from 3 to 7% over the same time period.

Maintaining healthy body weight is a critical part of readiness in the military. The many possible consequences of being overweight include decreased fitness, poor public perception of military readiness, increased medical costs, and numerous administrative costs. Annual obesity-related hospitalization costs in the U.S. Navy have been estimated at $5,842,627 for the top 10 obesity-related diagnoses (Bradham et al., 2001). Also, it was estimated that the yearly costs of weight problems in the Air Force top $28 million, with about $24 million in direct medical costs and $4 million in indirect costs because of lost workdays (Robbins, Chao, Russ, & Fonseca, 2002). A 2007 study of TRICARE-PRIME enrollees revealed annual expenditures of $1.1 billion on obesity-related disease and close to $1 billion each year on nonmedical programs targeting obesity, tobacco use, and alcohol use (Dall et al., 2007). Excessive weight may be of particular concern for critical military operations since it is associated with increased daytime sleepiness, even without sleep apnea (Vgontzas et al., 1998). This may be due to the lack of physical fitness and/or eating habits characterized by excessive intake of high-fat foods, both of which have been shown to be a cause of low perceived energy. Also, the excessive administrative pressure to maintain or lose weight in the military is associated with disordered eating behaviors (McNulty, 2001; Peterson, Talcott, Kelleher, & Smith, 1995).

In-depth details of evidence-based behavioral interventions for weight management are beyond the scope of this chapter. Behavioral interventions provide a methodology for systematically modifying eating, exercise, or other behaviors that are thought to contribute to or to maintain excessive weight (Stunkard, 2001). Most of the various behavior therapies have several factors in common, including the use of self-monitoring and goal setting, stimulus control and modification of eating styles and habits, cognitive restructuring strategies that focus on challenging and modifying unrealistic or maladaptive thoughts or expectations, stress reduction and management strategies, and the use of social support (Foreyt & Goodrick, 1994; Perri & Fuller, 1995). The best published review of the current state of knowledge on overweight and obesity is the National Institutes of Health (1998) book *Clinical Guidelines on the Identification, Evaluation, and Treatment of Overweight and Obesity*. The best manualized intervention with significant empirical evidence of its efficacy is the *LEARN Program for Weight Management* (Brownell, 2004). This is a 16-week program emphasizing lifestyle, education, attitude, relationships, and nutrition. The Tripler Army Medical Center LE3AN Program (emphasizing healthy lifestyles, reasonable exercise, realistic expectations, emotions, attitudes, and nutrition) gives active-duty service members a treatment strategy that involves a reasonable low-intensity exercise regimen, behavior modification, intensive nutritional counseling, healthy meal planning, relapse prevention strategies, cognitive coping strategies, and healthy lifestyle principles for weight loss and maintenance. Several articles have demonstrated that this program is associated with significant weight loss for active-duty military participants (James et al., 1997; James, Folen, Page, et al., 1999; Simpson, Earles, Folen, Trammel, & James, 2004). There is good evidence that behavioral interventions for weight management can be administered over the Internet (Tate, Wing,

& Winett, 2001), including data from a large randomized controlled trial of this approach conducted in an active-duty military population in San Antonio through Wilford Hall (Hunter et al., 2008).

The increase in overweight and obesity among active-duty personnel, retirees, and their dependents has led to a rise in the use of bariatric surgery options to help obese individuals lose excess weight. Although surgical options may vary among military treatment facilities, three common surgical procedures include the Roux-en-Y gastric bypass, adjustable LAP-BAND® procedure, and sleeve gastrectomy. From a medical perspective, surgery should be considered for individuals with a BMI of 35–40 with comorbidities or a BMI > 40 (National Institutes of Health, 1991).

As weight loss surgeries proliferate, clinical health psychologists in the military are increasingly being challenged with meeting the need for psychosocial screenings of bariatric surgery candidates (Santry, Gillen, & Lauderdale, 2005). Many agree that these presurgical screenings contribute to the likelihood that candidates will benefit from the surgery (Bauchowitz et al., 2005; National Institutes of Health, 1991), although there is still some question as to the most significant domains for assessment. Bauchowitz and colleagues note that psychosocial exclusion criteria seem to vary widely among different institutions, and they suggest the need for improved assessment guidelines and more research on psychosocial predictors of postsurgical success. Areas of assessment tend to include details about eating behaviors and food choices, emotional symptoms that may contribute to "emotional eating" or poor coping after the procedure, familiarity with the weight loss surgery procedure itself, knowledge of side effects of the surgery (e.g., dumping syndrome), plans for managing/coping with these side effects, social support resources for recovery after surgery, the presence of eating disorders that may impact treatment success (e.g., binge eating), and exercise or other health behaviors that impact response to the surgery. Apart from screening for surgical candidates, the military clinical health psychologist may also be asked to follow up with surgery patients to help with coping and adherence to behavioral recommendations after the surgery.

Tobacco Cessation and Weight Gain in Military Personnel

One of the limitations of tobacco cessation is that many people gain weight afterward. This can be particularly problematic for military personnel because of the potential negative impact it can have on their military careers. Studies show that smokers lose weight after starting to smoke, weigh less than nonsmokers, and gain weight when they quit (French & Jeffery, 1995; Gritz, Klesges, & Meyers, 1989; Klesges, Myers, Klesges, & La Vasque, 1989; Perkins, 1993). A U.S. surgeon general's report (U.S.

Department of Health and Human Services, 1990) indicates that 80% of smokers who quit gain an average of 5 pounds. The results of the second NHANES indicate that female smokers who quit tend to gain more weight than their male counterparts (8.4 vs. 6.2 pounds; Williamson et al., 1991). Furthermore, about 10% of male and 13% of female ex-smokers gained more than 28 pounds. A study of active-duty military personnel indicates that they gained about the same amount of weight after smoking cessation as their civilian counterparts (Peterson & Helton, 2000). Therefore, it should not be surprising that the potential for weight gain is seen as a primary deterrent to smoking cessation.

Postcessation weight gain has been attributed to a variety of factors, including changes in metabolism, activity level, taste preferences, and energy storage and increases in food intake, especially sweet, fat, and salty foods (Klesges et al., 1989; Perkins, 1993; Williamson et al., 1991). Current practice guidelines for tobacco cessation include strategies to prevent weight gain (American Psychiatric Association, 1996), even though interventions designed specifically for that problem have generally been unsuccessful (Hall, Tunstall, Vila, & Duffy, 1992). One recent study (Spring et al., 2004) compared the effects of adding a diet and exercise intervention to a tobacco cessation program either concurrently or after smoking cessation. The weight management intervention was added to the first 8 weeks or the final 8 weeks of a 16-week tobacco cessation program. The results indicated that behavioral weight control did not undermine smoking cessation and produced better weight gain suppression when initiated after the smoking quit date.

Only one study to date has reported no weight gain after smoking cessation (Talcott et al., 1995). The authors evaluated U.S. Air Force recruits who were forced to quit smoking as part of their basic military training. The results indicated that smokers who quit in basic training did not gain weight during their 6-week training program. However, this investigation was conducted in a very controlled environment (i.e., limited access to sweet and fatty foods, no access to alcohol, and significantly increased levels of exercise).

One important factor may be one's knowledge of body weight prior to cessation of smoking. A meta-analysis of 24 studies on self-reported weight compared with measured weight among the general population and individuals in a weight loss program found that for 84% of the sample the average self-report was lower than measured weights, typically by 2 to 5 pounds (Bowman & Delucia, 1992). Similarly, a study by Peterson (1999) found that about two-thirds of individuals entering a smoking cessation program significantly underestimated their body weight: females weighed about 9 pounds and males about 6 pounds more than their estimates. These weight differences are of the same magnitude found in controlled studies of weight gain after smoking cessation (Klesges et al., 1989; Perkins, 1993; Williamson et al., 1991). The significance of these results is that because many people underestimate their body weight prior to smoking cessation, they believe they have gained about twice as much weight as they actually have. This may be particularly true for those who weigh themselves only after they have quit smoking.

It has been suggested that a common reason for people to smoke is to help control their weight. One military study examined concern about weight gain and found that active-duty members, especially those who were close to or over their maximum allowable weight, had significantly higher levels of concern about weight gain with tobacco cessation and increased risk of anticipated relapse with weight gain than did civilians (Russ et al., 2001).

Despite the impact of tobacco use on the health and fitness of active-duty members, as well as the large direct medical costs and indirect costs (lost work days), there are no official negative consequences for tobacco use in the military (Robbins et al., 2000). In contrast, poor cardiovascular fitness and excess abdominal girth place active-duty individuals under immediate scrutiny by their commander. Should the members fail to make adequate improvements in fitness and/or abdominal circumference, they could be separated from the service. Given such consequences, military personnel are in a bind because, although they would like to quit smoking, it may have a negative impact on their military career.

Chronic Pain Management

Military clinical health psychologists treat a variety of chronic pain conditions, including musculoskeletal disorders (Guzman et al., 2001), headaches (Holroyd, 2002), arthritis (Keefe, Smith, et al., 2002), fibromyalgia (Baumstark & Buckelew, 1992), temporomandibular disorders (Bogart et al., 2007; Peterson, Dixon, Talcott, & Kelleher, 1993; Turk, Zaki, & Rudy, 1993), and abdominal pain (Blanchard & Scharff, 2002), to name just a few. Although there are many similarities in the behavioral treatment of various chronic pain conditions, there are also unique differences. A review of the specific treatment approaches for each pain condition is beyond the scope of this chapter. However, chronic musculoskeletal pain is of particular importance for military clinical health psychologists. Such pain conditions are the leading cause of medical discharge from active duty for the Army (53%), Navy and Marine Corps (63%), and Air Force (22%). Chronic musculoskeletal disorders are also a significant economic cost to the U.S. Department of Defense in terms of disability payments. For example, the Army paid $485 million for disability cases in 1993 alone (Amoroso & Canham, 1999). The discharge of one active-duty member for a musculoskeletal pain condition costs the U.S. government an estimated $250,000 in lifetime disability payments, not including potential additional healthcare costs (Feuerstein, Berkowitz, Pastel, & Huang, 1999).

The most effective treatment for chronic musculoskeletal disorders in terms of reducing pain and improving function in civilian populations is an interdisciplinary chronic pain rehabilitation program (Guzman et al., 2001; Turk & Okifuji, 2002). These programs, usually full time for several weeks, include an integrated program comprising a number of clinical services (e.g., physical therapy, occupational therapy, biofeedback, cognitive therapy, relaxation, and a gradually increasing self-managed physical exercise program).

Functional restoration (FR) is a model of interdisciplinary musculoskeletal pain management based on a sports medicine approach that uses a patient's physical and functional capacity as well as psychosocial assessments to organize an interdisciplinary team treatment plan whose primary goal is to restore patients to productivity (Mayer, McGeary, & Gatchel, 2003). Treatment is tailored around the patient's self-report of pain, medical history, personal goals, and functional capacity measurements. The role of the clinical health psychologist in an FR model can vary but typically includes quantifying the patient's social and emotional functioning, reactivating the deconditioned patient in preparation for exercise and restoration of function, reintegrating the patient into work and social life, feeding information about emotional and motivational adjustment to the rest of the team, and tracking patient outcome after treatment to evaluate continuing patient needs and treatment success. Although offering an excellent opportunity to learn from working closely with other disciplines, the FR approach offers unique challenges for psychologists and may leave them feeling alienated from the rest of their profession (Pieters & Baumgartner, 2002) or struggling to clearly identify their role in the new organization (McCallin, 2001). A functional restoration model was recently developed and utilized with a military musculoskeletal pain population with good results (Gatchel et al., 2009).

The current conflicts in Iraq and Afghanistan have resulted in an increased prevalence of musculoskeletal injuries, which could lead to chronic pain conditions. Because of the nature of most deployment-related injuries in Operation Iraqi Freedom/Operation Enduring Freedom (OIF/OEF), many deployers sustaining painful injuries are also subjected to posttraumatic stress disorder (PTSD) or traumatic brain injury (TBI). The combination of chronic musculoskeletal pain and PTSD/TBI offers significant challenges for pain treatment, making the role of the clinical health psychologist on pain treatment teams vital. Although there is a dearth of information about the prevalence of these comorbid conditions, one recent study found a 40–50% prevalence of pain and PTSD, pain and TBI, or all three conditions among a

Veterans Administration OIF/OEF combat-related trauma population (Lew et al., 2009). The combination of chronic pain and PTSD, in particular, is now receiving a great deal of attention (Otis, Keane, & Kerns, 2003).

There seems to be a high incidence of psychological distress and PTSD following general trauma (Holbrook, Anderson, Sieber, Browner, & Hoyt, 1999). A study conducted by Starr and colleagues in 2004 found a relatively high incidence of PTSD symptoms in an orthopedic pain population, with some estimates of the comorbidity of pain and PTSD at well over 50%. PTSD seems to affect patients' reports of physical complaints (Michaels et al., 1999) and is among the variables that are most predictive of functional outcome following injury. In a retrospective study examining persons with moderate traumatic injury, PTSD was found to contribute more to perceived general health than injury severity or the degree of physical functioning (Schnyder, Moergeli, Klaghofer, & Buddeberg, 2001).

Because posttraumatic stress may explain why some trauma patients report poor outcomes (even when traditional "objective" variables, such as wound healing or limb function, would lead a clinician to expect good results), it seems logical that psychological treatment might be a key component in improving pain patients' overall functioning. The WHO World Mental Health Survey Consortium in 2004 noted that treatments that improve psychological outcome, even if only slightly, should reduce the economic impact of trauma as well as improve functional outcomes for trauma survivors. Psychosocial trauma treatments have also been encouraged by the Centers for Disease Control and Prevention (2002) injury research agenda, calling for pain and trauma researchers to "develop and evaluate protocols that provide onsite interventions in acute care settings, or linkages to off-site services, for patients at risk of injury or psychosocial problems following injury."

The current conflicts in Iraq and Afghanistan have led to an increase in chronic pain prevalence (thanks to life-saving advancements in medical care and body armor). Additionally, the uniquely traumatic mechanisms of orthopedic injury in OIF/OEF are resulting in complex pain presentation as a result of the added impact of posttraumatic stress and TBI symptoms. As the problem of pain in the military grows, it has become increasingly clear that there is a role for military clinical health psychology in the effective treatment and long-term management of chronic pain. Although little information is currently available to guide the interdisciplinary treatment of complex trauma pain, efforts are already well under way to clarify effective pathways.

Insomnia and Nightmares

Insomnia is another common condition of significant importance to military clinical health psychologists because of its high prevalence rate and potential source of accidents, especially in deployed locations (Peterson, Goodie, Satterfield, & Brim, 2008). Insomnia has received increased attention since OEF and OIF/Operation New Dawn (OND) began, because insomnia is a common symptom among persons with PTSD. Chronic insomnia is one of the most common clinical symptoms in primary care settings, with an estimated prevalence rate of 32% (Kushida et al., 2000; National Heart, Lung, and Blood Institute Working Group on Insomnia, 1999). Insomnia is associated with increased healthcare utilization (Kapur et al., 2002) and decreased health-related quality of life (Katz & McHorney, 2002; Zammit, Weiner, Damato, Sillup, & McMillan, 1999). Another sleep concern often associated with insomnia is nightmares. Treatment of nightmares (a frequent sleep-related symptom of PTSD) has also garnered significant attention in recent years in military psychology.

Pharmacological treatments for insomnia are the most commonly used approaches (Morin, Colecchi, Stone, Stood, & Brink, 1999; Morin & Wooten, 1996), although such treatments are most helpful with acute insomnia (Smith, Perlis, et al., 2002). Behavioral approaches are the treatment of choice for chronic insomnia and include a combination of stimulus control, sleep restriction, relaxation, paradoxical intention, and cognitive-behavior therapy (Lichstein & Riedel, 1994; Morin et al., 2006; Morin, Colecchi, et al., 1999; Morin, Culbert, & Schwartz, 1994; Morin, Hauri, et al., 1999; Murtagh & Greenwood, 1995; Smith, Perlis, et al., 2002). These psychological and behavioral interventions have been documented to effectively treat not only primary insomnia but also insomnia associated with some medical conditions and to a lesser extent insomnia associated with psychiatric conditions (Morin et al., 2006). This finding is particularly important given the number of wounded warriors with physical, psychiatric, or combined injuries returning from OEF and OIF/OND. Group treatment for insomnia has also been demonstrated to be clinically effective in military healthcare settings (Hryshko-Mullen, Broeckl, Haddock, & Peterson, 2000) and to result in a significant reduction in overall healthcare utilization (Peterson, Hryshko-Mullen, Alexander, & Nelson, 1999).

Before initiating treatment for insomnia, it is important to have a patient complete a 1- to 2-week sleep diary. The sleep diary is the gold standard for the objective assessment of insomnia on an outpatient basis (Mimeault & Morin, 1999; Morin, 1993) and provides a relatively reliable picture of a patient's sleep patterns. A daily sleep diary allows for the calculation of total sleep time, sleep-onset latency, number of nighttime awakenings, sleep efficiency, and other sleep variables. These results can then be used for setting goals and planning treatment.

Sleep hygiene education instructs the patient to avoid caffeine consumption within 4–6 hours of bedtime, smoking near bedtime, alcohol after dinner, sleep medications, alcohol as a sleep aid, rigorous exercise within 2 hours of bedtime, and napping (Riedel, 2000). Although changes in such practices alone often do not lead to significant improvements in insomnia, poor sleep hygiene can aggravate it.

Stimulus control has been long recognized as a well-established behavioral treatment for insomnia (Bootzen & Epstein, 2000; Chesson et al., 1999; Morin et al., 2006). With stimulus control, the bed and bedroom should be reserved for sleep and sex only (e.g., do not watch television, listen to the radio, eat, or read in the bedroom). The general guidelines for stimulus control are to (1) set a reasonable bedtime and arising time and stick to them, (2) go to bed only when you are sleepy, (3) get out of bed when you can't fall asleep or go back to sleep in about 15 minutes, (4) return to bed only when you are sleepy, and (5) repeat steps 2–4 as often as necessary. Sleep restriction—now recognized as a well-established treatment for insomnia (Morin et al., 2006)—involves limiting or restricting the sleep window (established bedtime and awakening time) to the average total sleep time obtained from the sleep diary (Spielman, Saskin, & Thorpy, 1987).

For a case example of the use of sleep restriction, suppose that Petty Officer (PO) Smith's sleep diary indicates that he usually goes to bed at about 2000, takes about 90 minutes to fall asleep, wakes up about three times during the night, lies awake in bed for about 30 minutes each time he wakes up, and gets out of bed about 0600 immediately after he wakes up in the morning. In this case, PO Smith's total time in bed is 10 hours, his total sleep time 7 hours, and his sleep efficiency 70% [total sleep time (7 hours)/ total time in bed (10 hours) = 70%]. In this case, a sleep window of 7 hours would be recommended to PO Smith. The provider would then collaborate with him to establish the sleep window. Let's assume that PO Smith indicates that he would prefer to continue to wake up at 0600. His sleep window would then be set for 2300 to 0600. In this case, PO Smith would probably be shocked at the suggestion that he has to stay awake until 2300, 3 hours after his regular bedtime. The provider would then discuss the fact that he was already spending 3 hours awake in bed every night and then ask what kinds of activities he might engage in if he had an additional 3 hours of time available to him every day. In all likelihood, PO Smith would still not be convinced that the sleep restriction approach would work for him, and he would probably suggest that he did not think he could possibly stay up that late every night. In this case, a useful response by the provider might be to ask him, "Which do you think would be more difficult for you to do: force yourself to fall asleep or force yourself to stay awake?" To this question, PO Smith would most likely acknowledge that trying to force himself to fall asleep had not worked in the past. The provider might then suggest, "Would you be willing to try an experiment? Perhaps you could try this approach for just 4 weeks and see what happens? If your sleep gets worse after a few weeks of trying this, you can always stop and go back to your approach again."

Assuming that PO Smith agreed to give this approach a try, it would be important to encourage him to continue to maintain his sleep diary as a "scientific" way to see whether the experiment works. It would also be helpful to review the sleep hygiene and stimulus control procedures with him before starting the sleep restriction. If PO Smith was able to come up with a good plan to keep himself awake until 2300 each evening, he would probably be very tired by 2300, he would be looking forward to his bedtime (instead of dreading it), and he would probably fall asleep within about 15 minutes. If his sleep efficiency were to remain above 85% for the week, the duration of his sleep window would be increased by 20–30 minutes so that his bedtime was reset for 2230 or 2240. This same procedure of gradually increasing the sleep window each week that sleep efficiency remained above 85% would be repeated until sleep disruption occurred. This would indicate that the sleep window was too wide, and the duration of the window would be fine-tuned until PO Smith reached his optimum sleep window.

A sleep problem receiving increased attention within military psychology is nightmares. Although nightmares can occur as a stand-alone problem (i.e., nightmare disorder in the *Diagnostic and Statistical Manual*; American Psychiatric Association, 2000), they are also an example of the intrusion/reexperiencing symptom cluster of PTSD (American Psychiatric Association, 2000). In addition, nightmare frequency is known to be directly related to the risk of death by suicide (Tanskanen et al., 2001). Given the increased attention to PTSD and suicide in military psychology in recent years, nightmare treatment is an important tool for military psychologists. In most cases, nightmares decrease with evidence-based treatment for PTSD (Peterson, Luethcke, Borah, Borah, & Young-McCaughan, 2011). One study of exposure therapy for PTSD indicated that at posttreatment 24 of 27 participants (89%) no longer experienced nightmares, although 13 of 27 (48%) reported continued problems with insomnia (Zayfert & DeViva, 2004). These results suggest that effectively treating PTSD is likely to also help eliminate nightmares, but cognitive-behavioral treatment for insomnia may need to be added as an additional component.

Nightmares can also occur in the absence of PTSD, and imagery rehearsal therapy (IRT) has received the most empirical support for the independent treatment of nightmares (Krakow & Zadra, 2006). IRT has been used with individuals and groups and has been studied in combat settings (Moore & Krakow, 2007). IRT is composed of two components: The first addresses "nightmares as a learned sleep disorder" (akin to the learned behavioral theory on insomnia), and the second addresses "nightmares as the symptom of a damaged imagery system." Krakow and Zadra (2006) present a version of IRT that involves four 2-hour sessions in addition to follow-up sessions. The first two sessions focus predominantly on nightmares as a learned behavior that can promote insomnia. The latter two sessions focus predominantly on imagery work. Specifically, the imagery work includes writing down the recurring dream, changing it in any way desired, writing down the changed dream, and rehearsing the new dream using imagery for 5–20 minutes per day (Lamarche & Koninck, 2007). Participants sequentially apply this technique to various nightmares, typically starting with a nightmare of lesser intensity and one that does not exactly replay the trauma. IRT combined with CBT for insomnia has been found to significantly improve sleep disturbance among persons with PTSD (Lamarche & Koninck, 2007).

Primary Care Psychology

Most military clinical health psychologists work in a specialty mental health setting. In this type of setting, the psychology service is a separate, independent clinic that receives referrals from medical and dental providers. A recent development in the field of clinical health psychology is working in primary care settings as one of the primary care team members (Gatchel & Oordt, 2003).

There has been an increased emphasis over the past decade on the role of psychologists in primary care (Blount, 1998; Brantley, Veitia, Callon, Buss, & Sias, 1986; Cummings, Cummings, & Johnson, 1997; McDaniel, 1995; Strosahl, 1996). During 1999, the Air Force initiated the Primary Care Optimization Project. The purpose of this program was to reengineer primary care clinics and to optimize healthcare services in primary care settings throughout the Air Force medical service. This project called for psychologists to work as part of the primary care team. Similar programs have also been initiated in the Army (James, Folen, Porter, et al., 1999) and the Navy. Primary care physicians have long known that psychosocial problems are prevalent in the patients they treat, and they deliver nearly one-half of all formal mental healthcare in the United States (Narrow, Regier, Rae, Manderscheid, & Locke, 1993; Reiger et al., 1993). A growing body of research demonstrates that targeted behavioral health interventions integrated into primary care can lead to improved patient and provider satisfaction (Katon et al., 1996), decreased medical costs (Cummings, 1997), and improved patient outcomes (Hellman, Budd, Borysenko, McClelland, & Benson, 1990). Primary care psychology training programs have now been developed at Army, Navy, and Air Force internship sites (Hunter & Peterson, 2001).

Numerous models have been used to guide how psychologists operate in primary care settings (Blount, 1998; Brantley et al., 1986; Cummings et al., 1997; McDaniel, 1995; Strosahl, 1996). Primary care psychology is not simply locating psychologists in primary care settings to do the kind of work they would ordinarily do in an outpatient mental health setting.

Rather, it requires specific clinical skills and a comprehensive knowledge of behavioral assessment, applied behavioral analysis, behavior therapy, behavioral medicine, differential diagnosis, and psychopharmacology. All of these skills may be called on during a 15- to 30-minute primary care appointment.

The Army, Navy, and Air Force adopted the primary care psychology training program developed by Kirk Strosahl (1996). This model includes having a psychologist co-located in the primary care setting, working for the primary care manager as a behavioral health consultant. Appointment time slots are modeled after those of primary care managers. Psychologists provide brief behavioral health consultations and interventions with the medical patients but do not follow patients for outpatient therapy, as they might in a specialty mental health clinic (e.g., outpatient mental health clinic or clinical health psychology clinic). Patients can be seen as many times as needed but usually have three or fewer appointments. If more comprehensive assessment or treatment is required, the psychologist will refer the patient to a specialty mental health clinic.

Some initial data have been reported on the application of behavioral medicine and clinical health psychology treatment approaches in military primary care settings. In one study (Goodie et al., 2005), military clinical health psychologists collaborated with family practice physicians in an enhanced weight loss intervention program compared with a minimal-contact, standard care program. Providers followed brief, structured guidance derived from evidence-based practice guidelines. The results indicated that participants in the enhanced-care group lost a significant amount of weight, whereas there was no difference for the minimal-contact group.

Another study (Goodie, Isler, Hunter, & Peterson, 2009) evaluated the effectiveness of a brief behavioral treatment for insomnia in a military primary care setting. Participants were referred by their primary care manager to a clinical health psychologist working in the primary care clinic. The sessions consisted of brief behavioral treatment (Isler, Peterson, & Isler, 2005) and the use of a self-help book for insomnia (Zammit, 1997). The results indicated improvements in sleep efficiency and in sleep impairment of a magnitude similar to that obtained in specialty care.

A limitation of primary care psychology is that it requires additional staff to run the primary care and specialty care settings effectively. The Air Force Primary Care Optimization Project attempted to integrate psychologists into primary care without adding any staff. Unfortunately, this became a significant challenge at many locations, especially those in which the specialty care clinics were already booked full time with specialty care patients.

A new development that requires less time and yet addresses the needs of many primary care providers is the use of drop-in group medical appointments or shared medical appointments (Bronson & Maxwell, 2004). Shared medical visits are a new concept in patient care in which a physician and a behaviorist (usually a psychologist) collaborate in a group medical appointment. The physician performs a series of one-on-one patient encounters in a group setting during a 90-minute visit, and the psychologist facilitates group discussion, problem solving, and strategies for health behavior change between each individual patient encounter. Participation is voluntary, and patients agree to have their medical condition managed and to be advised in front of the other patients. Patients benefit from improved access to their physician, increased education, group support, and in most cases improved patient satisfaction. Providers can boost their access and productivity by 200–300% without increasing hours.

POPULATION HEALTH AND DISEASE MANAGEMENT

Clinical health psychologists in the military have much to contribute to population health management, that is, the management of the overall health of a population through surveillance, proactive delivery of prevention and intervention services, disease management, and outcome measurement (Peterson, 2003). Surveillance includes methods to measure the health status of a population, such as the review of population data from the universal assessment of tobacco use and weight in primary care clinics or from a health risk assessment completed during annual physical exams. Population health management includes a combination of primary, secondary, and tertiary prevention programs. Primary prevention includes strategies to prevent the onset of a targeted condition in asymptomatic individuals (i.e., tobacco use prevention in basic military training). Secondary prevention focuses on approaches to identify asymptomatic individuals who have known behavioral health risks or preclinical disease (i.e., overweight military members). Tertiary prevention treats symptomatic patients in order to mitigate untoward consequences of their disease (i.e., smoking cessation and weight management for active-duty diabetics).

"Disease management" is another term used to describe the spectrum of approaches, from primary prevention to intensive tertiary treatments. Disease management is a clinical management process that spans the continuum of care from primary prevention to ongoing and long-term health maintenance for individuals with chronic health conditions or diagnoses (Friedman, 2002). It involves the optimal management of the most common and costly acute and chronic disease states (e.g., diabetes) across the continuum of care. For example, the U.S. military healthcare system should not wait to be involved in services until after a patient is diagnosed with diabetes. Programs should be available to identify and intervene with high-risk individuals (e.g., overweight). On the other end of the spectrum, comprehensive and multidisciplinary diabetes treatment programs can help limit the progression of potential health consequences in insulin-dependent diabetics.

One limitation of many evidence-based, comprehensive treatment programs is that, although they are effective for those who participate, they have a minimal impact on the overall health of the population because of limited recruitment, enrollment, or participation. For example, many comprehensive tobacco cessation programs achieve high quit rates, but only a small percentage of the population of tobacco users enroll in such programs. Consider a population of 1,000 smokers; a 30-second primary care tobacco cessation intervention universally applied to every patient seen in a clinic as part of the annual preventive health assessment might result in an annual quit rate of 3% (1,000 × 3% = 30 quits). By comparison, a comprehensive, multisession tobacco cessation program that yields a 40% quit rate would result in less overall successful quits if only 5% of the population participated (1,000 × 5% = 50; 50 × 40% = 20 quits). This example demonstrates the potential impact on population health of intervention programs that are brief, population based, and focused on a behavioral risk factor. Improving the overall health of a population requires the use of creative behavioral medicine and clinical health psychology interventions. These approaches often extend outside of the healthcare organization to include families, schools, employers, communities, health policy changes, and environmental improvements (Epping-Jordan, 2004; Keefe, Buffington, Studts, & Rumble, 2002).

CONCLUSIONS

It is anticipated that clinical health psychology and behavioral medicine will continue to grow at a rapid pace. One area of expected growth is the use of technology for behavioral medicine assessment, treatment, and prevention programs (Keefe, Buffington, et al., 2002). A number of areas have already employed Internet-based behavioral interventions in such areas as weight management (Hunter et al., 2008; Tate et al., 2001) and tobacco cessation (Andrews et al., 2011). Other technological applications deserving continued attention include the use of telemedicine, smart phones, and interactive websites.

The financial aspects of healthcare for clinical health psychologists will become even more important in the future. The possibility of reducing costs and healthcare utilization by improving health and lifestyle behaviors make clinical health psychologists a valuable asset in healthcare organizations (Rasu, Hunter, Peterson, Maruska, & Foreyt, 2010). However, it can be very challenging to evaluate the financial aspects of behavioral interventions (Kaplan & Groessl, 2002). Future studies of treatment outcomes should evaluate the cost-effectiveness of interventions and the potential impact of medical cost offset.

Some clinical health psychologists have boldly suggested that in the future clinical and counseling psychology will be considered subspecialties under the broader umbrella of clinical health psychology. This model posits that in the future clinical health psychology will be thoroughly integrated throughout the entire healthcare setting to include all primary care and most specialty medical care. Most patients will seek healthcare from their primary care or specialty care physician, who will have a clinical health psychologist as part of the primary or specialty healthcare team. This model also assumes that the majority of patients will be able to be treated successfully by clinical health psychologists embedded into these healthcare settings. Those individuals who cannot be successfully treated by the clinical health psychologist will then be referred to a mental health specialty clinic staffed by clinical and counseling psychologists and other mental health specialists. The overall number of patients needing referral to these specialty clinics will be a minority of the overall patient population seen throughout the entire healthcare system. This bold model is a bit extreme, and only the future will tell whether or not the field of clinical health psychology develops to this extent. Nevertheless, clinical health psychology and behavioral medicine have great potential to continue to significantly influence the future of healthcare in both military and civilian settings.

ACKNOWLEDGMENTS

The views expressed in this chapter are solely those of the author(s) and do not reflect an endorsement by or the official policy of the U.S. Air Force or the Department of Defense.

REFERENCES

Abrams, D. B., Niaura, R., Brown, R. A., Emmons, K. M., Goldstein, M. G., & Monti, P. M. (2003). *The tobacco dependence treatment handbook: A guide to best practices.* New York: Guilford Press.

Altarac, M., Gardner, J. W., Popovich, R. M., Potter, R., Knapik, J. J., & Jones, B. H. (2000). Cigarette smoking and exercise-related injuries among young men and women. *American Journal of Preventive Medicine, 18,* 96–102.

American Psychiatric Association. (1996). Practice guideline for the treatment of patients with nicotine dependence. *American Journal of Psychiatry, 153*(Suppl.), 1–31.

American Psychiatric Association. (2000). *Diagnostic and statistical manual of mental disorders* (4th ed., text rev.). Washington, DC: Author.

American Psychological Association. (2002). Ethical principles of psychologists and code of conduct. *American Psychologist, 57,* 1060–1073.

American Psychological Association. (2012). *Public description of clinical health psychology.* Retrieved from *www.apa.org/ed/graduate/specialize/health. aspx.*

Amoroso, P. J., & Canham, M. L. (1999). Disabilities related to the musculoskeletal system: Physical Evaluation Board data. In B. H. Jones, P. J. Amoroso, & M. L. Canham (Eds.), Atlas of injuries in the U.S. Armed Forces [Special issue]. *Military Medicine, 164*(4), 1–73.

Andrews, J. A., Gordon, J. S., Hampson, S. E., Christiansen, S. M., Gunn, B., Slovic, P., et al. (2011). Short-term efficacy of Click City®: Tobacco: Changing etiological mechanisms related to the onset of tobacco use. *Prevention Science, 12,* 89–102.

Association of Psychology Postdoctoral and Internship Centers. (2010). *Postdoctoral programs directory.* Retrieved October 3, 2010, from *www.appic.org/ directory/search_dol_postdocs.asp.*

Bauchowitz, A. U., Gonder-Frederick, L. A., Olbrisch, M. E., Azarbad, L., Ryee, M. Y., Woodson, M., et al. (2005). Psychosocial evaluation of bariatric surgery candidates: A survey of present practices. *Psychosomatic Medicine, 67,* 825–832.

Baum, A., Revenson, T. A., & Singer, J. E. (Eds.). (2001). *Handbook of health psychology.* Mahwah, NJ: Erlbaum.

Baumstark, K. E., & Buckelew, S. P. (1992). Fibromyalgia: Clinical signs, research findings, treatment implications, and future directions. *Annals of Behavioral Medicine, 14,* 282–291.

Belar, C. D., & Deardorff, W. W. (2009). *Clinical health psychology in medical settings: A practitioner's guidebook* (2nd ed.). Washington, DC: American Psychological Association.

Blanchard, E. B. (1982). Behavioral medicine: Past, present, and future. *Journal of Consulting and Clinical Psychology, 50,* 795–796.

Blanchard, E. B. (1992). Behavioral medicine: An update for the 1990s. *Journal of Consulting and Clinical Psychology, 60,* 537–551.

Blanchard, E. B., & Scharff, L. (2002). Psychosocial aspects of assessment and treatment of irritable bowel syndrome in adults and recurrent abdominal pain in children. *Journal of Consulting and Clinical Psychology, 70,* 725–738.

Blount, A. (Ed.). (1998). *Integrated primary care: The future of medical and mental health collaboration.* New York: Norton.

Bogart, R. K., McDaniel, R. J., Dunn, W. J., Hunter, C. M., Peterson, A. L., & Wright, E. F. (2007). Efficacy of group cognitive behavior therapy for the treatment of masticatory myofascial pain. *Military Medicine, 172,* 169–174.

Boll, T. J., Johnson, S. B., Perry, N., & Rozensky, R. H. (2002). *Handbook of clinical health psychology: Volume 1. Medical disorders and behavioral applications.* Washington, DC: American Psychological Association.

Bootzin, R. R., & Epstein, D. R. (2000). Stimulus control. In K. L. Lichstein & C. M. Morin (Eds.), *Treatment of late-life insomnia* (pp. 167–184). Thousand Oaks, CA: Sage.

Bowman, R. L., & Delucia, J. L. (1992). Accuracy of self-reported weight: A meta-analysis. *Behavior Therapy, 23*, 637–655.

Bradham, D. D., South, B. R., Saunders, H. J., Heuser, M. D., Pane, K. W., & Dennis, K. E. (2001). Obesity-related hospitalization costs to the U.S. Navy, 1993–1998. *Military Medicine, 166*, 1–10.

Brantley, P. J., Veitia, M. C., Callon, E. B., Buss, R. R., & Sias, C. R. (1986). Assessing the impact of psychological intervention on family practice clinic visits. *Family Medicine, 18*, 351–354.

Bray, R. M., Hourani, L. L., Rae, K. L., Dever, J. A., Brown, J. M., Vincus, A. A., et al. (2003). *2002 Department of Defense survey of health related behaviors among military personnel.* Retrieved from *www.dtic.mil/cgi-bin/GetTRDoc?AD=ADA431566.*

Bronson, D. L., & Maxwell, R. A. (2004). Shared medical appointments: Increasing patient access without increasing physician hours. *Cleveland Clinic Journal of Medicine, 71*, 369–370.

Brownell, K. D. (2004). *The LEARN Program for weight management.* Dallas: American Health.

Centers for Disease Control and Prevention. (1997). Perspectives in disease prevention and health promotion: Smoking—attributable mortality and years of potential life lost—United States, 1984. *Morbidity and Mortality Weekly Report, 46*, 444–451.

Centers for Disease Control and Prevention. (2000). Cigarette smoking among adults—United States, 1998. *Morbidity and Mortality Weekly Report, 49*, 881–884.

Centers for Disease Control and Prevention. (2002). *CDC injury fact book.* Washington, DC: U.S. Department of Health and Human Services.

Centers for Disease Control and Prevention. (2004). *Behavioral risk factor surveillance system prevalence data.* Retrieved November 22, 2004, from *http://apps.nccd.cdc.gov/brfss.*

Chesson, A. L., Anderson, W. M., Littner, M., Davila, D., Hartse, K., Johnson, S., et al. (1999). Practice parameters for the nonpharmacologic treatment of insomnia. *Sleep, 22*, 1128–1133.

Cigrang, J. A., Severson, H. H., & Peterson, A. L. (2002). Pilot evaluation of a population-based health intervention for reducing use of smokeless tobacco. *Nicotine and Tobacco Research, 4*, 127–131.

Conway, T. L., Woodruff, S. I., Edwards, C. C., Elder, J. P., Hurtado, S. L., & Hervig, L. K. (2004). Operation Stay Quit: Evaluation of two smoking relapse prevention strategies for women after involuntary cessation during US Navy recruit training. *Military Medicine, 169*, 236–342.

Cummings, N. A. (1997). Behavioral health in primary care: Dollars and sense. In N. A. Cummings, J. L. Cummings, & J. N. Johnson (Eds.), *Behavioral health in primary care: A guide for clinical integration* (pp. 3–21). Madison, CT: Psychosocial Press.

Cummings, N. A., Cummings, J. L., & Johnson, J. N. (Eds.). (1997). *Behavioral health in primary care.* Madison, CT: Psychosocial Press.

Dall, T. M., Zhang, Y., Chen, Y. J., Wagner, A. R. C., Hogan, P. F., Fagan, N. K., et al. (2007). Cost associated with being overweight and with obesity, high alcohol consumption, and tobacco use within the military health system's TRICARE prime-enrolled population. *American Journal of Health Promotion, 22,* 120–139.

Epping-Jordan, J. E. (2004). Research to practice: International dissemination of evidence-based behavioral medicine. *Annals of Behavioral Medicine, 28,* 81–87.

Faue, M., Folen, R. A., James, L. C., & Needels, T. (1997). The Tripler Tobacco-Cessation Program: Predictors for success and improved efficacy. *Military Medicine, 162,* 445–449.

Feuerstein, M., Berkowitz, S. M., Pastel, R., & Huang, G. D. (1999, July). *Secondary prevention program for occupational low back pain-related disability.* Paper presented at the meeting of the Worker's Compensation Research Group, New Brunswick, NJ.

Fiore, M. C., Jaén, C. R., Baker, T. B., Bailay, W. C., Benowitz, N. L., Curry, S. J., et al. (2008). *Treating tobacco use and dependence: 2008 update* (Clinical Practice Guideline, AHRQ Publication No. 08-0050-1). Rockville, MD: U.S. Department of Health and Human Services, Public Health Service.

Fiore, M. C., Smith, S. S., Jorenby, D. E., & Baker, T. B. (1994). The effectiveness of the nicotine patch for smoking cessation: A meta-analysis. *Journal of the American Medical Association, 27,* 1940–1947.

Flegal, K. M., Carroll, M. D., Ogden, C. L., & Johnson, C. L. (2002). Prevalence and trends in obesity among US adults, 1999–2000. *Journal of the American Medical Association, 288,* 1723–1727.

Foreyt, J. P., & Goodrick, G. K. (1994). Attributes of successful approaches to weight loss and control. *Applied and Preventive Psychology, 3,* 209–215.

France, C. R., Masters, K. S., Belar, C. D., Kerns, R. D., Klonoff, E. A., Larkin, K. T., et al. (2008). Application of the competency model to clinical health psychology. *Professional Psychology: Research and Practice, 39,* 573–580.

Frank, R. G., Baum, A., & Wallander, J. L. (2004). *Handbook of clinical health psychology: Volume 3. Models and perspectives in health psychology.* Washington, DC: American Psychological Association.

Frank, R. G., & Elliott, T. R. (2000). *Handbook of rehabilitation psychology.* Washington, DC: American Psychological Association.

French, S. A., & Jeffery, R. W. (1995). Weight concerns and smoking: A literature review. *Annals of Behavioral Medicine, 17,* 234–244.

Fried, V. M., Prager, K., MacKay, A. P., & Xia, H. (2003). Chartbook on trends in the health of Americans. In *Health, United States, 2003* (p. 471). Hyattsville, MD: National Center for Health Statistics.

Friedman, N. (2002). Evidence-based medicine: The key to guidelines, disease and care management programmes. *Annals Academy of Medicine Singapore, 31,* 446–451.

Gatchel, R. J., McGeary, D. D., Peterson, A. L., Moore, M., LeRoy, K., Isler, W.

C., et al. (2009). Preliminary findings of a randomized controlled trial of an interdisciplinary military pain program. *Military Medicine, 174,* 270–277.

Gatchel, R. J., & Oordt, M. S. (2003). *Clinical health psychology and primary care: Practical advice and clinical guidance for successful collaboration.* Washington, DC: American Psychological Association.

Goldberg, G. M., Carlson, E., & Paige-Dobson, B. (1994). Health psychology in the Navy: Emergence of a new discipline. *Navy Medicine, 85*(1), 15–77.

Goodie, J. L., Hunter, C. L., Hunter, C. M., McKnight, T., Leroy, K., & Peterson, A. L. (2005, March). *Comparison of weight loss interventions in a primary care setting: A pilot investigation.* Poster presented at the 26th annual meeting of the Society of Behavioral Medicine, Boston, MA.

Goodie, J. L., Isler, W. C., Hunter, C. L., & Peterson, A. L. (2009). Using behavioral health consultants to treat insomnia in primary care: A clinical case series. *Journal of Clinical Psychology, 65*(3), 294–304.

Gritz, E. R., Klesges, R. C., & Meyers, A. W. (1989). The smoking and body weight relationship: Implications for intervention and post-cessation weight control. *Annals of Behavioral Medicine, 11,* 144–153.

Guzman, J., Esmail, R., Karjalinen, K., Malmivaara, A., Irvin, E., & Bombadier, C. (2001). Multidisciplinary rehabilitation for chronic low back pain: Systematic review. *British Medical Journal, 322,* 1511–1516.

Hall, S. M., Tunstall, C. D., Vila, K. L., & Duffy, J. (1992). Weight gain prevention and smoking cessation: Cautionary findings. *American Journal of Public Health, 82,* 799–803.

Hatsukami, D. K., Grillo, M., Boyle, R., Allen, S., Jensen, J., Bliss, R., et al. (2000). Treatment of spit tobacco users with transdermal nicotine system and mint snuff. *Journal of Consulting and Clinical Psychology, 68,* 241–249.

Hellman, C. J. C., Budd, M., Borysenko, J., McClelland, D. C., & Benson, H. (1990). A study of the effectiveness of two group behavioral medicine interventions for patients with psychosomatic complaints. *Behavioral Medicine, 16,* 165–173.

Holbrook, T. L., Anderson, J. P., Sieber, W. J., Browner, D., & Hoyt, D. B. (1999). Outcome after major trauma: 12-month and 18-month follow-up results from the Trauma Recovery Project. *Journal of Trauma, 46,* 765–771.

Holroyd, K. A. (2002). Assessment and psychological management of recurrent headache disorders. *Journal of Consulting and Clinical Psychology, 70,* 656–677.

Hryshko-Mullen, A. S., Broeckl, L. S., Haddock, C. K., & Peterson, A. L. (2000). Behavioral treatment of insomnia: The Wilford Hall insomnia program. *Military Medicine, 165,* 200–207.

Hsu, L. L., Nevin, R. L., Tobler, S. K., & Rubertone, M. V. (2007). Trends in overweight and obesity among 18-year-old applicants to the United States military, 1993–2006. *Journal of Adolescent Health, 41,* 610–612.

Hunter, C. L., & Peterson, A. L. (2001). Primary care training at Wilford Hall Medical Center. *The Behavior Therapist, 24,* 220–222.

Hunter, C. M., Peterson, A. L., Alvarez, L., Poston, W. C., Brundige, A., Haddock, C. K., et al. (2008). Weight management using the Internet: A randomized controlled trial. *American Journal of Preventive Medicine, 34,* 119–126.

Hurt, R. D., Sachs, D. P. L., Glover, E. D., Offord, K. P. J., Johnston, A., Dale, L. C., et al. (1997). A comparison of sustained-release bupropion and placebo for smoking cessation. *New England Journal of Medicine, 337*, 1195–1202.

Isler, W. C., Peterson, A. L., & Isler, D. (2005). Behavioral treatment of insomnia in primary care settings. In L. James (Ed.), *The primary care consultant: The next frontier for psychologists in hospitals and clinics* (pp. 121–151). Washington, DC: American Psychological Association.

James, L. C., Folen, R. A., Garland, F. N., Edwards, C., Noce, M., Gohdes, D., et al. (1997). The Tripler Army Medical Center LEAN Program: A healthy lifestyle model for the treatment of obesity. *Military Medicine, 162*, 328–332.

James, L. C., Folen, R. A., Page, H., Noce, M., Brown, J., & Britton, C. (1999). The Tripler LE3AN Program: A two-year follow-up report. *Military Medicine, 164*, 389–395.

James, L. C., Folen, R. A., Porter, R. I., & Kellar, M. A. (1999). A conceptual overview of a proactive health psychology service: The Tripler health psychology model. *Military Medicine, 164*, 396–400.

Jorenby, D. E., Leischow, S. J., Nides, M. A., Rennard, S. I., Johnston, A. J., Hughes, A. D., et al. (1999). A controlled trial of sustained-release bupropion, a nicotine patch, or both for smoking cessation. *New England Journal of Medicine, 340*, 685–691.

Kaplan, R. M., & Groessl, E. J. (2002). Applications of cost-effectiveness methodologies in behavioral medicine. *Journal of Consulting and Clinical Psychology, 70*, 482–493.

Kapur, V. K., Redline, S., Nieto, F. J., Young, T. B., Newman, A. B., & Henderson, J. A. (2002). The relationship between chronically disrupted sleep and health care use. *Sleep, 25*, 289–296.

Katon, W., Robinson, P., Von Korff, M., Lin, E., Bush, T., Ludman, E., et al. (1996). A multifaceted intervention to improve treatment of depression in primary care. *Archives of General Psychiatry, 53*, 924–932.

Katz, D. A., & McHorney, C. A. (2002). The relationship between insomnia and health-related quality of life in patients with chronic illness. *Journal of Family Practice, 51*, 229–235.

Keefe, F. J., Buffington, A. L. H., Studts, J., & Rumble, M. (2002). Behavioral medicine: 2002 and beyond. *Journal of Consulting and Clinical Psychology, 70*, 852–856.

Keefe, F. J., Smith, S. J., Buffington, A. L. H., Gibson, J., Studts, J., & Caldwell, D. S. (2002). Recent advances and future directions in the biopsychosocial assessment and treatment of arthritis. *Journal of Consulting and Clinical Psychology, 70*, 640–655.

Kerns, R. D., Berry, S., Frantsve, L. M. E., & Linton, J. C. (2009). Life-long competency development in clinical health psychology. *Training and Education in Professional Psychology, 3*, 212–217.

Klesges, R. C., Haddock, C. K., Chang, C. F., Talcott, G. W., & Lando, H. (2001). The association of smoking and the cost of military training. *Tobacco Control, 10*, 43–47.

Klesges, R. C., Haddock, C. K., Lando, H., & Talcott, G. W. (1999). Efficacy of forced smoking cessation and an adjunctive behavioral treatment on long-term smoking rates. *Journal of Consulting and Clinical Psychology, 67,* 952–958.

Klesges, R. C., Myers, A. W., Klesges, L. M., & La Vasque, M. E. (1989). Smoking, body weight, and their effects on smoking behavior: A comprehensive review of the literature. *Psychological Bulletin, 106,* 204–230.

Krakow, B., & Zadra, A. (2006). Clinical management of chronic nightmares: Imagery rehearsal therapy. *Behavioral Sleep Medicine, 4,* 45–70.

Kushida, C. A., Nichols, D. A., Simon, R. D., Young, T., Grauke, J. H., Britzmann, J. B., et al. (2000). Symptom-based prevalence of sleep disorders in an adult primary care population. *Sleep and Breathing, 4,* 9–14.

Lamarche, L., & Koninck, J. (2007). Sleep disturbance in adults with posttraumatic stress disorder: A review. *Journal of Clinical Psychiatry, 68,* 1257–1270.

Larkin, K. T. (2009). Variations in doctoral training programs in clinical health psychology: Lessons learned at the box office. *Training and Education in Professional Psychology, 3,* 202–211.

Lew, H. L., Otis, J. D., Tun, C., Kerns, R. D., Clark, M. E., & Cifu, D. X. (2009). Prevalence of chronic pain, posttraumatic stress disorder, and persistent post-concussive symptoms in OIF/OEF veterans: Polytrauma clinical triad. *Journal of Rehabilitation Research and Development, 46,* 697–702.

Lichstein, K. L., & Riedel, B. W. (1994). Behavioral assessment and treatment of insomnia: A review with an emphasis on clinical application. *Behavior Therapy, 25,* 659–688.

Lincoln, A. E., Smith, G. S., Amoroso, P. J., & Bell, N. S. (2003). The effect of cigarette smoking on musculoskeletal-related disability. *American Journal of Industrial Medicine, 43,* 337–349.

Lipowski, Z. J., Lipsitt, D. R., & Whybrow, P. C. (1977). *Psychosomatic medicine: Current trends and clinical applications.* New York: Oxford University Press.

Llewelyn, S., & Kennedy, P. (2003). *Handbook of clinical health psychology.* Indianapolis, IN: Wiley.

Masters, K. S., France, C. R., & Thorn, B. E. (2009). Enhancing preparation among entry-level clinical health psychologists: Recommendations for "best practices" from the first meeting of the Council of Clinical Health Psychology Training Programs (CCHPTP). *Training and Education in Professional Psychology, 3,* 193–201.

Matarazzo, J. D. (1980). Behavioral health and behavioral medicine. *American Psychologist, 35,* 807–817.

Matarazzo, J. D., Weiss, S. M., Herd, J. A., Miller, N. E., & Weiss, S. M. (Eds.). (1984). *Behavioral health: A handbook of health enhancement and disease prevention.* New York: Wiley.

Mayer, T. G., McGeary, D., & Gatchel, R. J. (2003). Chronic pain management through functional restoration for spinal disorders. In J. Frymoyer & S. Wiesel (Eds.), *Adult and pediatric spine* (3rd ed., pp. 323–333). Philadelphia: Lippincott, Williams & Wilkins.

McCallin, A. (2001). Interdisciplinary practice—a matter of teamwork: An integrated literature review. *Journal of Clinical Nursing, 10,* 419–428.

McDaniel, S. (1995). Collaboration between psychologists and family PCMs: Implementing the biopsychosocial model. *Professional Psychology: Research and Practice, 26,* 117–122.

McNulty, P. A. (2001). Prevalence and contributing factors of eating disorder behaviors in active duty service women in the Army, Navy, Air Force, and Marines. *Military Medicine, 166,* 53–58.

Michaels, A. J., Michaels, C. E., Moon, C. H., Smith, J. S., Zimmerman, M. A., Taheri, P. A., et al. (1999). Posttraumatic stress disorder after injury: Impact on general health outcome and early risk assessment. *Journal of Trauma, 47,* 460–466.

Millon, T. (1982). On the nature of clinical health psychology. In T. Millon, C. Green, & J. Meagher (Eds.), *Handbook of clinical health psychology* (pp. 1–28). New York: Plenum Press.

Mimeault, V., & Morin, C. M. (1999). Self-help treatment for insomnia: Bibliotherapy with and without professional guidance. *Journal of Consulting and Clinical Psychology, 67,* 511–519.

Mokdad, A. H., Marks, J. S., Stroup, D. F., & Gerberding, J. L. (2004). Actual causes of death in the United States, 2000. *Journal of the American Medical Association, 291,* 1238–1245.

Moore, B. A., & Krakow, B. (2007). Imagery rehearsal therapy for acute posttraumatic nightmares among combat soldiers in Iraq. *American Journal of Psychiatry, 164,* 683–684.

Morin, C. M. (1993). *Insomnia: Psychological assessment and management.* New York: Guilford Press.

Morin, C. M., Bootzin, R. R., Buysse, D. J., Edinger, J. D., Espie, C. A., & Lichstein, K. L. (2006). Psychological and behavioral treatment of insomnia: Update of the recent evidence (1998–2004). *Sleep, 29,* 1398–1414.

Morin, C. M., Colecchi, C., Stone, J., Stood, R., & Brink, D. (1999). Behavioral and pharmacological therapies for late-life insomnia: A randomized controlled trial. *Journal of the American Medical Association, 281,* 991–999.

Morin, C. M., Culbert, J. P., & Schwartz, S. M. (1994). Nonpharmacological interventions for insomnia: A meta-analysis of treatment efficacy. *American Journal of Psychiatry, 151,* 1172–1180.

Morin, C. M., Hauri, P. J., Espie, C. A., Speilman, A. J., Buysse, D. J., & Bootzin, R. R. (1999). Nonpharmacological treatment of chronic insomnia. *Sleep, 22,* 1134–1156.

Morin, C. M., & Wooten, V. (1996). Psychological and pharmacological approaches to treating insomnia. *Clinical Psychology Review, 16,* 521–542.

Murtagh, D. R., & Greenwood, K. M. (1995). Identifying effective psychological treatments for insomnia: A meta-analysis. *Journal of Consulting and Clinical Psychology, 63,* 79–89.

Narrow, W. E., Regier, D. A., Rae, D. S., Manderscheid, R. W., & Locke, B. Z. (1993). Use of services by persons with mental and addictive disorders: Findings from the National Institute of Mental Health epidemiologic catchment area program. *Archives of General Psychiatry, 50,* 95–107.

National Heart, Lung, and Blood Institute Working Group on Insomnia. (1999).

Insomnia: Assessment and management in primary care. *American Family Physician, 59*, 3029–3038.

National Institutes of Health. (1991). Gastrointestinal surgery for severe obesity: Proceedings of a National Institutes of Health Consensus Development Conference. *American Journal of Clinical Nutrition, 55*, 487S–619S.

National Institutes of Health. (1998). *Clinical guidelines on the identification, evaluation, and treatment of overweight and obesity: The evidence report.* Washington, DC: U.S. Government Printing Office.

Niaura, R., & Abrams, D. B. (2002). Smoking cessation: Progress, priorities, and prospectus. *Journal of Consulting and Clinical Psychology, 70*, 494–509.

Nicassio, P. M., & Smith, T. W. (1995). *Managing chronic illness: A biopsychosocial perspective.* Washington, DC: American Psychological Association.

Otis, J. D., Keane, T. M., & Kerns, R. D. (2003). An examination of the relationship between chronic pain and post-traumatic stress disorder. *Journal of Rehabilitation and Research Development, 40*, 397–406.

Perkins, K. A. (1993). Weight gain following smoking cessation. *Journal of Consulting and Clinical Psychology, 61*, 768–777.

Perri, M. G., & Fuller, P. R. (1995). Success and failure in the treatment of obesity: Where do we go from here? *Medicine, Exercise, Nutrition, and Health, 4*, 255–272.

Peterson, A. L. (1999). Inaccurate estimation of body weight prior to smoking cessation: Implications for quitting and weight gain. *Journal of Applied Biobehavioral Research, 4*, 79–84.

Peterson, A. L. (2003, March). *Population health management: Building healthy communities with behavioral medicine.* Paper presented at the 24th annual meeting of the Society of Behavioral Medicine, Salt Lake City, UT.

Peterson, A. L., Dixon, D. C., Talcott, G. W., & Kelleher, W. J. (1993). Habit reversal treatment of temporomandibular disorders: A pilot investigation. *Journal of Behavior Therapy and Experimental Psychiatry, 24*, 49–55.

Peterson, A. L., Goodie, J. L., Satterfield, W., & Brim, W. (2008). Sleep disturbance during military deployment. *Military Medicine, 173*, 230–235.

Peterson, A. L., & Helton, J. (2000). Smoking cessation and weight gain in the military. *Military Medicine, 165*, 536–538.

Peterson, A. L., Hryshko-Mullen, A. S., Alexander, R. W., & Nelson, L. (1999, November). *Evaluation of health care utilization after behavior therapy for insomnia.* Paper presented at the 33rd Annual Convention of the Association for Advancement of Behavior Therapy, Toronto, Ontario, Canada.

Peterson, A. L., Luethcke, C. A., Borah, E. V., Borah, A. M., & Young-McCaughan, S. (2011). Assessment and treatment of combat-related PTSD in returning war veterans. *Journal of Clinical Psychology in Medical Settings, 18*, 164–175.

Peterson, A. L., Severson, H. H., Andrews, J. A., Gott, S. P., Cigrang, J. A. Gordon, J. S., et al. (2007). Smokeless tobacco use in military personnel. *Military Medicine, 172*, 1300–1305.

Peterson, A. L., Talcott, G. W., Kelleher, W. J., & Smith, S. D. (1995). Bulimic weight-loss behaviors in mandatory versus voluntary weight management programs. *Military Medicine, 160*, 616–620.

Peterson, A. L., Vander Weg, M. W., & Jaén, C. R. (2011). *Advances in psychotherapy—Evidence-based practice—Vol. 21. Nicotine and tobacco dependence.* Cambridge, MA: Hogrefe.

Pieters, R., & Baumgartner, H. (2002). Who talks to whom? Intra- and interdisciplinary communication of economics journals. *Journal of Economic Literature, 40,* 483–509.

Prokop, C., & Bradley, A. A. (1981). *Medical psychology: Contributions to behavioral medicine.* New York: Academic Press.

Raczynski, J. M., & Leviton, L. C. (2004). *Handbook of clinical health psychology: Volume 2. Disorders of behavior and health.* Washington, DC: American Psychological Association.

Rasu, R. S., Hunter, C. M., Peterson, A. L., Maruska, H. M., & Foreyt, J. P. (2010). Economic evaluation of an Internet-based weight management program. *American Journal of Managed Care, 16,* 98–104.

Reiger, D., Narrow, W., Rae, D., Manderschied, R., Locke, B., & Goodwin, F. (1993). The de facto U.S. mental and addictive disorders service system: Epidemiologic catchment area prospective 1-year prevalence rates of disorders and services. *Archives of General Psychiatry, 50,* 85–94.

Riedel, B. W. (2000). Sleep hygiene. In K. L. Lichstein & C. M. Morin (Eds.), *Treatment of late-life insomnia* (pp. 125–146). Thousand Oaks, CA: Sage.

Robbins, A. S., Chao, S. Y., Coil, G. A., & Fonseca, V. P. (2000). Costs of smoking among active duty U.S. Air Force personnel in 1997. *Morbidity and Mortality Weekly Reports, 49,* 441–445.

Robbins, A. S., Chao, S. Y., Russ, C. R., & Fonseca, V. P. (2002). Costs of excess body weight among active duty personnel, U.S. Air Force, 1997. *Military Medicine, 167,* 393–397.

Rodolfa, E., Bent, R., Eisman, E., Nelson, P., Rehm, L., & Ritchie, P. (2005). A cube model for competency development: Implications for psychology educators and regulators. *Professional Psychology: Research and Practice, 36,* 347–354.

Russ, C. R., Fonseca, V. P., Peterson, A. L., Blackman, L. R., & Robbins, A. S. (2001). Weight gain as a barrier to smoking cessation among military personnel. *American Journal of Health Promotion, 16,* 79–84.

Santry, H. P., Gillen, D. L., & Lauderdale, D. S. (2005). Trends in bariatric surgical procedures. *Journal of the American Medical Association, 294,* 1909–1917.

Schnyder, U., Moergeli, H., Klaghofer, R., & Buddeberg, C. (2001). Incidence and prediction of posttraumatic stress disorder symptoms in severely injured accident victims. *American Journal of Psychiatry, 158,* 594–599.

Severson, H. H., Peterson, A. L., Andrews, J. A., Gordon, J. S., Cigrang, J. A., Danaher, B. G., et al. (2009). Smokeless tobacco cessation in military personnel: A randomized clinical trial. *Nicotine and Tobacco Research, 11,* 730–738.

Sheridan, E. P. (1999). Psychology's future in medical schools and academic health care centers. *American Psychologist, 54,* 267–271.

Sheridan, E. P., Matarazzo, J. D., Boll, T. J., Perry, N. W., Jr., Weiss, S. M., & Belar, C. D. (1988). Postdoctoral education and training for clinical service providers in health psychology. *Health Psychology, 7,* 1–17.

Simpson, M., Earles, J., Folen, R., Trammel, R., & James, L. (2004). The Tripler Army Medical Center's LE3AN program: A six-month retrospective analysis of program effectiveness for African-American and European-American females. *Journal of the National Medical Association, 96,* 1332–1336.

Smith, M. T., Perlis, M. L., Park, A., Smith, M. S., Pennington, J., Giles, D. E., et al. (2002). Comparative meta-analysis of pharmacotherapy and behavior therapy for persistent insomnia. *American Journal of Psychiatry, 159,* 5–10.

Smith, T. W., Kendall, P. C., & Keefe, F. (2002). Behavioral medicine and clinical health psychology: Introduction to the special issue. *Journal of Consulting and Clinical Psychology, 70,* 459–462.

Society of Behavioral Medicine. (2012). *About the Society of Behavioral Medicine.* Retrieved May 17, 2012, from *www.sbm.org/about.*

Spielman, A. J., Saskin, P., & Thorpy, M. J. (1987). Treatment of chronic insomnia by restriction of time in bed. *Sleep, 10,* 45–56.

Spring, B., Doran, N., Pagoto, S., Schneider, K., Pingitore, R., & Hedeker, D. (2004). Randomized controlled trial for behavioral smoking and weight control treatment: Effect of concurrent versus sequential intervention. *Journal of Consulting and Clinical Psychology, 72,* 785–796.

Starr, A. J., Smith, W. R., Frawley, W. H., Borer, D. S., Morgan, S. J., Reinert, C. M., et al. (2004). Symptoms of posttraumatic stress disorder after orthopaedic trauma. *Journal of Bone and Joint Surgery, 86-A*(6), 1115–1121.

Stone, G., Weiss, S., Matarazzo, J., Miller, N., Rodin, J., Belar, C., et al. (1987). *Health psychology: A discipline and a profession.* Chicago: University of Chicago Press.

Strosahl, K. (1996). Confessions of a behavior therapist in primary care: The odyssey and the ecstasy. *Cognitive and Behavioral Practice, 3,* 1–28.

Stunkard, A. J. (2001). Current views on obesity. *American Journal of Medicine, 100,* 230–236.

Suls, J. (2010, Spring). What's spinning in health psychology. *Health Psychologist, 32*(1), 1, 4.

Talcott, G. W., Fiedler, E. R., Pascale, R. W., Klesges, R. C., Peterson, A. L., & Johnson, R. S. (1995). Is weight gain following smoking cessation inevitable? *Journal of Consulting and Clinical Psychology, 63,* 313–316.

Tanskanen, A., Tuomilehto, J., Viinamaki, H., Vartiainen, E., Lehtonen, J., & Puska, P. (2001). Nightmares as predictors of suicide. *Sleep, 24,* 845–848.

Tate, D. F., Wing, R. R., & Winett, R. A. (2001). Using Internet technology to deliver a behavioral weight loss program. *Journal of the American Medical Association, 285,* 1172–1177.

Turk, D. C., & Okifuji, A. (2002). Psychological factors in chronic pain: Evolution and revolution. *Journal of Consulting and Clinical Psychology, 70,* 678–690.

Turk, D. C., Zaki, H. S., & Rudy, T. E. (1993). Effects of intraoral appliance and biofeedback/stress management alone and in combination in treating pain and depression in patients with temporomandibular disorders. *Journal of Prosthetic Dentistry, 70,* 158–164.

U.S. Department of Health and Human Services. (1990). *The health benefits of smoking cessation: A report of the surgeon general.* Washington, DC: U.S. Government Printing Office.

Weddington, W. W., Jr., & Blindt, K. (1983). Behavioral medicine: A new development. *Hospital Community Psychiatry, 34,* 702–708.

Wetter, D. W., Fiore, M. C., Gritz, E. R., Lando, H. A., Stitzer, M. L., Hasselblad, V., et al. (1998). The Agency for Health Care Policy and Research Smoking Cessation clinical practice guideline: Findings and implications for psychologists. *American Psychologist, 6,* 657–669.

WHO World Mental Health Survey Consortium. (2004). Prevalence, severity, and unmet need for treatment of mental disorders in the World Health Organization world mental health surveys. *Journal of the American Medical Association, 291,* 2581–2590.

Williamson, D. F., Madans, J., Anda, R. F., Kleinman, J. C., Giovino, G. A., & Byers, T. (1991). Smoking cessation and severity of weight gain in a national cohort. *New England Journal of Medicine, 324,* 739–745.

Woodruff, S. I., Conway, T. L., & Edwards, C. C. (2000). Effect of an eight week smoking ban on women at US Navy recruit training command. *Tobacco Control, 9,* 40–46.

Yamane, G. K. (2007). Obesity in civilian adults: Potential impact on eligibility for U.S. military enlistment. *Military Medicine, 172,* 1160–1165.

Zammit, G. K. (1997). *Good nights: How to stop sleep deprivation, overcome insomnia, and get the sleep you need.* Kansas City, KS: Andrews McMeel.

Zammit, G. K., Weiner, J., Damato, N., Sillup, G. P., & McMillan, C. A. (1999). Quality of life in people with insomnia. *Sleep, 22,* S379–S385.

Zayfert, C., & DeViva, J. C. (2004). Residual insomnia following cognitive behavioral therapy for PTSD. *Journal of Traumatic Stress, 17,* 69–73.

CHAPTER 7

Military Roles
in Postdisaster Mental Health

Teresa M. Au
Teresa L. Marino-Carper
Benjamin D. Dickstein
Brett T. Litz

On Tuesday, January 12, 2010, a devastating, magnitude-7.0 earthquake struck Haiti, leveling houses and buildings, burying people under heaps of rubble, and engulfing the country in chaos. As one of the deadliest natural disasters in the past century, the earthquake killed more than 230,000 people, injured approximately 300,000, and left more than 1 million homeless. Within 24 hours, the U.S. military initiated Operation Unified Response to provide relief supplies and humanitarian aid to Haiti (Keen, Vieira Neto, Nolan, Kimmey, & Althouse, 2010). The U.S. Southern Command coordinated this response, immediately deploying Coast Guard and Air Force units, followed by the Navy, Marine Corps, and Army (U.S. Southern Command, 2010). At the peak of the U.S. military relief response, more than 22,000 U.S. troops had deployed to Haiti (U.S. Southern Command, 2010). Military personnel engaged in extremely varied relief activities: distributing food, water, and emergency supplies; saving lives through search and rescue; clearing the streets; preparing mass graves; and providing medical care (Keen et al., 2010). Military care providers offered support services to service members who were assisting with the relief effort and to civilians affected by the disaster (e.g., Warner, 2010).

As seen in Haiti, the U.S. military is often called to the frontlines of both international and domestic crises because of its logistical expertise, transportation capabilities, manpower, resources, and ability to mobilize swiftly (Keen, 2010; Mancuso, Price, & West, 2008). Other notable mass trauma events that utilized military relief operations include Hurricane Katrina in 2005 and the September 11, 2001, attacks on the World Trade Center and Pentagon. The nature of each crisis and its setting varies dramatically, from natural cataclysms (e.g., earthquakes, floods, tsunamis, hurricanes) to man-made disasters (e.g., terrorist attacks, transportation accidents). In humanitarian assistance and disaster relief (HA/DR) operations, all branches of the U.S. military may be involved in providing the following services: evacuation, search and rescue, medical services, translation services, transportation assistance, aid distribution, recovery of human remains, logistical coordination, water and sanitation assessments, disease control, movement of supplies, construction of field hospitals, and planning (Defense Security Cooperation Agency, 2009; Grieger & Lyszczarz, 2002; Hoge, Orman, & Robichaux, 2002; Mancuso et al., 2008). While engaging in this work, service members may be exposed to a variety of aversive sensory stimuli, large-scale devastation, and gruesome scenes of death and suffering (e.g., Keller & Bobo, 2004).

In the aftermath of disaster, military mental health practitioners, psychiatrists, social workers, nurses, corpsmen and medics, and chaplains provide services to U.S. military personnel, families of service members, and occasionally civilians. Most commonly, these care providers work with service personnel who are indirectly exposed to traumatic devastation, loss, and suffering while engaging in relief operations (e.g., Amundson, Lane, & Ferrara, 2008; Joyce, 2006; McGuiness, 2006). Military care providers also assist service personnel who have been directly affected by a disaster, including acts of terrorism (e.g., the September 11 attack on the Pentagon in 2001) and noncombat military accidents (e.g., helicopter and submarine accidents; Cozza, Huleatt, & James, 2002; Grieger & Lyszczarz, 2002; Jankosky, 2008). Supportive services may be offered to families of service members as well (Hoge et al., 2002). Military care providers also provide services to civilians affected by disaster-related trauma, from the humanitarian efforts of Navy hospital ships to deployed providers working with families in the combat zone after war-related trauma (e.g., Grieger & Lyszczarz, 2002). Such scenarios require special consideration, since therapeutic techniques that draw on military culture and support systems may not generalize to civilians. Furthermore, interventions with civilians may be limited to single interactions, and clinical competence may require a working understanding of local norms and customs (for a review, see Wessells, 2009).

The training, preparation, and intervention strategies used by military care providers from disparate disciplines vary greatly. Some mental health teams within the military specialize in rapid response and receive specific training in disaster interventions (e.g., the Navy's Special Psychiatric Rapid Intervention Teams; Grieger & Lyszczarz, 2002). However, often military care providers with less experience and training are also mobilized to respond to disasters, particularly in circumstances where the need for services overwhelms existing capacities. Even among those with specialized disaster response training, there is no clear consensus on which psychological interventions should be delivered. This ambiguity may be due in part to the relative dearth of empirical studies testing the effectiveness of disaster interventions. There is, however, growing awareness that these interventions must be guided by solid, evidence-based practices and systematically evaluated.

This chapter addresses topics relevant to military care providers who provide services to military personnel and civilians in the days and weeks following a disaster. We first examine the historical and present-day context of military-led humanitarian missions. We then provide an overview of the nature of trauma, typical reactions to disaster-related trauma and stressors, and critical issues involved in identifying individuals who would benefit from intervention. Next, we address training recommendations and specific interventions employed in the immediate wake of disasters to alleviate acute distress, prevent the development of psychological disorders, and promote long-term adaptive functioning. Finally, we end with a discussion of current best practices in the field.

HISTORICAL CONTEXT OF MILITARY-LED HUMANITARIAN MISSIONS

The U.S. Department of Defense's (DoD) role in providing HA/DR has evolved dramatically over the years. Historically, international relief organizations and nongovernmental organizations (NGOs) have served as the primary providers of humanitarian aid. When the DoD began overseeing humanitarian assistance missions in 1986, military relief efforts primarily focused on transporting privately donated materials to countries in need (USAID Office of Military Affairs, 2010). However, spurred by the events of September 11, 2001, the U.S. military has begun to devote more resources and attention toward worldwide humanitarian assistance and disaster relief operations. Consequently, the DoD humanitarian assistance program has undergone significant changes, including a surge in the number of humanitarian initiatives implemented as well as changes to the goals and overall purpose of these initiatives. Recognizing that humanitarian assistance can play a crucial role in promoting foreign diplomacy, the DoD expanded the military's involvement in HA/DR in 2005 with the directive "Military Support for Stability, Security, Transition, and Reconstruction Operations." This directive focuses on bolstering U.S. security objectives, including countering ideological support for terrorism (Amundson et al., 2008; DoD, 2005). There is evidence that such initiatives have been effective at improving perceptions of the United States, as seen following the 2004 Indian Ocean tsunami and the 2005 Pakistani earthquake, when positive opinion of the United States doubled among local populations after the U.S. military participated in relief efforts (Amundson et al., 2008).

As mutual civilian and military aid operations have become increasingly common, many NGOs have voiced concerns about the U.S. military's general involvement in relief missions. Opponents of military involvement claim that civilian relief agencies are generally more effective than military personnel in delivering aid, in part because civilian organizations are not affiliated with the U.S. government and thus do not pose a threat to the authority of local governments. In addition, it is argued that local populations may have difficulty distinguishing NGOs from military personnel who are involved in relief efforts. In areas where hostile groups are present, this ambiguity may endanger the lives of civilian aid workers. In light of these concerns, some NGOs suggest that the U.S. military limit its role to providing ambient security to civilian relief agencies (see Patrick, 2009). Regardless of whether this recommendation is ultimately heeded, it is fair to say that tensions exist between the DoD and various NGOs, and that the provision of military disaster relief is an ongoing topic of debate. Having provided some context for the DoD's humanitarian assistance program, we now turn our attention to the nature of disasters and the populations they affect.

DEFINING DISASTER AND THE AFFECTED POPULATIONS

Disaster is a term used to encompass a variety of incidents associated with sudden, widespread destruction, human loss, and devastation to community infrastructure (Halpern & Tramontin, 2007). Disasters are inherently unpredictable and entail a series of unfolding emergencies and traumas. Although certain commonalities exist, each disaster event differs with regard to setting, scope, duration, and populations affected. Domestically, the Federal Emergency Management Agency (FEMA) estimates that, on average, 4,000 national disasters—56 of which are presidentially declared national disasters—have occurred each year over the past decade (FEMA, 2010a; Reyes & Elhai, 2004). These disasters have ranged from transportation disasters to acts of terrorism.

Military care providers must be prepared to provide supportive services to military personnel and civilians directly or indirectly exposed to a variety of disaster-related stressors. It is worth noting that, in some cases, the distinction between direct and indirect exposure may be unclear, such as incidents in which service members are assigned to recover human remains or asked to perform duties that evoke significant distress or discomfort (e.g., Keller & Bobo, 2004). Moreover, this distinction may not be useful when predicting psychological outcomes among emergency responders. For instance, in one study examining members of the Norwegian military, rescuers responding to an avalanche were as symptomatic as directly exposed victims 2 and 4 months after the event (Johnsen, Eid, Lovstad, & Michelsen, 1997).

Given the large number of individuals impacted by disasters, military care providers cannot be expected to provide treatment to all of those exposed to disaster-related traumas. It is, therefore, necessary for military care providers to systematically identify those individuals most in need of services. However, assessment of risk is often difficult in the immediate aftermath of trauma, as acute trauma reactions are normative, often transient, and not necessarily predictive of subsequent psychiatric morbidity and role impairment (e.g., Bryant, 2004). Next, we take a closer look at the ways in which individuals often respond to potentially traumatic events and subsequently discuss strategies for identifying those most in need of treatment.

RESPONSES AND REACTIONS TO DISASTER AND TRAUMA

In the early aftermath of disasters and other potentially traumatic events, individuals often experience a variety of marked physiological, behavioral, cognitive, and emotional reactions. Research studies investigating acute reactions to trauma have consistently identified a constellation of symptoms consisting of heightened sympathetic arousal (e.g., increased heart rate and skin conductance), avoidance of trauma cues, maladaptive cognitions about the self and the world, dissociative symptomatology, emotional numbing, and depressed and anxious mood (e.g., Bryant, Sackville, Dang, Moulds, & Guthrie, 1999; Elsesser, Freyth, Lohrmann, & Sartory, 2009; Yahav & Cohen, 2007). In addition, a number of other trauma-related symptoms specific to bereavement and traumatic loss have been well recognized, and these may be particularly prevalent in postdisaster populations. These symptoms include grief reactions (e.g., preoccupation with the deceased and profound feelings of loneliness and longing) and survivor guilt (e.g., Gray, Prigerson, & Litz, 2004).

It appears, however, that in the wake of even highly traumatic events, including disasters, a significant percentage of those exposed do not exhibit acute stress reactions or do so only transiently (e.g., Bonanno et al., 2008; Bonanno, Galea, Bucciarelli, & Vlahov, 2006). Trauma researchers have long been aware of this phenomenon and have been in active pursuit of risk and resilience prediction models for nearly two decades. Beginning with DSM-IV, acute stress disorder (ASD) was added to the psychiatric nosology as a way of calling attention to this subject and identifying those at high risk for chronic posttraumatic stress disorder (PTSD; e.g., Bryant, 2004). Although ASD has been found to have moderate sensitivity and specificity in predicting PTSD (Bryant, Harvey, Guthrie, & Moulds, 2003), researchers have acknowledged the disorder's overemphasis on dissociative features and its overall predictive inefficiency (Harvey & Bryant, 2002).

To aid in the development of more sophisticated prediction models, a new line of research is under way that presupposes qualitatively distinct, prototypical patterns of response to trauma (i.e., trajectories of adaptation) and that seeks to identify risk and resilience factors associated with prototypical symptom trajectories rather than simple, cross-sectional symptom measurements. This area of research is built on Bonanno's (2004) theoretical model, which hypothesizes four prototypical patterns, or classes, of response to trauma: resilience, recovery, delayed, and chronic. Whereas resilient individuals are described as never developing clinically significant symptoms at any point following trauma exposure, those in the recovery class are said to exhibit a marked acute reaction followed by a steady decrease in symptoms. The delayed response is posited to consist of an initial asymptomatic presentation followed by an abrupt increase in symptoms, and the chronic class is described as having the strongest initial response followed by sustained chronicity.

Although a handful of studies utilizing variants of a sophisticated analytic approach (latent class growth modeling) have succeeded in validating Bonanno's model either in part or in full (e.g., Bonanno et al., 2008; deRoon-Cassini, Mancini, Rusch, & Bonanno, 2010; Dickstein, Suvak, Litz, & Adler, 2010; Orcutt, Erickson, & Wolfe, 2004), this line of research remains in its infancy. Few robust predictors of trajectory (i.e., class) assignment have been identified, and a number of trauma populations have yet to be examined. In addition to these limitations, relatively little attention has been paid to psychological sequelae other than PTSD. In particular, it appears that few studies have assessed for symptoms of depression or generalized anxiety prior to labeling trauma survivors as resilient. Given recent epidemiological research suggesting that these forms of psychopathology may be equally if not more prevalent than PTSD in the wake of trauma (Bryant et al., 2010), this omission is problematic.

PREDICTORS OF PTSD

Although researchers have yet to produce reliable prediction models of PTSD, they have succeeded in identifying a number of pre-, peri-, and posttrauma risk and resilience variables that may be used to inform early intervention efforts. Unfortunately, taken together, it appears that these variables are able to account for only about 20% of the overall variance in PTSD symptom severity (Ozer, Best, Lipsey, & Weiss, 2003).

To date, two meta-analyses examining predictors of PTSD, have been published (Brewin, Andrews, & Valentine, 2000; Ozer et al., 2003). Both studies concluded that, overall, predictors occurring more proximally to traumatic events (e.g., trauma severity and peritraumatic reactions) were better predictors of subsequent PTSD than variables occurring more distally (e.g., pretrauma history), and that the predictive power associated with given predictors varied significantly as a function of moderating variables, such as gender and military status. Brewin and colleagues found lack of social support, life stress, and trauma severity to best predict PTSD, whereas Ozer and colleagues found peritraumatic dissociation and perceived support to be the best predictors. Brewin et al. compared effect sizes between military and civilian samples, and found that among military samples the best predictors of PTSD were lack of social support, life stress, trauma severity, and adverse childhood experiences. Among civilians, the best predictors were life stress, lack of social support, trauma severity, and low socioeconomic status. Although teasing apart these differences is helpful, other moderators (e.g., gender) bear meaningfully on effect size, and researchers caution against the creation of general vulnerability models (Brewin et al., 2000). Thus, although the extant risk and resilience literature may be used to inform best practices for identifying high-risk individuals, further research is needed to maximize the utility of screening tools. Still, these results offer some guidance to early interventionists seeking to prevent the development of psychopathology among high-risk individuals.

PREVENTION STRATEGIES AND CRITICAL ISSUES

Traditionally, three types of prevention strategies have been described in the early intervention literature: universal, selective, and indicated (e.g., Gordon, 1987). *Universal prevention* entails providing services to an entire population and does not involve assessing differences in risk across individuals. *Selective prevention*, in contrast, refers to the provision of services to high-risk subgroups (e.g., all individuals exposed to a given traumatic event), but does not involve assessing differences in risk among individuals in the subgroup. *Indicated prevention* entails the provision of services to individuals exhibiting early, subsyndromal or preclinical symptoms that indicate risk of illness. The best available evidence shows that selective interventions are ineffective and waste resources, while indicated preventions are the optimal methodology in acute trauma contexts (Roberts, Kitchiner, Kenardy, & Bisson, 2009).

However, currently there is no consensus in the military on how to define, let alone screen for the presence of, preclinical distress, which would warrant indicated prevention strategies. Only the Navy–Marine Corps stress continuum model (U.S. Department of the Navy, 2000) describes a preclinical state of combat or operational stress injury, which indicates that early prevention is needed. In the stress continuum model, four zones of psychiatric functioning are used to determine the type of intervention, if any, that is appropriate for a given individual: green (ready), yellow (reacting), orange (injured), and red (ill). Individuals within the green zone are described as operating at optimal levels of functioning and wellness. This is typified by high mission focus, physical fitness, and self-control. Those in the yellow zone are described as experiencing mild and transient forms of distress and impairment, such as feelings of irritability, loss of focus, and sleep dysregulation. In the orange zone, individuals are said to experience more severe and persistent stress reactions, such as loss of control, panic, disorganization, withdrawal, emotion dysregulation, depressive symptoms, and excessive guilt or shame. Last, individuals are considered to be in the red zone after the onset of a clinical mental disorder (e.g., PTSD, depression, anxiety, substance abuse).

According to the model, yellow zone stress reactions are normal, and a natural course of recovery is expected. In the yellow zone, natural supports and respite are sufficient to return an individual back to the green (ready) zone. In contrast, orange zone preclinical states entail a sufficient degree of distress, symptoms, and impairment that make a service member nonmission ready. In the Navy and Marine Corps, orange zone reactions signal the need for combat and operational stress first aid, which can be administered by military care providers, leaders, peers, and other social supports (Nash, Westphal, Watson, & Litz, 2010; Watson, Nash, Westphal, & Litz, 2010). The Navy and Marine Corps have developed an observational screening tool, the Peritraumatic Behavior Questionnaire (Nash, 2010), which Navy Corpsmen and leaders can use in situ to identity orange zone stress injuries. At the more severe end of the stress continuum, service members experiencing red zone stress reactions require assessment and treatment by a mental health professional.

In addition to the challenge of identifying individuals who require indicated prevention, there are several other important considerations surrounding prevention strategies. It remains unclear how the scope, intensity, and duration of disasters affect survivors' reactions and how this should inform the provision of aid. Furthermore, there is some concern that intervening too soon after trauma could disrupt individuals' natural recovery processes or produce other negative effects (van Emmerik, Kamphuis, Hulsbosch, & Emmelkamp, 2002). Further research is needed to determine an optimal time frame for administering early interventions (Litz & Gray, 2004). Despite these limitations, however, various early intervention strategies have been developed that are believed to mitigate the pernicious effects of disaster-related trauma, and that have been tailored to meet the needs of military populations. The remainder of this chapter is spent discussing the competencies needed for administering these strategies, their respective treatment components, and the status of their empirical support.

TRAINING FOR MILITARY CARE PROVIDERS

Within the military, there are few formal models for training care providers in disaster preparedness. Military training in disaster response is often idiosyncratic to each team and occurs primarily through informal consultation with practitioners who have worked in disaster settings (e.g., Reeves, 2002; Schwerin, Kennedy, & Wardlaw, 2002). This lack of formalized training means that levels of experience and expertise vary greatly within mental health teams (Cozza et al., 2002). Accordingly, there have been calls for the DoD to develop more extensive, evidence-based training programs for military care providers responding to disaster (Amundson et al., 2008; Mancuso et al., 2008). Outside of the military, the field of disaster mental health (DMH) suffers from a similar lack of coordination and consensus regarding training requirements and best practices (Reyes & Elhai, 2004; Wickramage, 2006; Young, Ruzek, Wong, Salzer, & Naturale, 2006).

Generally, military care providers receive most of their training through civilian institutions and organizations (Johnson et al., 2007). Specialized DMH training can be obtained through various governmental and nongovernmental relief agencies. The American Red Cross provides the most well-established DMH training (e.g., American Red Cross of the Greater Lehigh Valley, 2010). The following organizations also offer disaster training: the National Child Traumatic Stress Network (2010), the National Organization for Victim Assistance (n.d.), FEMA (2010b), and the North Carolina Disaster Response Network (2010). Recognizing the need for more extensive training, several universities now offer short trainings as well as specialized DMH doctoral training and certification courses (e.g., the University of Rochester's [n.d.] Disaster Mental Health Program and the University of South Dakota's [2010] Disaster Mental Health Institute).

Training programs emphasize that working in disaster settings requires not only skill in assessing risk and administering interventions but also several other important proficiencies. Key competencies include the ability to coordinate care, work effectively with people of different backgrounds and cultures, and manage personal reactions. Given the heterogeneous nature of disasters, care providers must be proficient in quickly assessing situations and evaluating current needs and resources, even in disorganized settings with limited infrastructure (Reyes & Elhai, 2004; Young et al., 2006). Knowledge of trauma and posttraumatic stress can be helpful for conceptualizing reactions to disaster and informing interventions. However, a background in trauma work is not always necessary, nor sufficient, for responding effectively in disaster settings. Indeed, applying a posttraumatic stress framework to disaster interventions may constrain the view of care providers and lead them to overlook significant individual or communitywide disaster-related problems (Reyes & Elhai, 2004). Moreover, the posttraumatic stress framework does not address the practical constraints and ongoing sources of stress that survivors face in a disaster setting. Before engaging in disaster work, care providers should accurately assess their skills and capacities, as self-awareness of one's strengths and limitations is crucial for this work (Haskett, Scott, Nears, & Grimmett, 2008; Merchant, Leigh, & Lurie, 2010).

On top of these general competencies for disaster work, uniformed care providers must have a thorough understanding of the military context in which they perform their duties. The military culture and organizational structure may contribute to certain problems, such as stigma, while also serving as useful tools for promoting recovery (Nash et al., 2010). In delivering postdisaster interventions to service members, coordinating efforts and conferring with command structure are essential for providing a unified response (Amundson et al., 2008; Cozza et al., 2002). Compared with NGOs that provide disaster relief and humanitarian assistance, military care providers often encounter additional challenges, such as greater organizational fluctuations as commanders are frequently transferred to different posts (Amundson et al., 2008).

When providing care to civilians, it is important to establish effective communication systems and coordinate care not only within the military but also between the military and other relief organizations. Considering that delivery of disaster relief and humanitarian aid has historically been the domain of other governmental and nongovernmental organizations such as USAID and Red Cross, military care providers must recognize when such organizations may be faster or more effective at providing services (Amundson et al., 2008; Mancuso et al., 2008). Coordinating efforts with these organizations can pose a substantial challenge, with the potential to either impede or facilitate delivery of services. If relief efforts are not well coordinated, the military risks contributing to a "carnival of interventions" (Wickramage, 2006) that squanders resources, duplicates services, and may overwhelm, confuse, or overpathologize the civilians they intend to help (Cozza et al., 2002; Dodgen, LaDue, & Kaul, 2002). Military care providers must also be skilled in coordinating care with local authorities and attend closely to requests from the affected community (Merchant et al., 2010).

Providing services to civilian populations also requires that care providers adapt their interventions to the specific context and culture. Within both domestic and foreign populations, diverse cultural beliefs and practices often influence how psychological disorders and interventions are viewed and received (Haskett et al., 2008). Providers must, therefore, understand that psychosocial interventions cannot be universally delivered in the same manner as hygiene kits or relief supplies (Wickramage, 2006). Rather, respect and awareness of the context and culture are critical. For instance, Haitians who subscribe to voodoo beliefs and practices may attribute mental disorders to spells or displeased spirits (Pierre et al., 2010). As a result, psychological problems may be seen as a family or religious affair, requiring treatment from traditional healers and priests. More generally, perceptions of disclosure and Western-style individual counseling often vary greatly among cultures (Wessells, 2009). Ethical challenges may also arise regarding informed consent, which may be difficult to obtain in a disaster setting with language and literacy barriers, autonomy issues, disparities in access to information and resources, and different cultural norms about rejecting help (Wessells, 2009).

Disaster response teams must avoid creating dependency among civilians and undermining existing supports. Inadvertently, providers may compete with and weaken existing informal support systems or local governmental structures. Although it may appear more expedient to create a parallel system of care that does not require the input of local government, free-standing programs are unlikely to confer sustainable benefits to the community and may leave civilians dependent on them (Wessells, 2009). Rather than introducing competing systems, the emphasis should be on bolstering and improving existing supports, which can be sustained after military care providers depart (Merchant et al., 2010).

In addition to developing competencies for working with individuals and institutions, it is necessary for care providers to monitor and manage their own personal reactions to the emotionally and physically taxing work. Care providers working in disaster settings are vulnerable to a host of negative effects, including compassion fatigue, burnout, and vicarious trauma, which may result in decreased patient care quality and high worker turnaround (for an in-depth discussion of these phenomena, see Halpern & Tramontin, 2007). As such, care providers should be aware of these hazards and actively engage in protective measures. Preventive plans that allow care providers to take breaks to recharge physically and mentally, connect with social supports, and obtain professional support from colleagues are vital for maintaining morale and promoting high-quality delivery of services (Cozza et al., 2002; Schwerin et al., 2002).

While adequate training and preparation for disaster work is essential, it is also impossible to fully prepare for and predict all of the contingencies surrounding a disaster (Amundson et al., 2008; Cozza et al., 2002). Considering this reality, it is critical for mental health providers to receive rigorous training in specific interventions while also learning how to adapt and flexibly apply these strategies. We now turn our attention to specific psychological interventions employed in the immediate aftermath of a disaster.

EARLY INTERVENTIONS

The interventions employed by military care providers in disaster settings vary tremendously (Reyes & Elhai, 2004). Although trauma research has identified effective interventions for preventing and treating PTSD and other long-term trauma-related sequelae (Ponniah & Hollon, 2009; Roberts et al., 2009), there has been very little systematic research on acute interventions administered in the immediate aftermath of disaster (Orner, Kent, Pfefferbaum, Raphael, & Watson, 2006). This lack of rigorous postdisaster research is due in part to the logistical difficulties of conducting research where entire communities and existing organizational structures have been thrown into disarray. In addition, postdisaster research has lacked adequate theoretical models for understanding acute responses to mass trauma (Shalev, 2006). The following section examines the utility of five different forms of early interventions: psychoeducation, psychological debriefing, psychological first aid, combat and operational stress first aid, and cognitive-behavioral therapy.

Psychoeducation

Historically, the term *psychoeducation* has been loosely defined and somewhat generic. Wessely et al. (2008) proposed defining psychoeducation as "the provision of information, in a variety of media, about the nature of stress, posttraumatic and other symptoms, and what to do about them" (p. 287). Such information typically includes a description of normative reactions to a stressful event, a review of the nature and symptoms of stress disorders (i.e., ASD and PTSD), suggestions for adaptive coping strategies, and information on when and how to seek professional help.

Although psychoeducation is a component of most postdisaster interventions for both military service members and civilians, it is also commonly used as a discrete method (Creamer & O'Donnell, 2008). Psychoeducation as an acute, stand-alone intervention can be delivered in a variety of ways, including via educational pamphlets, informational and self-help websites, bibliotherapy, group sessions with a provider, or individual, face-to-face meetings. Given the ubiquity with which such information is disseminated following disasters, there is a general belief that psychoeducation is beneficial for trauma survivors. Wessely et al. (2008) identified five theoretically based assumptions that appear to serve as the basis for this conjecture: (1) Symptoms will be less disturbing if they are expected; (2) normalization of psychological sequelae is reassuring; (3) awareness of traumatic stress symptoms facilitates help-seeking behaviors; (4) psychoeducation helps to correct inaccurate beliefs; and (5) the self-help aspect of psychoeducation promotes a sense of empowerment.

Despite these plausible theoretical underpinnings, there is insufficient evidence suggesting that psychoeducation prevents the development of PTSD. In fact, some research suggests that individuals who receive posttrauma psychoeducation are equally or more likely to experience PTSD symptoms than those receiving no intervention (Scholes, Turpin, & Mason, 2007; Turpin, Downs, & Mason, 2005). In a review article that sparked considerable debate, Wessely et al. (2008) concluded that no evidence exists that psychoeducation is an effective stand-alone posttrauma intervention and challenged the aforementioned assumptions supporting its use. The authors further suggested that the paradoxical effects of psychoeducation may be accounted for by the "nocebo effect"; that is, individuals' expectations of possible future symptoms may trigger the development of these phenomena. Additionally, they argue that psychoeducation may inadvertently increase sensitivity to and pathologize normal responding. However, proponents of psychoeducation dispute these assertions (e.g., Kilpatrick, Cougle, & Resnick, 2008; Krupnick & Green, 2008; Southwick, Friedman, & Krystal, 2008), arguing that the question of whether psychoeducation prevents psychological distress is too broad and that more circumscribed research is needed to evaluate potential moderators of treatment outcome (e.g., modes of intervention delivery, target populations).

Psychological Debriefing

Compared with psychoeducation, psychological debriefing (PD) is a more specific framework for delivering posttrauma intervention. PD refers to any intervention, delivered shortly following a crisis, that encourages survivors to recount and emotionally process their experiences with the ultimate goal of minimizing maladaptive psychological sequelae (Bisson, McFarlane, Rose, Ruzek, & Watson, 2009). Although alternate variations have emerged, PD is generally delivered in a single session, using a semistructured group format, within 24 hours to a few days following traumatic exposure. Although several frameworks exist (e.g., Dunning, 1988; National Organization for Victim Assistance, 1987), the most common form of PD is critical incident stress debriefing (CISD; e.g., Mitchell, 1983; Mitchell & Everly, 1995). CISD guides survivors to "emotionally ventilate" by disclosing the thoughts and feelings that they experienced during the traumatic event. It also provides information on posttraumatic stress symptoms and prompts survivors to identify current symptoms. Although it was originally intended for use with crisis responders (e.g., emergency workers, disaster response teams), CISD is now often used with primary victims as well (Mitchell, 2004). Despite the recommendation that CISD be used within the context of the comprehensive, multicomponent, critical incident stress management intervention (Mitchell, 2004), it is most frequently administered as an independent intervention (McNally, Bryant, & Ehlers, 2003).

CISD has been highly debated in the literature, as a preponderance of research has emerged suggesting that it is at best ineffective and at worst detrimental (Bisson et al., 2009; Bisson, Jenkins, Alexander, & Bannister, 1997; Hobbs, Mayou, Harrison, & Worlock, 1996). Moreover, meta-analyses indicate that CISD does not improve distress, PTSD, depression, or anxiety symptoms above and beyond what can be accounted for by natural recovery (Rose, Bisson, Churchill, & Wessely, 2002; van Emmerik et al., 2002). Some researchers speculate that CISD may produce iatrogenic effects because it approximates an exposure paradigm without allowing time for subsequent habituation and may impede individuals from utilizing their own established social networks (Bisson et al., 1997; Devilly, Gist, & Cotton, 2006; van Emmerik et al., 2002).

Proponents of CISD argue that conclusions of its ineffectiveness are unfounded, citing methodological issues such as inappropriate participant inclusion, protocol deviations, and inappropriate generalization of findings in the studies showing null or negative results (Everly, Flannery, & Mitchell, 2000; Robinson, 2004). However, a recent randomized controlled trial involving U.S. peacekeeping soldiers addressed these concerns and did not find that CISD reduced symptoms and impairment compared with no treatment or a psychoeducational stress management class (Adler et al., 2008). In light of these studies, strong recommendations have been made against the use of CISD (e.g., Bisson et al., 2009), and most current guidelines now advocate using psychological first aid instead (Litz, 2008; McNally et al., 2003). At the same time, some U.S. military care providers have continued to administer group debriefings modeled after CISD that retain the basic format but omit the requirement to discuss thoughts and reactions in great detail (Cozza et al., 2002; Peterson, Nicolas, McGraw, Englert, & Blackman, 2002). Further research is needed to fully define non-CISD debriefing strategies and examine their effectiveness.

Psychological First Aid

Broadly defined, psychological first aid (PFA) is an approach that is initiated as soon after a traumatic event as possible, with the goal of allaying
distress and buffering against the development of PTSD or other psychological disorders among civilian populations (Brymer et al., 2006; Ruzek
et al., 2007). Whereas PD is a more structured intervention that typically
does not occur until at least 1 day posttrauma, PFA is a system for providing immediate and often on-scene support that varies in response to the
nature of the situation and the idiosyncratic needs of each individual. In
response to the need for empirically refined relief efforts to fill the gap left
by CISD, Hobfoll et al. (2007) delineated five evidence-based principles that
are essential for effective immediate interventions. These elements include
promoting a sense of safety, calmness, self- and collective efficacy, connectedness, and hope. Although several frameworks have been proposed for
structuring PFA, here we review in detail the psychological first aid field
operations guide (Brymer et al., 2006).

The psychological first aid field operations guide, developed through
a joint effort by the National Child Traumatic Stress Network and the
National Center for PTSD, was created and refereed by an international
cohort of experts in the field (Vernberg et al., 2008). Designed to formalize
PFA and more explicitly inform its delivery, the guide identifies eight empirically informed components, or "core actions," of PFA that are appropriate
for the heterogeneity of disaster settings. The first component, contact and
engagement, guides providers to introduce themselves in a calm manner,
communicate compassion, and consider cultural factors. In triaging their
services, providers should first respond to individuals who are seeking out
care and then offer services to other survivors. Confidentiality considerations also fall under this first component. Although disaster settings are
typically not conducive to protecting confidentiality, rescue workers should
strive to maximize privacy to the greatest extent possible.

In delivering the second component, safety and comfort, the focus is
on ensuring physical safety, optimizing physical comfort, and providing
emotional support. Specific ways for mental health responders to address
immediate safety needs may involve creating an inventory of those with
special requirements (e.g., medications), continuously scanning the environment for threats to safety, and communicating with medical or law
enforcement officials as appropriate. After maximizing the survivors'
physical safety, rescue workers should then begin to relay information on
the disaster itself, services that are available to survivors, possible stress
reactions that may be expected, and the importance of self-care. However,
in consideration of the survivors' current psychological states, it is crucial
that providers use clinical judgment in determining when and how much

information to reveal. Emotional support and comfort can be facilitated by promoting social engagement among trauma survivors and shielding them from further traumatization (e.g., exposure to media reports, severely injured individuals and bodies, or attorney solicitations). Responders must also be prepared to assist with acute grief responses of individuals who have been informed that a loved one is missing or has died.

The third component, stabilization, may be required if a survivor is in a disoriented state. Although atypical, some trauma reactions may involve severe emotional numbing or arousal that will interfere with basic functioning and safety. In such situations, grounding techniques and/or medication referrals may be warranted. The fourth component, information gathering, is integral in tailoring PFA to the unique needs and circumstances of each individual. Important information to ascertain includes the survivor's objective and subjective experience of the event, unresolved questions and concerns, physical and mental health status, and available social supports. During the fifth component, practical assistance, relief workers help survivors clarify pressing issues and carry out immediate pragmatic needs. Some needs (e.g., placing a phone call) can be quickly resolved; for those that cannot (e.g., submitting an insurance claim), providers can assist by helping to develop an action plan. The sixth component of PFA, connection with social supports, involves helping survivors to reach out to their primary supports (e.g., family, close friends, clergy), and facilitating connectedness with those individuals who are more immediately available (e.g., other survivors and relief workers). Survivors may not want to socialize or discuss their experiences, and any resistance toward doing so should be validated and normalized. However, physical isolation should be discouraged, as merely being in the presence of others, even in the absence of any conversation, can be helpful.

Information on coping, the seventh component of PFA, involves educating individuals about normative reactions to traumatic events and identifying adaptive coping strategies. Information on symptoms of stress disorders can be useful in helping survivors to identify future symptoms that may arise. Additionally, discussions about grief responses, depression, and bodily reactions can be beneficial in alerting individuals to these potential sequelae. Survivors may particularly benefit from learning healthy, adaptive methods of coping with reactions to the trauma, which can reduce distress and prevent them from engaging in maladaptive coping behaviors. Finally, linkage with collaborative services is needed to establish ongoing care. Facilitating contact or placing referrals to community centers, support groups, and other such resources establishes the care network beyond PFA.

A wide range of healthcare providers, paraprofessionals, and even individuals without a background in mental health can be trained to deliver

PFA (Allen et al., 2010; Brymer et al., 2006; Ruzek et al., 2007). Supervision and consultation commensurate with the provider's background and competencies should be implemented to optimize care (Ruzek et al., 2007). Despite the high frequency with which PFA is implemented after traumatic events, little is known about its long-term efficacy in preventing posttraumatic mental disorders and role impairment (Vernberg et al., 2008).

Combat and Operational Stress First Aid

While PFA shows promise as an early intervention strategy, it is intended primarily for civilians. In contrast to civilian victims, military personnel assume active roles in responding to disaster, expect to encounter severe stressors that are constant and cumulative, and function within a unique military context and culture. Thus, to meet the particular needs of service members, The U.S. Navy, Marine Corps, and National Center for PTSD have collaboratively adapted PFA to create combat and operational stress first aid (COSFA). Below we review the COSFA training manual for caregivers (Nash et al., 2010).

COSFA is an indicated prevention strategy comprising tools for restoring wellness and functioning in service members with subclinical stress symptoms, distress, and impairment after a disaster. It also seeks to prevent the further development of psychiatric symptoms. COSFA tools are multidimensional, targeting not only psychological components of recovery but also biological, social, and spiritual factors. Its assessment and intervention strategies are applied flexibly with respect to the needs of the individual service member and situational constraints. COSFA was developed to be used by anyone, including military leaders, individual service members, and family members. However, military care providers are considered the "champions" of COSFA, as they are best situated to provide expert care and delivery of services.

COSFA differs from PFA in several noteworthy ways. Whereas PFA is typically utilized after isolated traumatic events, COSFA addresses not only traumatic stress but also ongoing and cumulative stress (i.e., "wear and tear"), grief and loss, and internal, moral conflicts (Litz et al., 2009). It targets a number of disabling states, including guilt, shame, demoralization, hopelessness, withdrawal, exhaustion, disillusionment, moral injury, and betrayal. COSFA acknowledges that operational stress can impact all of these domains and that addressing multiple areas is essential for lasting recovery.

To identify service members in need of care, COSFA uses the aforementioned Navy–Marine Corps stress continuum. It emphasizes continuous monitoring of each service member's status along the stress continuum, so that those who require intervention are identified and treated expediently.

COSFA interventions focus primarily on orange zone stress, while providing guidance and recommendations for how military leadership can take charge of mitigating yellow zone stress. The overarching goal of COSFA is to return service members to the green zone, where they are functioning optimally: physically, mentally, and spiritually.

Another distinguishing feature of COSFA is that it capitalizes on existing military philosophies, practices, organizing frameworks, and social structures. In particular, it emphasizes the role of leaders in mentoring service members back to the green zone. It views service members not as passive victims but as effective, highly trained individuals who can draw on both personal and organizational resources to regain optimal functioning. As part of this approach, COSFA recommends that caregivers employ motivational interviewing, an empathic, nonjudgmental, collaborative counseling style (Miller & Rollnick, 2002). Motivational interviewing empowers individuals to take responsibility for making changes in their lives, to explore and resolve ambivalence, to systematically evaluate the options for enacting change, and to employ problem-solving strategies.

In addition, COSFA recognizes how military social structures, such as unit cohesion, can play a large role in either hindering or promoting healing and recovery (Wright et al., 2009). COSFA also addresses interactions between service members and other social supports in their lives, such as their families. It recognizes how one can impact the other and, therefore, seeks to promote recovery by repairing and strengthening relationships. Rather than competing with military medical care, religious ministry, peer support, or leadership, COSFA seeks to fortify and bolster these important, preexisting support structures. Interventions are seen as a joint effort to return a service member to optimal functioning, which is a goal that is shared among all parties. To this end, COSFA urges providers to consult frequently with colleagues and with the chain of command. It also emphasizes that military leaders should act deliberately and decisively to mitigate the effects of potential stressors, identify those who require additional help, and reintegrate stress-injured service members into their unit.

COSFA comprises seven core actions: check, coordinate, cover, calm, connect, competence, and confidence. These components are organized into three levels: continuous, primary, and secondary aid. Continuous aid, consisting of the check and coordinate components, describes ongoing, individualized aid that is administered throughout the deployment cycle. Check involves determining service members' current position in the stress continuum by assessing their current distress, functioning, and risk. It directs caregivers to assess psychological well-being as well as social and physical functioning, paying close attention to any changes in behavior or functioning. Self-report, information from collateral sources (e.g., family, peers, leadership), and questionnaires may be employed to assess these factors in a thorough manner. This assessment is then used to determine whether primary aid, secondary aid, or referral to a higher level of care is needed. The second component of continuous aid, coordinate, describes a two-step process of identifying who can help the individual and determining who needs to know about the service member's current state. Caregivers must carefully navigate the arduous territory of deciding what information should be given to which parties, taking into account possible repercussions such as stigmatization.

Primary aid, consisting of the cover and calm components, targets service members who are experiencing intense distress or an abrupt loss of functioning. The cover component describes actions that ensure the physical safety of service members and allow them to emotionally and physically "reset." It encourages service members to stay active by performing tasks that are practical and familiar, provides information that promotes feelings of safety and comfort, and defuses any potential threat to self or others. The other component of primary aid, calm, seeks to reduce damaging physiological and psychological reactions that are associated with long-term impairment (e.g., dissociation, elevated heart rate, intense negative emotions, social withdrawal). Techniques used to physically and emotionally stabilize service members include modeling a calming presence, engaging in empathic conversation, and teaching diaphragmatic breathing and grounding skills to orient individuals to sensations in the present.

Secondary aid, comprising the connect, competence, and confidence components, seeks to foster long-term recovery once the individual is no longer in acute crisis. The connect component helps service members identify and connect with trusted, helpful military and social supports. The aim is to create, maintain, strengthen, or repair lasting military and family supports that can provide service members with practical, informational, and emotional support as they work toward recovery. Service members are also empowered to support peers who are suffering. Competence, another part of secondary aid, entails helping service members regain confidence in their physical and mental capabilities. The focus here is on restoring stress-injured service members' sense of personal competence and gradually returning them to full functioning. Potential interventions include teaching skills for managing stress reactions, working with leaders to adjust work roles and adopt a supportive mentorship role, and retraining as needed. The final component of secondary aid, confidence, involves using mentorship relationships to promote a sense of mastery, create realistic expectations, and strengthen service members' belief in themselves and the leadership. Caregivers should work with leaders to restore trust within units, confront stigma, and create environments that nurture self-confidence.

COSFA principles and practices are informed by a strong evidence base, including the latest empirical findings on risk and resilience (e.g., Hobfoll et al., 2007; Nash & Baker, 2007). However, to date, COSFA lacks direct empirical support from treatment outcome studies. Recognizing this limitation, the COSFA manual explicitly leaves room for continually updating and improving its strategies. Systematic investigation is needed to assess COSFA's effectiveness, acceptance by service members, and ease of implementation.

Cognitive-Behavioral Therapy

Over the past two decades, cognitive-behavioral therapy (CBT) has steadily gained empirical support for preventing and treating PTSD (Ponniah & Hollon, 2009; Roberts et al., 2009). When used as an indicated preventive intervention, CBT is normally administered several weeks to several months after the traumatic event. Preventive CBT typically involves psychoeducation, anxiety management techniques such as diaphragmatic breathing, imaginal and situational exposures to habituate patients to feared memories and stimuli, and cognitive restructuring to challenge distorted thought patterns associated with the traumatic event.

Meta-analyses suggest that exposure-based CBT is an effective indicated preventive intervention and treatment for PTSD (Ponniah & Hollon, 2009; Roberts et al., 2009). Randomized controlled trials have found that when CBT is employed as a preventive intervention within 3 months of traumatic exposure, it is more effective at reducing traumatic stress symptoms and preventing chronic PTSD than supportive counseling (Bryant, Harvey, Dang, Sackville, & Basten, 1998; Bryant, Moulds, & Nixon, 2003), relaxation training (Echeburua, de Corral, Sarasua, & Zubizarreta, 1996), and no-intervention control groups (Bisson, Shepherd, Joy, Probert, & Newcombe, 2004; Ehlers et al., 2003).

Given that preventive CBT interventions usually entail four- to five-sessions of structured, individual therapy conducted by a specialty care provider in a safe place, it is inappropriate as an acute intervention for individuals in the immediate aftermath of a disaster. In the chaos of disaster, military care providers may lack the time, resources, and infrastructure needed to administer multiple sessions of CBT. Moreover, civilian survivors may require assistance attending to more urgent, basic needs (e.g., food, shelter, safety). Military personnel engaging in postdisaster relief operations are unlikely to have the time to deliver a more intensive preventive intervention like CBT.

Nevertheless, military care providers administering PFA to civilians or COSFA to service members may find it helpful to be familiar with CBT, so that they can educate individuals about this resource, screen for those who may later benefit from an early CBT intervention, and direct those individuals to the appropriate resources if their symptoms persist.

SUMMARY AND CONCLUSIONS

As the DoD continues to enlarge its HA/DR program, an increasing number of military care providers will be called upon to support military personnel and civilians who are affected by disaster. Exposure to disaster-related trauma and stressors can cause great distress and long-term suffering among both survivors and responders. Military care providers are well situated to prevent and mitigate these negative sequelae and promote long-term adaptive functioning. In disaster settings, military care providers must quickly identify which individuals require services and decide when to intervene and which interventions to use. They must be skilled not only in screening individuals and delivering interventions, but also in adapting intervention strategies to each unique disaster context, incorporating cultural considerations (both military and local civilian culture), and coordinating care. To operate effectively in this capacity, a high degree of self-knowledge and humility are crucial. Training in disaster response—both formal and informal—can assist care providers in developing these competencies. It is encouraging that an increasing number of institutions offering DMH courses appear to recognize the need for more formalized and comprehensive training, but further development, dissemination, and evaluation of this training is needed.

The lack of empirical research prohibits any clear conclusions regarding the most effective disaster interventions, but several evidence-based early interventions seem promising. For military care providers providing early interventions to service personnel, COSFA offers the most comprehensive, evidence-based form of intervention. Importantly, COSFA leverages military culture and social structures, thereby capitalizing on existing support systems. In situations where military care providers are called upon to deliver acute services to civilians, PFA emerges as the preferred intervention. PFA's flexibility and empirically supported underpinnings represent an improvement over psychological debriefing. COSFA, PFA, and psychoeducation as a stand-alone intervention await evaluation. For individuals who need services beyond those provided immediately after a disaster, CBT may be a helpful resource, given its demonstrated efficacy at preventing and treating PTSD.

It should be emphasized that these recommendations emerge from our current knowledge base on disaster inventions, a still nascent field. As such, there is a clear need for further empirical investigation to expand upon the existing literature, broaden our understanding of the type of clinical work that is most essential following a disaster, systematically evaluate and refine current best practices, and develop a larger repertoire of interventions. Unfortunately, myriad issues inherent to disaster research limit its feasibility and pose unique logistical and ethical challenges. By definition, disasters occur without warning; thus, practical barriers preclude our ability to minimize the time between the initial event and the beginning of data collection. Furthermore, special attention needs to be given to the informed consent process, considering that individuals exposed to trauma are in a vulnerable state and may have impaired decision-making capacities. The extent to which participating in research offers any direct benefit to disaster survivors needs to be carefully considered (e.g., Collogan, Tuma, Dolan-Sewell, Borja, & Fleischman, 2004; Rosenstein, 2004). Fortunately, emerging research in DMH has demonstrated that it is possible to conduct such research in an ethical and methodologically rigorous manner (e.g., Adams & Boscarino, 2006). These developments have fueled enthusiasm among researchers and care providers alike for evaluating, disseminating, and adopting evidence-based disaster interventions.

REFERENCES

Adams, R. E., & Boscarino, J. A. (2006). Predictors of PTSD and delayed PTSD after disaster: The impact of exposure and psychosocial resources. *Journal of Nervous and Mental Disease, 194,* 485–493.

Adler, A. B., Litz, B. T., Castro, C. A., Suvak, M., Thomas, J. L., Burrell, L., et al. (2008). A group randomized trial of critical incident stress debriefing provided to U.S. peacekeepers. *Journal of Traumatic Stress, 21,* 253–263.

Allen, B., Brymer, M., Steinberg, A., Vernberg, E., Jacobs, A., Speier, A., et al. (2010). Perceptions of psychological first aid among providers responding to Hurricanes Gustav and Ike. *Journal of Traumatic Stress, 23,* 509–513.

American Red Cross of the Greater Lehigh Valley. (2010). *Disaster response training courses.* Retrieved November 24, 2010, from *www.redcrosslv.org/disaster/disasterclass.html.*

Amundson, D., Lane, D., & Ferrara, E. (2008). The U.S. military disaster response to the Yogyakarta earthquake May through June 2006. *Military Medicine, 173,* 236–240.

Bisson, J. I., Jenkins, P., Alexander, J., & Bannister, C. (1997). A randomized controlled trial of psychological debriefing for victims of acute burn trauma. *British Journal of Psychiatry, 171,* 78–81.

Bisson, J. I., McFarlane, A. C., Rose, S., Ruzek, J. I., & Watson, P. J. (2009). Psychological debriefing for adults. In E. B. Foa, T. M. Keane, M. J. Friedman, & J. A. Cohen (Eds.), *Effective treatments for PTSD: Practice guidelines from the International Society for Traumatic Stress Studies* (2nd ed., pp. 83–105). New York: Guilford Press.

Bisson, J. I., Shepherd, J. P., Joy, D., Probert, R., & Newcombe, R. G. (2004). Early cognitive-behavioural therapy for post-traumatic stress symptoms after physical injury: Randomised controlled trial. *British Journal of Psychiatry, 184,* 63–69.

Bonanno, G. A. (2004). Loss, trauma, and human resilience: Have we underestimated the human capacity to thrive after extremely aversive events? *American Psychologist, 59,* 20–28.

Bonanno, G. A., Galea, S., Bucciarelli, A., & Vlahov, D. (2006). Psychological resilience after disaster: New York City in the aftermath of the September 11th terrorist attack. *Psychological Science, 17,* 181–186.

Bonanno, G. A., Ho, S. M. Y., Chan, J. C. K., Kwong, R. S. Y., Cheung, C. K. Y., Wong, C. P. Y., et al. (2008). Psychological resilience and dysfunction among hospitalized survivors of the SARS epidemic in Hong Kong: A latent class approach. *Health Psychology, 27,* 659–667.

Brewin, C. R., Andrews, B., & Valentine, J. D. (2000). Meta-analysis of risk factors for posttraumatic stress disorder in trauma-exposed adults. *Journal of Consulting and Clinical Psychology, 68,* 748–766.

Bryant, R. A. (2004). Acute stress disorder: Course, epidemiology, assessment, and treatment. In B. T. Litz (Ed.), *Early intervention for trauma and traumatic loss* (pp. 15–33). New York: Guilford Press.

Bryant, R. A., Harvey, A. G., Dang, S. T., Sackville, T., & Basten, C. (1998). Treatment of acute stress disorder: A comparison of cognitive-behavioral therapy and supportive counseling. *Journal of Consulting and Clinical Psychology, 66,* 862–866.

Bryant, R. A., Harvey, A. G., Guthrie, R. M., & Moulds, M. L. (2003). Acute psychophysiological arousal and posttraumatic stress disorder: A two-year prospective study. *Journal of Traumatic Stress, 16,* 439–443.

Bryant, R. A., Moulds, M. L., & Nixon, R. V. (2003). Cognitive behavior therapy of acute stress disorder: A four-year follow-up. *Behaviour Research and Therapy, 41,* 489–494.

Bryant, R. A., O'Donnell, M. L., Creamer, M., McFarlane, A. C., Clark, C. R., & Silove, D. (2010). The psychiatric sequelae of traumatic injury. *American Journal of Psychiatry, 167,* 312–320.

Bryant, R. A., Sackville, T., Dang, S. T., Moulds, M., & Guthrie, R. (1999). Treating acute stress disorder: An evaluation of cognitive behavior therapy and supporting counseling techniques. *American Journal of Psychiatry, 156,* 1780–1786.

Brymer, M., Jacobs, A., Layne, C., Pynoos, R., Ruzek, J., Steinberg, A., et al. (2006). *Psychological first aid field operations guide.* Washington, DC: National Child Traumatic Stress Network and National Center for PTSD.

Collogan, L. K., Tuma, F., Dolan-Sewell, R., Borja, S., & Fleischman, A. R. (2004). Ethical issues pertaining to research in the aftermath of disaster. *Journal of Traumatic Stress, 17,* 363–372.

Cozza, S. J., Huleatt, W. J., & James, L. C. (2002). Walter Reed Army Medical Center's mental health response to the Pentagon attack. *Military Medicine, 167*(Suppl. 9), 12–16.

Creamer, M., & O'Donnell, M. (2008). The pros and cons of psychoeducation following-trauma: Too early to judge? *Psychiatry: Interpersonal and Biological Processes, 71,* 319–321.

Defense Security Cooperation Agency. (2009). *Department of Defense fiscal year 2008 report on humanitarian assistance.* Washington, DC: Author.

deRoon-Cassini, T. A., Mancini, A. D., Rusch, M. D., & Bonanno, G. A. (2010). Psychopathology and resilience following traumatic injury: A latent growth mixture model analysis. *Rehabilitation Psychology, 55*, 1–11.

Devilly, G. J., Gist, R., & Cotton, P. (2006). Ready! Fire! Aim! The status of psychological debriefing and therapeutic interventions: In the work place and after disasters. *Review of General Psychology, 10*, 318–345.

Dickstein, B. D., Suvak, M., Litz, B. T., & Adler, A. B. (2010). Heterogeneity in the course of posttraumatic stress disorder: Trajectories of symptomatology. *Journal of Traumatic Stress, 23*, 331–339.

Dodgen, D., LaDue, L. R., & Kaul, R. E. (2002). Coordinating a local response to a national tragedy: Community mental health in Washington, DC after the Pentagon attack. *Military Medicine, 167*(Suppl. 9), 87–89.

Dunning, C. (1988). Intervention strategies for emergency workers. In M. Lystad (Ed.), *Mental health response to mass emergencies* (pp. 284–307). New York: Brunner/Mazel.

Echeburua, E., de Corral, P., Sarasua, B., & Zubizarreta, I. (1996). Treatment of acute posttraumatic stress disorder in rape victims: An experimental study. *Journal of Anxiety Disorders, 10*, 185–199.

Ehlers, A., Clark, D. M., Hackmann, A., McManus, F., Fennell, M., Herbert, C., et al. (2003). A randomized controlled trial of cognitive therapy, a self-help booklet, and repeated assessments as early interventions for posttraumatic stress disorder. *Archives of General Psychiatry, 60*, 1024–1032.

Elsesser, K., Freyth, C., Lohrmann, T., & Sartory, G. (2009). Dysfunctional cognitive appraisal and psychophysiological reactivity in acute stress disorder. *Journal of Anxiety Disorders, 23*, 979–985.

Everly, G. S., Flannery, R. B., & Mitchell, J. T. (2000). Critical incident stress management (CISM): A review of the literature. *Aggression and Violent Behavior, 5*, 23–40.

Federal Emergency Management Agency. (2010a, November 24). *Declared disasters by year or state*. Retrieved November 24, 2010, from *www.fema.gov/news/disaster_totals_annual.fema*.

Federal Emergency Management Agency. (2010b, November 5). *National training and education division*. Retrieved November 24, 2010, from *www.firstrespondertraining.gov*.

Gordon, R. (1987). An operational classification of disease prevention. In J. A. Steinberg & M. M. Silverman (Eds.), *Preventing mental disorders: A research perspective* (pp. 20–26). Rockville, MD: National Institute of Mental Health.

Gray, M. J., Prigerson, H. G., & Litz, B. T. (2004). Conceptual and definitional issues in complicated grief. In B. T. Litz (Ed.), *Early intervention for trauma and traumatic loss* (pp. 65–84). New York: Guilford Press.

Grieger, T. A., & Lyszczarz, J. L. (2002). Psychiatric responses by the U.S. Navy to the Pentagon attack. *Military Medicine, 167*, 24–25.

Halpern, J., & Tramontin, M. (2007). *Disaster mental health: Theory and practice*. Belmont, CA: Thomson Brooks/Cole.

Harvey, A. G., & Bryant, R. A. (2002). Acute stress disorder: A synthesis and critique. *Psychological Bulletin, 128*, 886–902.

Haskett, M., Scott, S., Nears, K., & Grimmett, M. (2008). Lessons from Katrina: Disaster mental health service in the Gulf Coast region. *Professional Psychology: Research and Practice, 39,* 93–99.

Hobbs, M., Mayou, R., Harrison, B., & Worlock, P. (1996). A randomized controlled trial of psychological debriefing for victims of road traffic accidents. *British Medical Journal, 313,* 1438–1439.

Hobfoll, S. E., Watson, P., Bell, C. C., Bryant, R. A., Brymer, M. J., Friedman, M. J., et al. (2007). Five essential elements of immediate and mid-term mass trauma intervention: Empirical evidence. *Psychiatry, 70,* 283–315.

Hoge, C. W., Orman, D. T., & Robichaux, R. J. (2002). Operation Solace: Overview of the mental health intervention following the September 11, 2001 Pentagon attack. *Military Medicine, 167,* 44–47.

Jankosky, C. J. (2008). Mass casualty in an isolated environment: Medical response to a submarine collision. *Military Medicine, 173,* 734–737.

Johnsen, B. H., Eid, J., Løvstad, T., & Michelsen, L. T. (1997). Posttraumatic stress symptoms in nonexposed, victims, spontaneous rescuers after an avalanche. *Journal of Traumatic Stress, 10,* 133–140.

Johnson, S. J., Sherman, M. D., Hoffman, J. S., James, L. C., Johnson, P. L., Lochman, J. E., et al. (2007, February). *The psychological needs of U.S. military service members and their families: A preliminary report.* Washington, DC: APA Presidential Task Force on Military Deployment Services for Youth, Families and Service Members.

Joyce, N. (2006). Civilian-military coordination in the emergency response in Indonesia. *Military Medicine, 171,* 66–70.

Keen, P. K. (2010, March 15). *As humanitarian assistance transitions, so does U.S. military.* Message posted to *www.dodlive.mil/index.php/2010/03/as-humanitarian-assistance-transitions-so-does-u-s-military.*

Keen, P. K., Vieira Neto, F. P., Nolan, C. W., Kimmey, J. L., & Althouse, J. (2010, May–June). Relationships matter: Humanitarian assistance and disaster relief in Haiti. *Military Review.* Retrieved November 23, 2010, from *usacac.army.mil/cac2/call/docs/11-23/ch_16.asp.*

Keller, R. T., & Bobo, W. V. (2004). Handling human remains: Exposure may result in severe psychological responses among rescue workers. *Psychiatric Annals, 34,* 635–640.

Kilpatrick, D. G., Cougle, J. R., & Resnick, H. S. (2008). Reports of the death of psychoeducation as a preventative treatment for posttraumatic psychological distress are exaggerated. *Psychiatry: Interpersonal and Biological Processes, 71,* 322–328.

Krupnick, J. L., & Green, B. L. (2008). Psychoeducation to prevent PTSD: A paucity of evidence. *Psychiatry, 71,* 329–331.

Litz, B. T. (2008). Early intervention for trauma: Where are we and where do we need to go? A commentary. *Journal of Traumatic Stress, 21,* 503–506.

Litz, B. T., & Gray, M. J. (2004). Early intervention for trauma in adults: A framework for first aid and secondary prevention. In B. T. Litz (Ed.), *Early intervention for trauma and traumatic loss* (pp. 87–111). New York: Guilford Press.

Mancuso, J. D., Price, E. O., & West, D. F. (2008). The emerging role of preventive medicine in health diplomacy after the 2005 earthquake in Pakistan. *Military Medicine, 173,* 113–118.

McGuiness, K. M. (2006). The USNS *Mercy* and the changing landscape of humanitarian and disaster response. *Military Medicine, 171,* 48–52.

McNally, R. J., Bryant, R. A., & Ehlers, A. (2003). Does early psychological intervention promote recovery from posttraumatic stress? *Psychological Science in the Public Interest, 4,* 45–79.

Merchant, R. M., Leigh, J. E., & Lurie, N. (2010). Health care volunteers and disaster response: First, be prepared. *New England Journal of Medicine, 362,* 872–873.

Miller, W. R., & Rollnick, S. (2002). *Motivational interviewing: Preparing people for change* (2nd ed.). New York: Guilford Press.

Mitchell, J. T. (1983). When disaster strikes . . . The critical incident stress debriefing. *Journal of Emergency Medical Services, 8,* 36–39.

Mitchell, J. T. (2004). A response to the Devilly and Cotton article, "Psychological debriefing and the workplace. . . . " *Australian Psychologist, 39,* 24–28.

Mitchell, J. T., & Everly, G. S. (1995). *Critical incident stress debriefing: An operations manual for the prevention of traumatic stress among emergency services and disaster workers.* Ellicott City, MD: Chevron.

Nash, W. P. (2010, May). *Peritraumatic Behavior Questionnaire (PBQ): Initial validation of a new tool to recognize orange zone stress injuries in theater.* Paper presented at the U.S. Marine Corps Combat and Operational Stress Control Conference, San Diego, CA.

Nash, W. P., & Baker, D. G. (2007). Competing and complementary models of combat stress injury. In C. R. Figley & W. P. Nash (Eds.), *Combat stress injuries: Theory, research, and management* (pp. 65–96). New York: Routledge.

Nash, W. P., Westphal, R., Watson, P., & Litz, B. T. (2010). *Combat and operational stress first aid training manual.* Washington, DC: U.S. Navy, Bureau of Medicine and Surgery.

National Child Traumatic Stress Network. (2010, November 8). *Training and education.* Retrieved November 24, 2010, from *www.nctsn.org/nccts/nav.do?pid=ctr_train.*

National Organization for Victim Assistance. (1987). *The National Organization for Victim Assistance debriefing.* Washington, DC: Author.

National Organization for Victim Assistance. (n.d.). *Crisis response training.* Retrieved November 24, 2010, from *www.trynova.org/crt/training.*

North Carolina Disaster Response Network. (2010). *North Carolina Disaster Response Network (NC DRN) training.* Retrieved November 24, 2010, from *cphp.sph.unc.edu/training/nc_drn.*

Orcutt, H. K., Erickson, D. J., & Wolfe, J. (2004). The course of PTSD symptoms among Gulf War veterans: A growth mixture modeling approach. *Journal of Traumatic Stress, 17,* 195–202.

Orner, R. J., Kent, A. T., Pfefferbaum, B. J., Raphael, B., & Watson, P. J. (2006). The context of providing immediate postevent intervention. In E. C. Ritchie, P. J. Watson, & M. J. Friedman (Eds.), *Interventions following mass violence and disasters: Strategies for mental health practice* (pp. 121–133). New York: Guilford Press.

Ozer, E. J., Best, S. R., Lipsey, T. L., & Weiss, D. S. (2003). Predictors of posttraumatic stress disorder and symptoms in adults: A meta-analysis. *Psychological Bulletin, 129,* 52–73.

Patrick, S. (2009). Impact of the Department of Defense initiatives on humanitarian assistance. *Prehospital and Disaster Medicine, 24,* 238–243.

Peterson, A., Nicolas, M., McGraw, K., Englert, D., & Blackman, L. (2002). Psychological intervention with mortuary workers after the September 11 attack: The Dover behavioral health consultant model. *Military Medicine, 167*(Suppl. 9), 83–86.

Pierre, A., Minn, P., Sterlin, C., Annoual, P. C., Jaimes, A., Raphaël, F., et al. (2010). Culture and mental health in Haiti: A literature review. *Santé Mentale en Haïti, 1,* 13–42.

Ponniah, K., & Hollon, S. D. (2009). Empirically supported psychological treatments for adult acute stress disorder and posttraumatic stress disorder: A review. *Depression and Anxiety, 26,* 1086–1109.

Reeves, J. J. (2002). Perspectives on disaster mental health intervention from the USNS *Comfort. Military Medicine, 167*(Suppl.), 90–92.

Reyes, G., & Elhai, J. (2004). Psychosocial interventions in the early phases of disasters. *Psychotherapy: Theory, Research, Practice, Training, 41,* 399–411.s

Roberts, N. P., Kitchiner, N. J., Kenardy, J., & Bisson, J. I. (2009). Systematic review and meta-analysis of multiple-session early interventions following traumatic events. *American Journal of Psychiatry, 166,* 293–301.

Robinson, R. (2004). Counterbalancing misrepresentations of critical incident stress debriefing and critical incident stress management. *Australian Psychologist, 39,* 29–34.

Rose, S., Bisson, J., Churchill, R., & Wessely, S. (2002). Psychological debriefing for preventing post traumatic stress disorder (PTSD). *Cochrane Database of Systematic Reviews, 2,* CD000560.

Rosenstein, D. L. (2004). Decision-making capacity and disaster research. *Journal of Traumatic Stress, 17,* 373–381.

Ruzek, J. I., Brymer, M. J., Jacobs, A. K., Layne, C. M., Vernberg, E. M., & Watson, P. J. (2007). Psychological first aid. *Journal of Mental Health Counseling, 29,* 17–49.

Scholes, C., Turpin, G., & Mason, S. (2007). A randomised controlled trial to assess the effectiveness of providing self-help information to people with symptoms of acute stress disorder following a traumatic injury. *Behaviour Research and Therapy, 45,* 2527–2536.

Schwerin, M. J., Kennedy, K., & Wardlaw, M. (2002). Counseling support within the Navy Mass Casualty Assistance Team post-September 11. *Military Medicine, 167,* 76–78.

Shalev, A. Y. (2006). Interventions for traumatic stress: Theoretical basis. In E. C. Ritchie, P. J. Watson, & M. J. Friedman (Eds.), *Interventions following mass violence and disasters: Strategies for mental health practice* (pp. 103–120). New York: Guilford Press.

Southwick, S., Friedman, M., & Krystal, J. (2008). Does psychoeducation help prevent post-traumatic psychological stress disorder? In reply. *Psychiatry, 71,* 303–307.

Turpin, G., Downs, M., & Mason, S. (2005). Effectiveness of providing self-help information following acute traumatic injury: Randomised controlled trial. *British Journal of Psychiatry, 187,* 76–82.

U.S. Department of Defense. (2005, November 28). *Military support for stability, security, transition, and reconstruction (SSTR) operations.* Retrieved November 29, 2010, from *www.fas.org/irp/doddir/dod/d3000_05.pdf.*

U.S. Department of the Navy. (2000). *Combat stress* (Marine Corps Reference Publication 6-11C). Washington, DC: Author.

United States Southern Command. (2010, May 25). *Narrative history of Operation Unified Response.* Retrieved March 15, 2012, from *www.southcom. mil/newsroom/Pages/Operation-Unified-Response-Support-to-Haiti-Earthquake-Relief-2010.aspx.*

University of Rochester Medical Center. (n.d.). *Finger Lakes Regional Resource Center: Training.* Retrieved March 14, 2012, from *www.urmc.rochester.edu/ flrrc/training.cfm.*

University of South Dakota. (2010). *DMHI home.* Retrieved November 24, 2010, from *www.usd.edu/arts-and-sciences/psychology/disaster-mental-health-institute/index.cfm.*

USAID Office of Military Affairs. (2010, April 27). *Civilian-Military Operations Guide.* Retrieved March 14, 2012, from *pdf. usaid. gov/pdf_docs/PNADS. 180. pdf*

van Emmerik, A. A. P., Kamphuis, J. H., Hulsbosch, A. M., & Emmelkamp, P. M. G. (2002). Single session debriefing after psychological trauma: A meta-analysis. *The Lancet, 360,* 766–771.

Vernberg, E. M., Steinberg, A. M., Jacobs, A. K., Brymer, M. J., Watson, P. J., Osofsky, J. D., et al. (2008). Innovation in disaster mental health: Psychological first aid. *Professional Psychology: Research and Practice, 39,* 381–388.

Warner, S. (2010, January 22). Hospital ship *Comfort* to support Operation Unified Response Haiti. *Navy and Marine Corp Medical News,* pp. 1, 3. Retrieved November 24, 2010, from *www.dtic.mil/cgi-bin/GetTRDoc?AD=ADA5175 91&Location=U2&doc=GetTRDoc.pdf.*

Watson, P., Nash, W. P., Westphal, R., & Litz, B. T. (2010, November). *Combat and operational stress first aid (COSFA).* Workshop presented at the annual convention of the International Society for Traumatic Stress Studies, Montreal, Quebec.

Wessells, M. G. (2009). Do no harm: Toward contextually appropriate psychosocial support in international emergencies. *American Psychologist, 64,* 842–854.

Wessely, S., Bryant, R. A., Greenberg, N., Earnshaw, M., Sharpley, J., & Hughes, J. H. (2008). Does psychoeducation help prevent post traumatic psychological distress? *Psychiatry: Interpersonal and Biological Processes, 71,* 287–302.

Wickramage, K. (2006). Sri Lanka's post-tsunami psychosocial playground: Lessons for future psychosocial programming and interventions following disasters. *Intervention, 4,* 163–168.

Wright, K. M., Cabrera, O. A., Bliese, P. D., Adler, A. B., Hoge, C. W., & Castro,

C. A. (2009). Stigma and barriers to care in soldiers postcombat. *Psychological Services, 6,* 108–116.

Yahav, R., & Cohen, M. (2007). Symptoms of acute stress in Jewish and Arab Israeli citizens during the second Lebanon War. *Social Psychiatry and Psychiatric Epidemiology, 42,* 830–836.

Young, B. H., Ruzek, J. I., Wong, M., Salzer, M. S., & Naturale, A. J. (2006). Disaster mental health training: Guidelines, considerations, and recommendations. In E. C. Ritchie, P. J. Watson, & M. J. Friedman (Eds.), *Interventions following mass violence and disasters: Strategies for mental health practice* (pp. 54–79). New York: Guilford Press.

CHAPTER 8

Neuropsychological Practice in the Military

Louis M. French
Victoria Anderson-Barnes
Laurie M. Ryan
Thomas M. Zazeckis
Sally Harvey

Military neuropsychology's roots date back to World War I when early assessment and neurological rehabilitative efforts were first undertaken as a result of the many head injuries sustained by service members during combat (Boake, 1989). Throughout World Wars I and II, several neuropsychological assessment tools were developed and implemented into routine practice within the military (Driskell & Olmstead, 1989). Since that time, military neuropsychology has grown and neuropsychological assessment practices continue to play a key role in operational readiness and maintenance of peak performance of military members (for a history of military neuropsychology, see Kennedy, Boake, & Moore, 2010; see also Chapter 1, this volume).

In today's conflicts in Iraq and Afghanistan, neuropsychologists are heavily involved in the identification, assessment, and treatment of neuropsychological disorders that arise as a result of deployment and combat. Head and neck injuries continue to be prevalent in the present-day conflicts, with traumatic brain injury (TBI) being described as the signature injury of these conflicts (McCrea et al., 2008). Additionally, postconcussive symptoms and posttraumatic stress symptoms frequently result in the military population following combat exposure (McCrea et al., 2008). Consequently, the need for military neuropsychologists is ever present. This chapter provides an overview of this specialized field, with brief discussions of requisite training; common areas of clinical practice; fitness-for-duty evaluations; symptom validity and military neuropsychological evaluations; the role of neuropsychology in assessing and treating brain injury, posttraumatic stress disorder (PTSD), attention-deficit/hyperactivity disorder (ADHD), and learning disorders (LD); aerospace neuropsychology; and various operational applications.

NEUROPSYCHOLOGY TRAINING IN THE MILITARY

Practicing as an active-duty neuropsychologist requires specialty training, and competitive fellowships in neuropsychology are provided through the U.S. Army, Navy, and Air Force. The Army trains active-duty neuropsychologists at Walter Reed National Military Medical Center in Bethesda, Maryland (MRNMMC-B), as well as at Tripler Army Medical Center in Honolulu, Hawaii. The Navy and Air Force generally contract with accredited universities (e.g., University of Virginia and University of California at San Diego) for neuropsychology fellowships, although the Walter Reed and Tripler fellowships are open to all service branches. Additionally, Brooke Army Medical Center in San Antonio, Texas, trains civilian neuropsychology fellows in a military setting, thereby promoting the competencies important for civilians working in a U.S. Department of Defense (DoD) or Department of Veterans Affairs setting (Reger, Etherage, Reger & Gahm, 2008).

The fellowship curriculum, regardless of program location or supervisor, places a strong emphasis on the development of an extensive knowledge base in brain–behavior relationships as well as specific skill sets in evaluation, diagnosis, consultation, and research. Military neuropsychology fellows training at either military or civilian facilities have the opportunity to study under experienced neuropsychologists and receive exposure to a wide variety of conditions affecting cerebral function, such as concussion/TBI, dementia, brain tumors, and epilepsy. The goal of this training is to prepare clinicians capable of providing the best neuropsychological services to active-duty members, retirees, and their families. Military neuropsychologists and civilian neuropsychologists working in a military setting must be prepared to assess the gamut of disorders and populations, make viable and informed recommendations regarding fitness for duty, rehabilitation, and treatment, and engage in state-of-the-art research activities.

MILITARY CLINICAL PRACTICE
IN NEUROPSYCHOLOGY

Military neuropsychology mirrors, in many respects, that of civilian practice. Within military medical treatment settings, a military neuropsychologist can expect to evaluate individuals experiencing the full range of neurocognitive disorders across the lifespan, to include concussion/TBI, learning disorders, toxic exposure, stroke, dementia, epilepsy, neoplasms, central nervous system infections, and other medical conditions, given that military neuropsychologists see not only active-duty personnel but also retired service members and dependents.

Within the active-duty population, referrals are often made following neurological diagnosis or other critical medical illnesses as well as for evaluation of possible learning or attentional problems or cognitive decline in older service members in relation to fitness-for-duty decisions. In addition, there are several specific situations requiring the administration of a neuropsychological assessment, to include disposition of individuals with special jobs demanding peak cognitive performance (e.g., individuals who handle explosives or have flight status, submarine duty, diving duty, or parachute duty). Generally, an acquired neurological condition precludes continued involvement in these professions, although some of these occupations are willing to consider waivers, on a case-by-case basis, in the event that neuropsychological assessment indicates appropriate neurocognitive functioning.

Although the neuropsychological evaluation practices in all military settings adhere to the standards of the field, there are differing medical regulations specific to each service branch in relation to various jobs that must be taken into consideration when an evaluation is completed and recommendations are made. Interested readers are encouraged to review each service's regulation (U.S. Department of the Air Force, 2001; U.S. Department of the Army, 2007; U.S. Department of the Navy, 1996; U.S. Department of Homeland Security, 2004).

Military neuropsychological assessment practices are slightly different from that of civilian practice in the areas of baseline assessment data and measures for special populations (i.e., aviation). One distinct advantage of military neuropsychology is the availability of premorbid or baseline assessment data for most military members. Given that premorbid functioning guides determinations of the extent of cognitive impairment, progress in rehabilitation, prognosis, and ultimate fitness for duty, this is a fundamental component of the military neuropsychological evaluation. In the case of enlisted personnel, military neuropsychologists are fortunate to have a reliable indicator of premorbid general ability in the form of the

Armed Services Vocational Aptitude Battery, or ASVAB (Welsh, Kucin-kas, & Curran, 1990; Kennedy, Kupke, & Smith, 2000). Orme, Ree, and Rioux (2001) also report good reliability when estimating premorbid ability using the Air Force Officer Qualifying Test (AFOQT). In addition to this information, military neuropsychologists have available to them all individual service records, which include documentation of military educational attainment and job performance. Neuropsychologists often rely on these various soruces of information to guide their interpretations of neuropsychological test findings.

Moreover, since 2008, the military has required that all service members receive a predeployment neuropsychological assessment, typically the Automated Neuropsychological Assessment Metrics (ANAM; Ivins, Kane, & Schwab, 2009). The ANAM was originally developed in response to a DoD initiative to examine the effects of pharmaceutical agents on cognitive performance (Reeves et al., 2006; Reeves, Winter, Bleiberg, & Kane, 2007), but has since been used in a variety of settings, including fitness for duty, military operational medicine, and aerospace medicine (Ivins et al., 2009; Reeves et al., 2007). The ANAM is a computer-based neuropsychological instrument that assesses attention, concentration, reaction time, memory, processing speed, and decision making (Vista Life Sciences, 2011). The ANAM may prove to be a useful tool that will assist military neuropsychologists to appropriately determine a service member's level of premorbid ability (Kelly, Mulligan, & Monahan, 2010).

Another divergence from traditional neuropsychological practice is the development of neuropsychological tests for use in specific military populations. For example, continuous performance tasks are commonly used in the assessment of attentional difficulties to include components of vigilance, discrimination, and impulsivity. To meet the needs of the military, the Aeromedical Vigilance Test was developed and normed on Navy pilots at the Naval Operational Medicine Institute (Almond, Harris, & Almond, 2005).

FITNESS-FOR-DUTY EVALUATIONS

Military neuropsychologists are asked to assess fitness for duty as a result of multiple disorders, especially brain disorders. Some neurological conditions, such as epilepsy, are grounds for automatic disqualification from military service, but others allow for a careful assessment of impairment, level of functioning, and prognosis given rehabilitation. Today's neuropsychologists are evaluating many war-related neurological injuries, including both penetrating head wounds and neurological blast injuries, which precipitate involvement of military neuropsychologists as well as the U.S. Department of Veterans Affairs and other rehabilitation neuropsychologists.

The military healthcare system has a long-established and methodical system for determining whether a service member is fit for duty (Kelly et al., 2010). Chapter 2 (this volume) discusses fitness-for-duty evaluations in greater detail, but a summary is provided here. According to Kelly et al. (2010), "DoD policy stipulates that a service member will be found unfit for duty if he or she has a disease or injury that prevents performance of the duties of his or her office, grade, rank, or rating." Kelly and colleagues (2010) go on to describe the multistep process that the DoD utilizes when determining fitness for duty. In summary, if a service member is at risk because of a medical or psychiatric condition, the command must first be informed and, subsequently, the process for determining fitness for duty is initiated. The first step in the process is to conduct a physical profile serial report (required by the Air Force and Army) or limited-duty board (required by the Navy and Marine Corps), outlining any duty limitations.

The next step is referred to as the Medical Evaluation Board (MEB). The MEB determines the severity of the injury or illness and whether the condition would interfere with the service member's ability to perform in his or her military occupation specialty (MOS, or rate). The neuropsychologist is heavily involved in the MEB process, and it is expected that a comprehensive neuropsychological evaluation will be performed. This evaluation, while not universal across all neuropsychologists, will likely include a description of the primary condition, including the history of the injury or illness; general medical and psychiatric history; social history; family history; any lab or imaging reports; medications; behavioral observations; a listing of the neuropsychological tests that were administered as well as the results; and a diagnostic conclusion and recommendations (Kelly et al., 2010).

If it is determined from the MEB that the necessary retention standards are not being met by the service member in question, the case is then passed on to the Physical Evaluation Board (PEB)—the final step in this process. The PEB consists of an informal evaluation followed by a formal evaluation. The informal PEB thoroughly reviews the documentation derived from the first two steps as well as any notes from the command and decides whether the service member is fit for duty. Those found unfit will be assigned a disability rating percentage and will have the opportunity to present supplemental information to the formal PEB on his or her status.

For many health conditions, the neuropsychological evaluation ultimately plays a key role in determining whether a service member is fit for duty. Consequently, the military neuropsychologist must have a thorough understanding of the issues surrounding fitness-for-duty evaluations and take the time to develop a comprehensive neuropsychological report.

SYMPTOM VALIDITY AND MILITARY NEUROPSYCHOLOGICAL EVALUATIONS

In addition to contributing to fitness-for-duty evaluations, the military neuropsychologist must also assess for "noncredible neuropsychological presentation," or effort. In order to ensure that the service member or veteran's neuropsychological test results are valid and, more importantly, to arrive at an accurate diagnosis, formal measures of effort are necessary.

Just as civilian neuropsychologists work with patients who may have motivation to simulate or dissimulate symptoms, military neuropsychologists must also evaluate effort of service members when conducting a neuropsychological evaluation. This should include an assessment of the individual's motivation for not only participation in the assessment but also involvement in rehabilitation and continued military retention. Under the Uniform Code of Military Justice, Article 115, any service member who attempts to feign an illness—or malinger—will be subject to court-martial punishment (Greiffenstein, 2010). While effort testing can only determine whether a test result is likely valid, and cannot determine the basis of an invalid performance, measuring effort is essential to the neuropsychologist's role.

Measurement of effort is standard neuropsychological practice (Bush et al., 2005). However, the extent to which the military or veteran population exaggerates symptoms is largely unknown, although rates in the civilian population are high. In one civilian study (Mittenberg, Patton, Canyock, & Condit, 2002), 29% of personal injury, 30% of disability claims, and 19% of criminal cases involved probable malingering. One study (Armistead-Jehle, 2010) using the Medical Symptom Validity Test (MSVT) in a veteran population showed 58% of the sample scoring below the MSVT cut scores. Those who were service connected and previously diagnosed with a depressive condition failed the measure at a higher rate than those who were not.

Service members undergoing neuropsychological evaluation may, wittingly or not, provide distorted or erroneous responses for any number of reasons, and there are indirect social and emotional rewards that can make the denial, exaggeration, or actual malingering of impairment and symptoms an attractive strategy. Regardless of the reason behind the distorted neuropsychological performance, the test data are not a valid measure of the individual's abilities. As noted in the American Academy of Clinical Neuropsychology Consensus Conference Statement on the Neuropsychological Assessment of Effort, Response Bias, and Malingering (Heilbronner et al., 2010), invalid neuropsychological test performance precludes the neuropsychologist from using those data as a basis for (1) attribution of the cause of symptoms and impairment (e.g., accident, injury), (2) the nature and extent of deficits and disability, and (3) guiding treatment or evaluating treatment effectiveness. Military neuropsychological evaluations must include both an assessment of the service member's motivation or effort on testing and an assessment of the validity of reported symptoms. A brief overview of symptom validity follows.

Symptom distortion can be cognitive, somatic, and/or psychological, and individuals may present noncredible symptoms in any or all of these domains. In the cognitive domain, methods for evaluating effort include stand-alone cognitive effort tests as well as embedded validity indicators within standard neuropsychological measures. The use of multiple methods to assess effort, including both stand-alone and embedded measures, is recommended (Heilbronner et al., 2010). Effort is not a static phenomenon. Effort is dynamic and may vary throughout the testing session and should be evaluated repeatedly during testing (Boone, 2009; Heilbronner et al., 2010). When poor effort is found at any point during an evaluation, all test performances and obtained test scores may underestimate the individual's actual abilities, even those obtained during apparent periods of adequate effort (Heilbronner et al., 2010).

In the somatic domain, symptoms of questionable validity may present as exaggerated or atypical symptom reports on general psychological measures, including personality measures, or on specialized rating scales such as pain measures. Many of these questionnaires include indices of validity. Somatic symptom exaggeration may also present as poor performance on measures of sensory perception, motor functioning, and strength (Greiffenstein, 2007; Greiffenstein, Fox, & Lees-Haley, 2007; Heilbronner et al., 2010).

Finally, in the psychological domain, symptoms of psychopathology may be exaggerated or fabricated. Symptoms reported during an interview on psychological measures or observed during evaluation should be compared with known symptomatology of the disorder in question for consistency (Heilbronner et al., 2010).

TRAUMATIC BRAIN INJURY AND POSTTRAUMATIC STRESS DISORDER

Traumatic Brain Injury

TBI is the principal cause of death and disability in active young adults today. Every 21 seconds, a person in the United States sustains a TBI; 5.3 million Americans live with disability as a result of brain injury, with an estimated cost to society of more than $48.3 billion annually (Lewin, 1992; Centers for Disease Control, 1999). The overall incidence of TBI-related hospitalization in the active-duty Army increased 105% from FY2000 to FY2006, and there was a 60-fold increase in the hospitalization rate for

TBIs attributed to weapons, suggesting that Operation Enduring Freedom and Operation Iraqi Freedom (OEF/OIF) may have had a substantial impact on the incidence of TBI-related hospitalization in the active-duty U.S. Army. However, during OEF/OIF, the Army's hospitalization rates for moderate and severe TBIs were actually lower than civilian rates. The Army's hospitalization rate for concussion/mild TBIs was higher than civilian rates (Ivins, 2010).

This chapter is not intended as a detailed overview of the pathophysiology or neuropsychology of TBI, and the interested reader can consult the websites and texts suggested at the end of the chapter for further information. TBI can result in a variety of cognitive, emotional, behavioral, and physical sequelae depending on the severity of the injury and location of the cerebral damage. The cognitive deficits associated with TBI often include problems with attention and concentration, speed of information processing, executive functioning (e.g., problem solving, mental flexibility, initiation, the ability to self-monitor), memory, and language. Possible emotional and behavioral problems include disinhibition, apathy, irritability, mood lability, depression, and anxiety. The physical symptoms after TBI may include dizziness, balance problems, sleep changes, vision changes, hearing changes, and headache. These symptoms demand thorough evaluation to monitor change and to ultimately make a fitness for duty decision. Unfortunately, even small decrements in abilities such as attention or processing speed deficits can have significant implications for the fighting force and its combat effectiveness during that recovery period. Fortunately, the majority of TBIs that occur both in civilian life and in the military, even during combat operations, are mild. These mild brain injuries (better known as concussions), are typically characterized by time-limited symptoms that improve and resolve over days or weeks. For some individuals (less than 5% in civilian populations), these symptoms may persist and evolve into a postconcussive syndrome (Iverson, 2005; Iverson, Zasler, & Lange, 2006).

Combat-Related TBI

The current conflicts in Iraq and Afghanistan have brought both increased training operations and increased exposure to battlefield conditions for our armed forces. More than 213,000 troops have been diagnosed with having suffered a brain injury, the vast majority of them mild (77%; Defense and Veterans Brain Injury Center, 2011). Additionally, following the trend in American warfare over the last 150 years, there have been ever increasing numbers of injuries related to explosion rather than gunshot wounds (Owens et al., 2008). This has also resulted in greater numbers of closed brain injuries relative to penetrating ones. Blast injury may have some characteristics that are different from other mechanisms, while other aspects do not appear to be different.

With regard to cognition, severity of injury is more predictive of neuropsychological functioning than is mechanism of injury. Analysis of neuropsychological test measures suggest that there are no differences in patterns of cognitive test performance in those who suffered TBI related to blast versus other mechanisms (Belanger, Kretzmer, Yoash-Gantz, Pickett, & Tupler, 2009). One recent study in a deployed setting (Luethcke, Bryan, Morrow, & Isler, 2011) evaluated concussive, psychological, and cognitive symptoms in military personnel and civilian contractors diagnosed with concussion. The results suggested that there are few differences in concussive symptoms, psychological symptoms, or neurocognitive performance between blast and nonblast mild TBIs, although clinically significant impairment in cognitive reaction time was measured for both blast and nonblast groups. A similar finding was observed in a sample of those with concussion being treated in a military hospital or a VA hospital (Belanger et al., 2011). In that study, mechanism of injury did not account for a significant amount of variance in postconcussion symptom reporting overall, nor did severity of mild TBI (i.e., brief loss of consciousness vs. an alteration of consciousness). Hearing difficulty was the only symptom that significantly varied between groups, with the blast-injured group reporting more severe difficulty with hearing.

Some differences in those injured through blast have been noted, however. These include high rates of sensory impairment (Lew, Jerger, Guillory, & Henry, 2007), pain issues (Lew et al., 2009; Smith, 2011), and polytrauma (Sayer et al., 2008; Smith, 2011). These differences have important rehabilitation considerations. In a civilian population, minimal extracranial injuries and low pain have been shown to predict better outcomes for return to work after mild TBI (Stulemeijer et al., 2006). Paradoxically, however, in one sample at Walter Reed Army Medical Center (WRAMC), where, intuitively, greater comorbid physical injuries would be expected to be associated with greater symptom burden, self-reported stress and postconcussive symptom burden significantly decreased as the severity of bodily injuries increased (French et al., 2012).

It can be expected that the vast majority of service members who suffer concussion on the battlefield will recover fully (Terrio et al., 2009). Nonetheless, even short-term symptoms may have operational consequences. Concerns over this, coupled with increased awareness and concerns of the potential morbidity associated with TBI, have increased military efforts in the assessment and evaluation of concussion both in garrison and on the battlefield. One tool, the Military Acute Concussion Evaluation (MACE; French, McCrea, & Baggett, 2008) was developed by the Defense and Veterans Brain Injury Center to better diagnose and characterize concussion on the battlefield (see Figure 8.1). The MACE has both a history and an evaluation component. The history component can confirm the diagnosis of concussion after establishing that a trauma has occurred, and that during the course of this traumatic event the service member experienced an alteration or loss of consciousness. The evaluation component, designed to be easily used by medics and corpsmen, can be administered within 5 minutes. It utilizes the Standardized Assessment of Concussion (SAC) to preliminarily document neurocognitive deficits in four cognitive domains: orientation, immediate memory, concentration, and delayed recall (McCrea et al., 2003). In sports concussion, the SAC has been shown to have validity in detecting and characterizing mental status abnormalities resulting from concussion (Barr & McCrea, 2001; McCrea, Kelly, Kluge, Ackley, & Randolph, 1997).

The MACE has limitations, however. One recent study using the MACE in a deployed population (Coldren, Kelly, Parish, Dretsch, & Russell, 2010) suggests that it lacks sufficient specificity and sensitivity to be useful when it is administered more than 12 hours after an injury event. The authors concluded that greater reliance should be placed on the history portion than the score when it is administered post acutely.

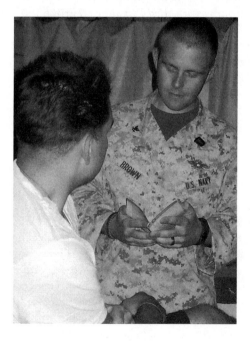

FIGURE 8.1. A Navy corpsman administers the MACE to a Marine injured by an IED. Photo courtesy of Carrie H. Kennedy.

Current policy guidance for in-theater concussion reporting and management is detailed in DTM 09-033, "Policy Guidance for Management of Concussion/Mild Traumatic Brain Injury in the Deployed Setting," compiled by Joint Mental Health Advisory Team 7 (2011). This document outlines event-driven protocols for reporting concussive events and the assessment and management of those exposed. Highlights include mandatory medical evaluation and downtime for those exposed to concussive events. The full text of the document can be found at *www.dtic.mil/whs/directives/ corres/pdf/DTM-09-033_placeholder.pdf* (note that DoD PKI certificate is required for access).

Another deployment-related health concern that has garnered significant attention is PTSD (see Figure 8.2). In the combat environment, exposure to potentially emotionally traumatic experiences is commonplace (Hoge et al., 2004). In a large population-based screening study of service members after deployment, the prevalence of reporting a mental health problem was 19.1% after returning from Iraq, 11.3% after returning from Afghanistan, and 8.5% after returning from other locations. Mental

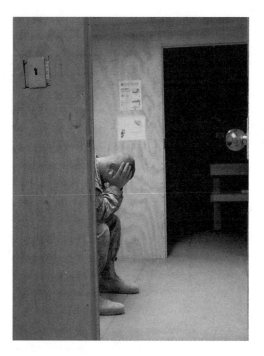

FIGURE 8.2. The interplay between blast concussion and combat stress symptoms is complicated. This soldier in Afghanistan is experiencing a severe headache from his very recent concussion. Photo courtesy of Keith Stuessi.

health problems were significantly associated with combat experiences, mental health care referral and utilization, and attrition from military service. About 35% of Iraq War veterans accessed mental health services in the year after returning home (Hoge, Auchterlonie, & Milliken, 2006). A more recent large study (Sandweiss et al., 2011) showed an 8.1% rate for PTSD at follow-up. The odds of screening positive for PTSD symptoms were more than 2.5 times greater for those with a baseline mental health disorder and 16% greater for every 3-unit increase in the Injury Severity Score, suggesting that baseline psychiatric status and deployment-related physical injuries were associated with screening positive for postdeployment PTSD.

Whether PTSD results in measurable cognitive deficits is not a resolved question. While some researchers have reported that patients with PTSD perform more poorly on neuropsychological tests than healthy adults (Buckley, Blanchard, & Neill, 2000; Jelinek et al., 2006; Jenkins, Langlais, Delis, & Cohen, 2000), especially on tests of verbal learning and memory (Bremner et al., 1993, 1995; Sutker, Allain, Johnson, & Butters, 1992; Vasterling, Brailey, Constans, & Sutker, 1998; Yehuda et al., 1995), other researchers have not found neurocognitive decrements associated with PTSD (Crowell, Kieffer, Siders, & Vanderploeg, 2002; Stein, Hanna, Vaerum, & Koverola, 1999; Twamley, Hami, & Stein, 2004). In a study of OIF/OEF veterans with comorbid mild TBI and PTSD, significant differences in processing speed and executive functioning were found on the basis of presence of comorbid PTSD. Those having comorbid PTSD and mild TBI scored significantly poorer than the mild TBI-only group (Nelson, Yoash-Gantz, Pickett, & Campbell, 2009). By contrast, Brenner et al. (2010) did not find any differences between those with and without PTSD and concurrent mild TBI in a military population on the Paced Auditory Serial Addition Test.

In-Theater Screening

The Mental Health Advisory Team 7, which issued its report in early 2011, described that prior to the implementation of DTM 09-033, rates of evaluation for concussion postincident were generally low, although they were expected to increase significantly with the implementation of the policy (Joint Mental Health Advisory Team 7, 2011). They did report value in neurocognitive testing postinjury, specifically the ANAM, as simple reaction time scores increased on average 150 msec (250–400 msec) from baseline to first evaluation postinjury. These scores normalized over serial evaluations in the course of several days. This observation is consistent with other recent work in theater (Luethcke et al., 2011) that suggests that ANAM reaction scores are affected by concussion and ANAM accuracy is related to duration of the associated loss of consciousness.

The ANAM, a library of computer-based cognitive assessment measures, was developed by the DoD. The ANAM4 TBI Battery was developed at the University of Oklahoma for the purposes of military concussion assessment. Since 2008, that instrument has been used for a predeployment baseline measure of cognition for comparison purposes as needed postinjury or postdeployment, although the latter use is infrequently done and may have limited clinical value (Ivins et al., 2009). While predeployment ANAM is required for all service members, other automated test measures may be used in some circumstances. The special operations community frequently uses the Immediate Post Concussion Assessment and Cognition tool (ImPACT), among other measures, to aid in return-to-duty decisions (Hettich, Whitfield, Kratz, & Frament, 2010).

With the ANAM, although performance is measured against a normative sample or an individual's own baseline, some cautions must be exercised on its interpretation. While the interpretive guidelines suggest that having two or more tests deviate significantly from baseline is "a serious cause for concern," patient characteristics and the environment must be considered in the interpretation. Reduced sleep/rest, distraction, dehydration, and mood state are among the factors that may influence performance. The test must be administered in the context of clinical judgment. The sleep and mood scales on the test, as well as a clinical interview, should be used in the decision-making process. Active engagement in the task is also crucial for accurate measure. Distraction, a conscious attempt to look bad, or other factors will also influence scores and the value of the testing.

There is no prescribed cognitive assessment instrument. Automated tests are used, as are pencil-and-paper tests, including the Repeatable Battery for the Assessment of Neuropsychological Status, tests drawn from the Wechsler Scales of Intelligence or Memory, the Trailmaking Test, or other measures. According to DTM 09-033, more comprehensive evaluations of cognition may be required in the case of multiple concussions over a deployment. When a comprehensive evaluation is required, assessments of attention, memory, processing speed, executive functioning, social pragmatics, and effort should all be administered. Input from physical and occupational therapy should also be considered when available.

Combat TBI Screening and Evaluation

The WRNMMC-B, which represents the combined facilities and staff of the former National Naval Medical Center and the WRAMC, is at the forefront in the treatment of service members injured in theater in recent conflicts, that is, OEF, OIF, and Operation New Dawn. Many of these service members have sustained injuries resulting from explosive devices. After treatment in the field and at combat support hospitals, the majority of the wounded needing further care are transported to Landstuhl Regional Medical Center in Germany and later transferred to the national capital area. There they are further assessed, treated, and transferred to other military and Veterans Administration medical sites as needed. Prior to their arrival, TBI clinicians identify all those at risk for brain injury based on the mechanism of injury. In some cases, a TBI has already been identified and, therefore, automatically receives further evaluation. For those at apparent risk (e.g., involved in blast, vehicle crashes, falls, gunshot/shrapnel wounds to the head or neck), clinical staff conduct brief interviews to assess current physical state, their recall of events surrounding the injury, loss (LOC) or alteration (AOC) of consciousness with the injury, alterations of recall surrounding the injury (retrograde amnesia, posttraumatic amnesia), and current cognitive or emotional symptoms. For those individuals at least meeting criteria for a concussion (Kay et al., 1993) and continuing to have postconcussive symptoms, more extensive evaluation is conducted. This evaluation includes cognitive screening, symptom questionnaires, neurological examination, a psychiatric interview, neuroimaging as clinically indicated, including magnetic resonance imaging of the brain to look for evidence of diffuse axonal injury or hemorrhage, among other abnormalities, and evaluation by rehabilitation specialties such as physical medicine and rehabilitation consult teams, physical and occupational therapy, and speech pathology. Additionally, all individuals screened receive educational materials alerting them to common postconcussive symptoms, information on the typical course of recovery, and the ways to receive further assistance if symptoms of concern emerge following hospital discharge. Patients are also assigned a TBI-specific case manager to further assist them in managing their TBI-related care.

ADHD AND LD

ADHD and LD are highly common neurodevelopmental disorders that affect cognition and frequently co-occur (Altarac & Saroha, 2007; Dopheide & Pliszka, 2009; Mayes, Calhoun, & Crowell, 2000). The actual prevalence of ADHD and LD within the military is not known, and while these conditions are generally disqualifying for military service, they are frequently encountered in military neuropsychological practice.

By regulation, individuals with a history of ADHD and/or LD are disqualified from entering military service unless they can demonstrate satisfactory academic performance and exhibit no need for medications for the condition within the preceding 12 months (DoD, 2004). If ADHD and/ or LD individuals have satisfactory academic and employment histories without recommendation or utilization of accommodations for 12 months or more, they may qualify for military service. In these circumstances, decisions are made on a case-by-case basis. Moreover, it is not uncommon for these diagnoses to be recognized for the first time in adulthood, particularly if the conditions are milder in nature. Thus, an individual may not be diagnosed with ADHD or an LD until entering the military. The section that follows gives a brief overview of these disorders within the military setting.

ADHD is a difficult diagnostic dilemma for the military, which requires individuals to maintain high levels of consistent attention and concentration in order to perform effectively and safely. Cigrang and colleagues (1998) found that 5% of mental health attrition among Air Force recruits was related to ADHD. Any history of ADHD will negate participation in jobs that have high attentional demands and other rigorous cognitive requirements, such as aviation and special operations forces, although a waiver may be obtained if the individual has not required medication for the past 12 months and does not show deficits on neuropsychological testing geared for these positions (Almond et al., 2005). Neuropsychological testing within the military is used to determine whether the service member has the functional capabilities to perform his or her duties.

Should individuals find themselves on active duty prior to the diagnosis of ADHD or an LD, depending on their specific military rate, retention is possible only if the disorder does not interfere with their capability of performing their job. As noted, it is not uncommon for these diagnoses to be recognized for the first time in adulthood, particularly in the military, given the complexity of task demands. Take the case of disorders of reading or written expression. Increases in rank equate to increases in administrative responsibilities no matter the MOS or rate of the individual. Individuals with disorders impacting primarily reading and writing (e.g., writing fitness reports, providing written briefs to committees) often reach a rank in which they can no longer compensate for the disorder, and it is not uncommon for individuals to be identified with a specific LD when this occurs. Anecdotally, the service generally makes a concerted effort to work with individuals who have a significant amount of time in service and are motivated to perform well. However, it should be noted that LD and ADHD are considered cause for administrative separation when individuals are unable to perform their military duties as a result of the condition. Because of the nature of the military environment, accommodations such as those one would receive in a school-based program are impossible to implement.

MILITARY AEROSPACE NEUROPSYCHOLOGY

Aerospace neuropsychology is the branch of clinical neuropsychology that manages the selection, assessment, and disposition of individuals in the armed services and National Aeronautics and Space Administration who are on flying status. It involves the unique integration of three fields of psychology (clinical, aviation, and neuropsychology) to maximize the functioning and safety of pilots and crew. Aviators must be carefully screened and selected for duty, both before entering service and after experiencing injury. Because the neuropsychology discipline provides a thorough analysis of brain and behavior relationships (Reitan & Wolfson, 1985), it is a logical choice for assessing aviation fitness and flying skills.

Historically, pilot selection was accomplished by a screening process that involved a review of records and a board decision. Aviators underwent a variety of tests that measured their balance, attention, reaction time, and decision-making capacity. These tests preceded modern neuropsychological measures and became the basis for some of the assessments used today. The neuropsychologist R. M. Reitan adapted portions of the Army alpha tests, and his early work eventually evolved into the Halstead–Reitan Neuropsychological Battery, which is widely used today in the assessment of neuropsychological impairment (Kennedy et al., 2010).

The early aerospace assessment process, especially in the astronaut program, was an attempt to "select in" the most capable individuals. At the time, the leaders in the field thought that "the best of the best" had to be selected to have the highest success rate in training and performance. However, with this strategy, the attrition rate for aviation cadets was between 45 and 75%. When the services shifted to a "select-out" stratagem, using base requirements of success in college, lack of disqualifying disorders, and absence of criminal record, the attrition rates dropped.

Aerospace neuropsychologists have since developed their assessments of aviator health and capability. Aside from the standard assessment of the individual (Stokes & Kite, 1994), the aerospace neuropsychologist may be asked to investigate human information processing (e.g., perception), cognition (e.g., spatial disorientation), sleep and fatigue (e.g., circadian rhythm), stress (e.g., effects), ergonomics (e.g., aircraft controls), toxicity (e.g., exposure to fuels, medications, or other substances), and personality (e.g., group decision making). In addition, the neuropsychologist typically remains involved in aviation issues such as pilot selection and retention, fitness for duty, motivation to fly, and stress reactions to flying. Recently, as aviation technologies have evolved, neuropsychologists have also helped develop policies for crew resource management, airsickness, gravity-induced loss of consciousness, hypoxia, air traffic control, mishap investigation, remote piloted aircrafts, and resident training, and have contributed to research in human factors.

Because of the specialization of this unique field, aerospace neuropsychologists deal with unique challenges. Aviators tend to be a rather healthy, young, and energetic group, but they may also gradually acquire the typical diseases of aging as they progress in their careers, such as cardiac disease and sleep apnea. Moreover, aviators tend to be "reverse malingerers" and will consciously or unconsciously minimize or hide their problems because of their high degree of motivation to fly. This requires neuropsychologists to create redundancy in the assessment battery to check for weaknesses that may interfere with flight safety, weaknesses the aviator may be attempting to hide. Additionally, military pilots generally exhibit intellectual functioning in the superior range and, therefore, assessments must be tailored to examine the relative decrement in performance rather than a level of impairment. Rarely, even in head-injured pilots, does performance fall in the impaired range on standardized neuropsychological tests. This produces a need for specific norms for this population to accurately assess any problems relative to flying function. Thus, approaches to neuropsychological testing that may be effective and accurate for other groups, including civilians or other military specialties, must be reappraised and adapted in aerospace neuropsychology.

There are many neuropsychological assessments used by aerospace neuropsychologists that take into account the needs and challenges of this unique population. Today, the U.S. Air Force School (USAF) of Aerospace Medicine, based out of Brooks City-Base in San Antonio, Texas, manages pilot selection. Prior to receiving specific training with aircrafts, potential pilots must pass the Flying Class (FC 1) physical exam as well as the Medical Flight Screening evaluation (MFS; Air Force Medical Service, 2011). The MFS evaluation consists of screening in ophthalmology, anthropometrics, and neuropsychology. The neuropsychological component of the MFS includes the following tests: (1) Multidimensional Aptitude Battery-II; (2) Armstrong Laboratory Aviator Personality Survey (ALAPS), (3) Neuroticism, Extraversion, and Openness Personality Inventory— Revised, and (4) MicroCog. Recently, the ALAPS was replaced by the Personality Assessment Inventory (Morey, 2010) to broaden the applicability of the personality profiles of aviators. In addition to the MFS evaluation, pilot aptitude tests are also administered. The two most common tests in the Air Force include the AFOQT and the Basic Attributes Test (Carretta, 2000).

After obtaining flying status, aviators continue to be monitored. The armed services highly regulate the screening and testing required for the assessment of individuals already on flying status. The U.S. Air Force standards are listed in AFI 48-123 (U.S. Department of the Air Force, 2001). The Army regulations are listed in AR40-501 (U.S. Department of the Army, 2007). The Navy lists its guidelines in NAVMED P-117 (U.S. Department of the Navy, 1996). In particular, all services require some form of standardized testing in the assessment of pilots for return to flying status after a neurological insult. In the case of head injuries, this testing is highly prescribed. AFI 48-123 indicates the length of LOC and post-traumatic amnesia (PTA) for the severity levels of TBI (mild, moderate, and severe). For a severe injury, for instance, the guidance is that the individual has a combined LOC/PTA of greater than 24 hours. The severe injury designation is also given to any pilot who has had a brain abscess, surgical or penetrating brain injury, focal signs of hematoma, central nervous system infection, and so on. The observation time is 5 years for active pilots, with a required evaluation of neuropsychological testing, as prescribed by the Aeromedical Consultation Services, within 30 days of the injury. The evaluation for return to flying minimally requires the Minnesota Multiphasic Personality Inventory, intelligence testing, formal memory assessment, and Halstead–Reitan Neuropsychological Battery in addition to a standard medical evaluation. The USAF has allowed individuals to return to duty in 2 years with MFS premorbid testing and good outcome on the current exam.

When making the aeromedical decision to allow an aviator to fly after an injury, the consulting neuropsychologist emphasizes to medical staff that one abnormal test does not disqualify the flyer. In the case of highly functioning individuals such as pilots, neuropsychological test performance is rarely in the impaired range (as described previously), so relative or task-specific lowering of functionality in the pilot is critical to assess. The neuropsychologist also emphasizes the need to look at the overall pattern of results and for multiple tests with overlapping measures. The critical elements of any sound neuropsychological assessment of an aviator must minimally include a good evaluation of speed and accuracy; attention and concentration; vigilance; memory and working memory; auditory, spatial, and kinesthetic processing; and new learning, multitasking, cognitive flexibility, and problem solving.

To accomplish these tasks, aerospace neuropsychologists generally work at the major evaluation centers in each of the services, and their reports are reviewed directly by the individual aeromedical consultation services. The aerospace neuropsychologist typically works through the flight surgeon, who combines all available data and makes a decision locally or prepares an aeromedical report that is then submitted for review for fitness for duty. The neuropsychologists in the field should confer with their specific aeromedical consultation services before attempting evaluations and interventions with flying personnel.

OPERATIONAL APPLICATIONS

The capacity for neuropsychological assessment to measure the effects of various environments, physical states, and medications makes it highly applicable to the operational functioning of the military. For example, neuropsychological assessment has been used as a means to guide recompression after deep dives as well as to study the impact of sleep deprivation on cognitive performance (Fishburn, 1991; Rabinowitz, Breitbach, & Warner, 2009). Additionally, cognitive testing is used regularly to determine the effects of prescription medications (e.g., lovastatin and pravastatin) on the performance of air crews in order to guide medication decisions (Gibellato, Moore, Selby, & Bower, 2001).

Stimulants have been used in the military since World War II (Bower & Phelan, 2003), and their effects on cognition have been studied in conjunction with military performance, particularly in cases of sustained military operations. Effects on cognition of various substances (e.g., modafinil, caffeine, nicotine, donepezil) are studied to allow for optimal dosing as well as provide guidelines for necessary sleep in such populations as aircrew, Navy SEALs, and medical personnel (Buguet, Moroz, & Radomski, 2003; Westcott, 2005; Lieberman, Tharion, Shukitt-Hale, Speckman, & Tulley, 2002; Mumenthaler et al., 2003). Other practical issues have also been studied, such as the effects of nicotine withdrawal in pilots in flight leading to conclusions that abrupt tobacco cessation in this population is detrimental and unsafe (Giannakoulas, Katramados, Melas, Diamantopoulos, & Chimonas, 2003).

SUMMARY

The military neuropsychologist is called upon to perform a wide variety of roles, both in garrison and in a deployed environment. Military neuropsychology is similar to civilian practice in many ways, but at the same time offers unique challenges in the assessment of active-duty service members, who must be fit to engage in physically rigorous and life-threatening activities. Neuropsychological assessment practices play a key role in fitness-for-duty evaluations; measuring effort; assessing deficits as a result of TBI, PTSD, ADHD, LD, or other injuries or illnesses; forensic evaluations; aerospace neuropsychology; and operational readiness and maintenance of peak performance of military members.

ADDITIONAL READING

Benedek, D. M., & Wynn, G. H. (Eds.). (2010). *Clinical management of PTSD.* Arlington, VA: American Psychiatric Publishing.

Defense and Veterans Brain Injury Center (DVBIC). (2011). *dvbic.org.*

Deployment Health Clinical Center. *www.pdhealth.mil.*

Kennedy, C., & Moore, J. (Eds.). (2010). *Military neuropsychology.* New York: Springer.

Pasquina, P. F., & Cooper, P. R. (Eds.). (2009). *Care of the combat amputee.* Washington, DC: Borden Institute.

Silver, J. M., McAllister, T. W., & Yudofsky, S. C. (Eds.). (2011). *Textbook of traumatic brain injury* (2nd ed.). Arlington, VA: American Psychiatric Publishing.

Traumatic Brain Injury: The Journey Home (CEMM traumatic brain injury website). *www.traumaticbraininjuryatoz.org.*

U.S. Army Medical Department, Rehabilitation and Reintegration Division (R2D). *www.amedd.army.mil/prr/index.html.*

VA/DoD Clinical Practice Guideline: Management of Concussion/Mild Traumatic Brain Injury. *www.healthquality.va.gov/mtbi/concussion_mtbi_full_1_0. pdf.*

REFERENCES

Air Force Medical Service. (2011). *U.S. Air Force School of Aerospace Medicine: Medical flight screening.* Retrieved January 26, 2011, from *airforcemedicine. afms.mil/idc/groups/public/documents/webcontent/knowledgejunction. hcst?functionalarea=MFS_USAFSAM&doctype=subpage&docname=CT B_071794.*

Almond, N., Harris, F., & Almond, M. (2005). You're the flight surgeon. *Aviation, Space, and Environmental Medicine, 76,* 601–602.

Altarac, M., & Saroha, E. (2007). Lifetime prevalence of learning disability among US children. *Pediatrics, 119,* S77–S83.

Armistead-Jehle, P. (2010). Symptom validity test performance in U.S. veterans referred for evaluation of mild TBI. *Applied Neuropsychology, 17,* 52–59.

Barr, W. B., & McCrea, M. (2001). Sensitivity and specificity of standardized neurocognitive testing immediately following sports concussion. *Journal of International Neuropsychological Society, 7*(6), 693–702.

Belanger, H. G., Kretzmer, T., Yoash-Gantz, R., Pickett, T., & Tupler, L. A. (2009). Cognitive sequelae of blast-related versus other mechanisms of brain trauma. *Journal of International Neuropsychological Society, 15*(1), 1–8.

Belanger, H. G., Proctor-Weber, Z., Kretzmer, T. S., Kim, M., French, L. M., & Vanderploeg, R. D. (2011). Symptom complaints following reports of blast versus non-blast mild TBI: Does mechanism of injury matter? *Clinical Neuropsychologist, 25,* 702–715.

Boake, C. (1989). A history of cognitive rehabilitation of head-injured patients, 1915–1980. *Journal of Head Trauma Rehabilitation, 4*(3), 1–8.

Boone, K. B. (2009). The need for continuous and comprehensive sampling of effort/response bias during neuropsychological examinations. *The Clinical Neuropsychologist, 23*(4), 729–741.

Bower, E. A., & Phelan, J. R. (2003). Use of amphetamines in the military environment. *Lancet, 362*(Suppl.), 18–19.

Bremner, J. D., Randall, P., Scott, T. M., Capelli, S., Delaney, R., McCarthy, G., et al. (1995). Deficits in short-term memory in adult survivors of childhood abuse. *Psychiatry Research, 59*(1–2), 97–107.

Bremner, J. D., Scott, T. M., Delaney, R. C., Southwick, S. M., Mason, J. W., Johnson, D. R., et al. (1993). Deficits in short-term memory in posttraumatic stress disorder. *American Journal of Psychiatry, 150*(7), 1015–1019.

Brenner, L. A., Terrio, H., Homaifar, B. Y., Gutierrez, P. M., Staves, P. J., Harwood, J. E., et al. (2010). Neuropsychological test performance in soldiers with blast-related mild TBI. *Neuropsychology, 24*(2), 160–167.

Buckley, T. C., Blanchard, E. B., & Neill, W. T. (2000). Information processing and PTSD: A review of the empirical literature. *Clinical Psychology Review, 20*(8), 1041–1065.

Buguet, A., Moroz, D. E., & Radomski, M. W. (2003). Modafinil: Medical considerations for use in sustained operations. *Aviation, Space, and Environmental Medicine, 74,* 659–663.

Bush, S. S., Ruff, R. M., Troster, A. I., Barth, J. T., Koffler, S. P., Pliskin, N. H., et al. (2005). Symptom validity assessment: Practical issues and medical necessity NAN policy and planning committee. *Archives of Clinical Neuropsychology, 20*(4), 419–426.

Carretta, T. R. (2000). U.S. Air Force pilot selection and training methods. *Aviation, Space, and Environmental Medicine, 71*(9), 950–956.

Centers for Disease Control. (1999). *Traumatic brain injury in the United States: A report to Congress, Centers for Disease Control.* Washington, DC: Author.

Cigrang, J. A., Carbone, E. G., Todd, S., & Fiedler, E. (1998). Mental health attrition from Air Force basic military training. *Military Medicine, 163,* 834–838.

Coldren, R. L., Kelly, M. P., Parish, R. V., Dretsch, M., & Russell, M. L. (2010). Evaluation of the Military Acute Concussion Evaluation for use in combat operations more than 12 hours after injury. *Military Medicine, 175*(7), 477–481.

Crowell, T. A., Kieffer, K. M., Siders, C. A., & Vanderploeg, R. D. (2002). Neuropsychological findings in combat-related posttraumatic stress disorder. *Clinical Neuropsychologist, 16*(3), 310–321.

Defense and Veterans Brain Injury Center (DVBIC). (2011). *dvbic.org.*

Dopheide, J. A., & Pliszka, S. R. (2009). Attention-deficit/hyperactivity disorder: An update. *Pharmacotherapy, 29*(6), 656–679.

Driskell, J. E., & Olmstead, B. (1989). Psychology and the military: Research applications and trends. *American Psychologist, 44*(1), 43–54.

Fishburn, F. J. (1991). Neuropsychological applications in military settings. In R. Gal & A. D. Mangelsdorff (Eds.), *Handbook of military psychology* (pp. 625–633). New York: Wiley.

French, L. M., Lange, R. T., Iverson, G. L., Ivins, B., Marshall, K., & Schwab, K. (2012). Influence of bodily injuries on symptom reporting following uncomplicated mild traumatic brain injury in U.S. military service members. *Journal of Head Trauma Rehabilitation, 27,* 63–74.

French, L. M., McCrea, M., & Baggett, M. (2008). The Military Acute Concussion Evaluation (MACE). *Journal of Special Operations Medicine, 8*(1), 68–77.

Giannakoulas, G., Katramados, A., Melas, N., Diamantopoulos, I., & Chimonas, E. (2003). Acute effects of nicotine withdrawal syndrome in pilots during flight. *Aviation, Space, and Environmental Medicine, 74,* 247–251.

Gibellato, M. G., Moore, J. L., Selby, K., & Bower, E. A. (2001). Effects of lovastatin and pravastatin on cognitive function in military aircrew. *Aviation, Space, and Environmental Medicine, 72,* 805–812.

Greiffenstein, M. F. (2007). Motor, sensory, and perceptual-motor pseudoabnormalities. In G. J. Larrabee (Ed.), *Assessment of malingered neuropsychological deficits* (pp. 100–130). New York: Oxford University Press.

Greiffenstein, M. F. (2010). Noncredible neuropsychological presentation in service members and veterans. In C. H. Kennedy & J. L. Moore (Eds.), *Military neuropsychology* (pp. 81–100). New York: Springer.

Greiffenstein, M. F., Fox, D., & Lees-Haley, P. R. (2007). The MMPI-2 Fake Bad Scale in detection of non-credible brain-injury claims. In K. B. Boone (Ed.), *Assessment of feigned cognitive impairment: A neuropsychological perspective* (pp. 210–235). New York: Guilford Press.

Heilbronner, R. L., Sweet, J. J., Morgan, J. E., Larrabee, G. J., Millis, S. R., & Conference Participants. (2010). American Academy of Clinical Neuropsychology Consensus Conference Statement on the Neuropsychological Assessment of Effort, Response Bias, and Malingering. *The Clinical Neuropsychologist, 23*(7), 1093–1129.

Hettich, T., Whitfield, E., Kratz, K., & Frament, C. (2010). Use of the Immediate Post Concussion Assessment and Cognitive Testing (ImPACT) to assist with return to duty determination of special operations soldiers who sustained mild traumatic brain injury. *Journal of Special Operations Medicine, 10*(4), 48–55.

Hoge, C. W., Auchterlonie, J. L., & Milliken, C. S. (2006). Mental health problems, use of mental health services, and attrition from military service after returning from deployment to Iraq or Afghanistan. *Journal of the American Medical Association, 295*(9), 1023–1032.

Hoge, C. W., Castro, C. A., Messer, S. C., McGurk, D., Cotting, D. I., & Koffman, R. L. (2004). Combat duty in Iraq and Afghanistan, mental health problems, and barriers to care. *New England Journal of Medicine, 351*(1), 13–22.

Iverson, G. L. (2005). Outcome from mild traumatic brain injury. *Current Opinion in Psychiatry, 18*(3), 301–317.

Iverson, G. L., Zasler, N. D., & Lange, R. T. (2006). Post-concussive disorder. In N. D. Zasler, D. I. Katz, & R. D. Zafonte (Eds.), *Brain injury medicine: Principles and practice* (pp. 373–405). New York: Demos Medical.

Ivins, B. J. (2010). Hospitalization associated with traumatic brain injury in the active duty US Army: 2000–2006. *NeuroRehabilitation, 26,* 199–212.

Ivins, B. J., Kane, R., & Schwab, K. A. (2009). Performance on the Automated Neuropsychological Assessment Metrics in a nonclinical sample of soldiers screened for mild TBI after returning from Iraq and Afghanistan: A descriptive analysis. *Journal of Head Trauma Rehabilitation, 24*(1), 24–31.

Jelinek, L., Jacobsen, D., Kellner, M., Larbig, F., Biesold, K. H., Barre, K., et al. (2006). Verbal and nonverbal memory functioning in posttraumatic stress disorder (PTSD). *Journal of Clinical and Experimental Neuropsychology, 28*(6), 940–948.

Jenkins, M. A., Langlais, P. J., Delis, D. A., & Cohen, R. A. (2000). Attentional dysfunction associated with posttraumatic stress disorder among rape survivors. *Clinical Neuropsychology, 14*(1), 7–12.

Joint Mental Health Advisory Team 7 (J-MHAT 7). (2011). *Operation Enduring Freedom 2010 Afghanistan.* Retrieved from *www.armymedicine.army.mil/reports/mhat/mhat_vii/J_MHAT_7.pdf.*

Kay, T., Adams, R., Anderson, T., Berrol, S., Cicerone, K., Dahlberg, C., et al. (1993). Definition of mild traumatic brain injury. *Journal of Head Trauma Rehabilitation, 8*, 86–87.

Kelly, M. P., Mulligan, K. P., & Monahan, M. C. (2010). Fitness for duty. In C. H. Kennedy & J. L. Moore (Eds.), *Military neuropsychology.* New York: Springer.

Kennedy, C. H., Boake, C., & Moore, J. L. (2010). A history and introduction to military neuropsychology. In C. H. Kennedy & J. L. Moore (Eds.), *Military neuropsychology* (pp. 1–28). New York: Springer.

Kennedy, C. H., Kupke, T., & Smith, R. (2000). A neuropsychological investigation of the Armed Service Vocational Aptitude Battery (ASVAB). *Archives of Clinical Neuropsychology, 15*, 696–697.

Lew, H. L., Jerger, J. F., Guillory, S. B., & Henry, J. A. (2007). Auditory dysfunction in traumatic brain injury. *Journal of Rehabilitation Research and Development, 44*(7), 921–928.

Lew, H. L., Otis, J. D., Tun, C., Kerns, R. D., Clark, M. E., & Cifu, D. X. (2009). Prevalence of chronic pain, posttraumatic stress disorder, and persistent postconcussive symptoms in OIF/OEF veterans: Polytrauma clinical triad. *Journal of Rehabilitation Research and Development, 46*(6), 697–702.

Lewin, I. (1992). *The cost of disorders of the brain.* Washington, DC: National Foundation for the Brain.

Lieberman, H. R., Tharion, W. J., Shukitt-Hale, B., Speckman, K. L., & Tulley, R. (2002). Effects of caffeine, sleep loss, and stress on cognitive performance and mood during U.S. Navy SEAL training. *Psychopharmacology, 164*, 250–261.

Luethcke, C. A., Bryan, C. J., Morrow, C. E., & Isler, W. C. (2011). Comparison of concussive symptoms, cognitive performance, and psychological symptoms between acute blast-versus nonblast-induced traumatic brain injury. *Journal of the International Neuropsychological Society, 17*, 1–10.

Mayes, S. D., Calhoun, S. L., & Crowell, E. W. (2000). Learning disabilities and ADHD: Overlapping spectrum disorders. *Journal of Learning Disabilities, 33*, 417–424.

McCrea, M., Guskiewicz, K. M., Marshall, S. W., Barr, W., Randolph, C., Cantu, R. C., et al. (2003). Acute effects and recovery time following concussion in collegiate football players: The NCAA Concussion Study. *Journal of the American Medical Association, 290*(19), 2556–2563.

McCrea, M., Kelly, J. P., Kluge, J., Ackley, B., & Randolph, C. (1997). Standardized assessment of concussion in football players. *Neurology, 48*(3), 586–588.

McCrea, M., Pliskine, N., Barth, J., Cox, D., Fink, J., French, L., et al. (2008). Official position of the military TBI task force on the role of neuropsychology and rehabilitation psychology in the evaluation, management, and research of military veterans with traumatic brain injury. *Clinical Neuropsychologist, 22*(1), 10–26.

Mittenberg, W., Patton, C., Canyock, E. M., & Condit, D. C. (2002). A national survey of symptom exaggeration and malingering base rates. *Journal of the International Neuropsychological Society, 8*(2), 247.

Morey, L. C. (2010). Personality Assessment Inventory (PAI). *PAR Catalog of Selected Testing Resources,* 6–7.

Mumenthaler, M. S., Yesavage, J. A., Taylor, J. L., O'Hara, R., Friedman, Lee, H., et al. (2003). Psychoactive drugs and pilot performance: A comparison of nicotine, donepezil, and alcohol effects. *Neuropsychopharmacology, 28,* 1366–1373.

Nelson, L. A., Yoash-Gantz, R. E., Pickett, T. C., & Campbell, T. A. (2009). Relationship between processing speed and executive functioning performance among OEF/OIF veterans: Implications for postdeployment rehabilitation. *Journal of Head Trauma Rehabilitation, 24*(1), 32–40.

Orme, D., Ree, M. J., & Rioux, P. (2001). Premorbid IQ estimates from a multiple aptitude test battery: Regression vs. equating. *Archives of Clinical Neuropsychology, 16,* 679–688.

Owens, B. D., Kragh, J. F., Wenke, J. C., Macaitis, J., Wade, C. E., & Holcomb, J. B. (2008). Combat wounds in Operation Iraqi Freedom and Operation Enduring Freedom. *Journal of Trauma Injury, Infection, and Critical Care, 64,* 295–299.

Rabinowitz, Y. G., Breitbach, J. E., & Warner, C. H. (2009). Managing aviator fatigue in a deployed environment: The relationship between fatigue and neurocognitive functioning. *Military Medicine, 174*(4), 358–362.

Reger, M. A., Etherage, J. R., Reger, G. M., & Gahm, G. A. (2008). Civilian psychologists in an Army culture: The ethical challenge of cultural competence. *Military Psychology, 20,* 21–35.

Reeves, D. L., Bleiberg, J., Roebuck-Spencer, T., Cernich, A. N., Schwab, K., Ivins, B., et al. (2006). Reference values for performance on the Automated Neuropsychological Assessment Metrics V3.0 in an active duty military sample. *Military Medicine, 171*(10), 982–994.

Reeves, D. L., Winter, K. P., Bleiberg, J., & Kane, R. L. (2007). ANAM genogram: Historical perspectives, description, and current endeavors. *Archives of Clinical Neuropsychology, 22*(S1), S15–S37.

Reitan, R. M., & Wolfson, D. (1985). *Neuroanatomy and neuropathology: A clinical guide for neuropsychologists.* Tucson, AZ: Neuropsychology Press.

Sandweiss, D. A., Slymen, D. J., Leardmann, C. A., Smith, B., White, M. R., Boyko, E. J., et al. (2011). Preinjury psychiatric status, injury severity, and postdeployment posttraumatic stress disorder. *Archives of General Psychiatry, 68*(5), 496–504.

Sayer, N. A., Chiros, C. E., Sigford, B., Scott, S., Clothier, B., Pickett, T., et al. (2008). Characteristics and rehabilitation outcomes among patients with blast and other injuries sustained during the Global War on Terror. *Archives of Physical Medicine and Rehabilitation, 89*(1), 163–170.

Smith, P. (2011). Discrepancies in clinical definitions of stress fractures: Implications for the United States Army. *Military Medicine, 176*(1), 60–66.

Stein, M. B., Hanna, C., Vaerum, V., & Koverola, C. (1999). Memory functioning in adult women traumatized by childhood sexual abuse. *Journal of Traumatic Stress, 12*(3), 527–534.

Stokes, A., & Kite, K. (1994). *Flight stress: Stress, fatigue, and performance in aviation.* Brookfield, VT: Ashgate.

Stulemeijer, M., van der Werf, S. P., Jacobs, B., Biert, J., van Vugt, A. B., Brauer, J. M., et al. (2006). Impact of additional extracranial injuries on outcome after mild traumatic brain injury. *Journal of Neurotrauma, 23*(10), 1561–1569.

Sutker, P. B., Allain, A. N., Jr., Johnson, J. L., & Butters, N. M. (1992). Memory and learning performances in POW survivors with history of malnutrition and combat veteran controls. *Archives of Clinical Neuropsychology, 7*(5), 431–444.

Terrio, H., Brenner, L. A., Ivins, B. J., Cho, J. M., Helmick, K., Schwab, K., et al. (2009). Traumatic brain injury screening: Preliminary findings in a US Army Brigade Combat Team. *Journal of Head Trauma Rehabilitation, 24*(1), 14–23.

Twamley, E. W., Hami, S., & Stein, M. B. (2004). Neuropsychological function in college students with and without posttraumatic stress disorder. *Psychiatry Research, 126*(3), 265–274.

U.S. Department of the Air Force. (2001). *Medical examinations and standards* (AFI 48-123). Washington, DC: Author.

U.S. Department of the Army. (2007). *Standards of medical fitness* (AR 40-501). Washington, DC: Author.

U.S. Department of Defense. (2004). *Criteria and procedure requirements for physical standards for appointment, enlistment, or induction in the armed forces* (DoDI 6130.4). Washington, DC: Author.

U.S. Department of Homeland Security. (2004). *Medical manual* (Commandant, United States Coast Guard Instruction M6000.1). Washington, DC: Author.

U.S. Department of the Navy. (1996). *Manual of the medical department* (NAVMED P-117). Washington, DC: Author.

Vasterling, J. J., Brailey, K., Constans, J. I., & Sutker, P. B. (1998). Attention and memory dysfunction in posttraumatic stress disorder. *Neuropsychology, 12*(1), 125–133.

Vista Life Sciences. (2011). ANAM4. Retrieved January 28, 2011, from *www.vistalifesciences.com/node/10.*

Walsh, J. R., Kucinkas, S. K., & Curran, L. T. (1990). *Armed Services Vocational*

Battery (ASVAB): Integrative review of reliability studies. San Antonio, TX: Air Force Systems Command.

Wescott, K. J. (2005). Modafinil, sleep deprivation, and cognitive function in military and medical settings. *Military Medicine, 170,* 333–335.

Yehuda, R., Keefe, R. S., Harvey, P. D., Levengood, R. A., Gerber, D. K., Geni, J., et al. (1995). Learning and memory in combat veterans with posttraumatic stress disorder. *American Journal of Psychiatry, 152*(1), 137–139.

★ CHAPTER 9 ★

Suicide Prevention in the Military

David E. Jones
Laurel L. Hourani
Mathew B. Rariden
Patricia J. Hammond
Aaron D. Werbel

The wars in Afghanistan and Iraq have been associated with an alarming rise in suicides among military troops (Christenson, 2010; Kovach, 2010). In the early years of these conflicts (2002–2006)—while increased suicide rates were noted particularly in the Army and Marine Corps—the military suicide rate remained below comparably matched demographic groups in the civilian sector. In 2009, however, Kuehn reported that the annualized suicide rate (20.2 per 100,000) for the military combined exceeded, for the first time in 28 years, the suicide rate in the civilian population. Although relationship problems, work performance, disciplinary issues, and mental health problems continue to be implicated as serious suicide risk factors, military leaders cannot attribute increased suicide rates to a single cause, such as a service member's deployment status, number of previous deployments, or even exposure to combat (Kruzel, 2009). To an organization that prizes decisive action, uncertainty about the underlying causes of suicide is a source of frustration for leaders at all levels of the military. While the current focus on suicide in the military is notable, the military has had major top-down reviews of suicide prevention policies and programs in the past (see Historical Context section). The purpose of this chapter is to provide an overview of suicide prevention efforts within the military, with sections devoted to historical context, epidemiological data, risk and protective factors, and resources for military members and their families. This chapter also offers information on practical matters in assessment, treatment, and consultation with military leaders regarding at-risk personnel (and family members). To keep the discussion grounded on the issues and concerns of leaders and service providers working in the field, best-practice information is integrated with experiences caring for suicidal patients in forward-deployed operational and hospital settings. The goal is to establish a resource for clinicians and leaders at all levels that provides practical ways to make a difference in preventing suicide and suicidal behavior across the entire military.

HISTORICAL CONTEXT

Given the impact of suicides on families and military units, efforts to prevent the loss of life and suffering have long been a part of military counseling, chaplaincy services, and medical treatment. A confluence of events in the mid-1990s brought increased attention within the U.S. Department of Defense (DoD) to suicide prevention. The suicide of Admiral Jeremy Boorda, Chief of Naval Operations, in 1996 led the DoD to commission a study to examine suicide prevention policies and programs across the services (Shaffer, 1997). At the same time, the U.S. Air Force was engaged in creating an interdisciplinary team to recommend organizational changes in response to an increase in suicides by airmen during the early 1990s (Knox, Litts, Talcott, Feig, & Caine, 2003; Litts, Moe, Roadman, Janke, & Miller, 1999). This team collaborated with the Centers for Disease Control and Prevention (CDC) to develop a communitywide approach. By the end of the decade, the Air Force received White House recognition for innovations in building community awareness and promoting help-seeking decisions as a means of reducing suicides (DoD, 1999). By the late 1990s, the Army, Navy, and Marine Corps had also engaged military and civilian experts to revitalize suicide prevention programs in keeping with the distinct organizational cultures and missions of those services (Army Chief of Public Affairs, 2000; Jones et al., 2001). At the national level, suicide prevention emerged as a major public health priority (U.S. Public Health Service, 1999), and this impetus energized joint service efforts to combat suicide. A decade later, with the continued rise in suicide rates related to Operations Enduring Freedom and Iraqi Freedom (OEF/OIF), the attention to suicide prevention within the military has only increased. The Army announced an unprecedented collaboration with the National Institute of Mental Health (2009) for a 5-year, $50,000,000 research project aimed at conducting an epidemiological study of mental health, psychological resilience, suicide risks, suicide-related behaviors, and suicide deaths in the U.S. Army. Further, a blue ribbon panel of nationally recognized experts has been appointed by the Secretary of Veterans Affairs (2008) to make recommendations for suicide prevention, research, and education among the veteran population. In August 2010, the DoD Task Force on the Prevention of Suicide by Members of the Armed Forces released a report that noted "extraordinary effort" has been made by the services in addressing suicide (more focus than any other employer in the nation). The report, however, criticized the lack of strategic planning among the services regarding suicide prevention activities and services and called for a new high-level office under the Secretary of Defense to coordinate strategy and programs (Viebeck, 2010).

EPIDEMIOLOGICAL ISSUES

Epidemiological investigations can promote the identification of individuals at risk and evaluate effective prevention and intervention strategies. Suicide surveillance in the military demands the best possible data on a difficult population. This section discusses both national and military-specific epidemiological issues to be considered when evaluating such suicide data.

National Profile of Suicide

Prevalence Rates

Despite a dramatic increase in prevention and treatment efforts in the 1990s, the lifetime prevalence of suicide attempts and ideation has remained unchanged (Kessler, Berglund, Borges, Nock, & Wang, 2005). As of 2006, suicide was the 11th leading cause of death in the United States and the fourth among males 18–60 years old (CDC, 2010). There were more than 33,000 suicides, with 11 of every 100,000 Americans killing themselves. This translates to about 91 suicides per day or one suicide every 16 minutes. For comparison, the homicide rate in 2006 was the fifth leading cause of death in the United States for males 18–60 years old, and the accidental death rate was more than twice as high. The rate of suicide in the general population varies with age, gender, and ethnicity. Men die in 79% of the suicides in the United States. Men have an early peak in rates in their 20s and a second peak in the elderly years. The overall risk of suicide rises with age, with white men over age 50—10% of the population—accounting for 30% of suicides. The age distribution of suicide is changing, however. People 15–24 years old, who once accounted for 5% of suicides, accounted for 14% in 2009 (McIntosh, 2012). A 16% increase in suicide among people ages 40–64 between 1999 and 2005 translated to an overall increase in the national suicide rate of 0.5% because this had traditionally been a low-risk group (Hu, Wilcox, Wissow, & Baker, 2008). This increase was seen in the proportion of women as well as in the methods of poisoning and hanging/suffocation.

In terms of ethnicity, the risk for suicide among young people is greatest among white males; however, from 1980 through 1995, suicide rates increased most rapidly (105%) among young African American males (CDC, 1998). Native Americans have the highest overall suicide rate of any racial or ethnic group. Divorced and widowed men and women have high rates of suicide at all ages, and single people are more likely to commit suicide than married people. From 1990–1994, both crude and adjusted (controlling for demographic differences) suicide rates were significantly higher in the West than in the South, Midwest, and Northeast (CDC, 1997). Twelve years later, the West (including mountain and Pacific areas) remains the highest risk region (McIntosh, 2012). Firearms are the most often utilized tool of suicide by all demographic groups, accounting for 51% of the total, and are the leading method in all regions, followed by suffocation/hanging (24%) and poisoning (17%). Although there are few official statistics on attempted (nonfatal) suicide, it is estimated that there are 25 attempts for each death by suicide and that about 10% of people who attempt suicide will succeed within 10 years. The risk of attempted suicide is greatest among women and the young. Women have generally been found to make three times as many attempts as males (McIntosh, 2012). Women also tend to use less reliable means of suicide than men (e.g., wrist cutting and drug overdose rather than gunshot) and are more likely to admit to a suicide attempt.

Risk and Protective Factors

It has been estimated that up to 90% of people who commit suicide have a psychiatric disorder, with mood disorders such as major depressive disorder and bipolar disorder constituting the most common diagnoses (Harvard Mental Health Letter, 2003). Other psychiatric disorders associated with suicide are alcohol and drug abuse/dependence, personality disorders, schizophrenia, and anxiety disorders. Feelings of hopelessness, however, are found to be more predictive of suicide risk than mental disorder per se. Social isolation (e.g., following bereavement, divorce, or unemployment), social disruption (e.g., victims of violence, family history of child maltreatment, incarceration), loss, physical illness, and barriers to or unwillingness to seek help are also associated with high risk for suicide (AAS, 2012; CDC, 2010; HMHL, 2003). In addition, a family history of suicide and suicide attempt greatly increases the risk of suicide, suggesting hereditary vulnerability or influence of a model. Protective factors that buffer individuals from suicidal thoughts and behaviors include easy access to and effective clinical care, family and community support, skills in problem solving, and cultural or religious beliefs that discourage suicide (CDC, 2010).

Military Rates of Suicide

Nationally, suicide rates have traditionally decreased in times of war and increased in times of economic crisis (AAS, 2012). In recent years, this observation has been challenged. Although individual demographic subgroups vary widely, the overall suicide rate in the U.S. military has historically approximated that of the total civilian population (10–13 deaths per 100,000). Since 2006, the total number of suicides has been rising across the DoD (see Figure 9.1). When adjusted for the demographic distribution of the United States, the military suicide rate has been generally lower than that of the nation as a whole. This was at least partially accounted for by the full-time employment status of military personnel, in contrast to the civilian population, and a lower rate of mental disorder as a result of screening practices and/or available counseling and healthcare services.

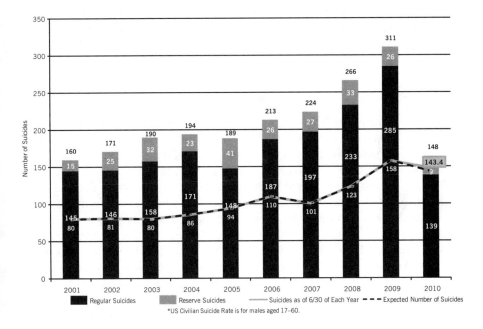

FIGURE 9.1. Active-duty and Reserve suicides for all branches and components between January 1, 2001, and June 30, 2010. U.S. civilian suicide rate is for males ages 17–60. Data from Mortality Surveillance Division Office of the Armed Forces Medical Examiner.

Suicide Rates by Service, 1991–2000

Between 1991 and 2000, the annual rates of suicide in the U.S. Army, Air Force, Navy, and Marine Corps were between 10 and 15 per 100,000 active-duty members. During the 1990s, these unadjusted rates sometimes exceeded the crude suicide rate for the entire United States (Jones, Kennedy, & Hourani, 2006, p. 133). The Army and Marine Corps frequently had higher annual rates than the Navy and Air Force, and as would be expected from the services with primarily ground combat troops, they also had higher death rates, including self-inflicted deaths during combat. In a study of all 1998 and 1999 military deaths, comparing official death reports and sources other than official records, 17% more suicides were found than were reported and an additional 4% of deaths suspicious for suicide. These data suggested that reporting and classification errors may account for 21% of additional suicides in the military, making rates comparable to those seen in civilian studies (Carr, Hoge, Gardner, & Potter, 2004). Several studies have examined the demographic distribution of suicide among military populations. A study of suicides from 1999–2001 using the joint Navy and Marine Corps suicide database showed that average gender-, age-, and race-specific suicide rates for Marines Corps personnel were higher than those for Navy personnel in almost all demographic groups and were frequently higher than for the U.S. population (Stander, Hilton, Kennedy, & Robbins, 2004).

Military Suicide Rates, 2001–2009

Since 2001, the military has seen a steady and alarming increase in the suicide rate, from a low of 9.1 per 100,000 personnel in 2001 to a high of 15.6 in 2009 (Defense Manpower Data Center, 2011), with soldiers surpassing the civilian rate since 2008 (Black, Gallaway, Bell, & Ritchie, 2011; Kuehn, 2009). The most alarming trend has taken place among active-duty Army and Marine Corps service members, whose rates have risen dramatically over those of the Navy and Air Force. Figures 9.2 and 9.3 illustrate the suicide rates per 100,000 and total number of suicides for all service branches, respectively, and are best understood when considered together. Recent data also show more than half of all veterans who took their own lives after returning from Iraq or Afghanistan were members of the National Guard or Reserves (Associated Press, 2008), and in the first 10 months of 2010, 86 non-active-duty National Guard soldiers killed themselves compared with 48 such suicides in 2009. Further, the Veterans Administration (VA) estimates about 18 veteran suicides a day, five by veterans who are receiving VA care (Association of the United States Navy, 2011). Indeed, the trends to date suggest that the OIF/OEF period may be the worst time to date for suicides in the military despite likely underreporting (Donnelly, 2011).

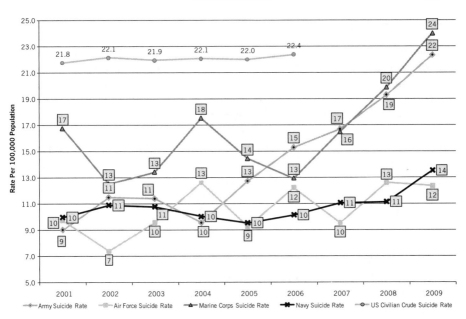

FIGURE 9.2. Active-duty suicide rates per 100,000 between January 2001 and December 2009. Data from Mortality Surveillance Division Office of the Armed Forces Medical Examiner. U.S civilian suicide rate is for males ages 17–60; data from CDC injury mortality reports (only up to 2006 information available).

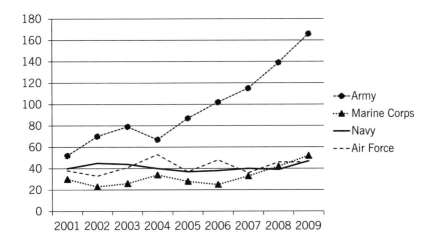

FIGURE 9.3. Active-duty and Reserve suicides by service branch and year (2001–2009). Data from Mortality Surveillance Division Office of the Armed Forces Medical Examiner.

Cross-Service Comparisons

There are several problems with past and current attempts to compare rates across services. Because the actual number of suicides is still relatively low in the military population, small fluctuations in the annual rate of different services may seem exaggerated when viewed across a limited number of years. As a result, caution must be exercised when making assumptions or drawing conclusions about a new risk factor or measuring the efficacy of suicide prevention efforts based on increases or decreases within a few years' time. One example may be the 2004 news release about the Army suicide rate during the Iraq War (Loeb, 2004). The focus on this discrete time period generated a good deal of both public policy and DoD concern at all levels. Soldiers accounted for 19 of 22 service members committing suicide in Iraq in 2003, a rate of 13.5 per 100,000 troops. Although this was a higher rate than in the previous 2 years, it was about the same rate as in 2000 (13.4) and lower than the rate in 1999. Indeed, it has taken several years of increased rates and comparable data to confirm the rising trend in rates among Army and Marine Corps personnel. To properly compare rates across services, it is also important to consider how many cases are pending final determination, to require consistent definitions and criteria for active-duty cases, and to encourage systematic investigations across service branches. Overall, the DoD as a whole as well as the individual services need comparable base populations or must satisfy or statistically control for sociodemographic differences. Other issues that have precluded a direct comparison of suicide rates across military services include nonstandardized methods of data collection and different definitions of the data elements collected. These issues include differences among services in investigation procedures and year-to-date extrapolation procedures to report projected annual rates. Finally, there were differences in the personnel categories that are included in the denominators used to calculate suicide rates. These differences contribute to variations that must be taken into account when making cross-service comparisons. For example, suicide rates for enlisted personnel in all services are double those for officers (Helmkamp, 1995). The proportion of officers in the Air Force is almost twice that of the Marine Corps, which has the highest proportion of enlisted personnel of all branches of service. Therefore, since suicides are more prevalent among the enlisted, the Marine Corps could be expected to have the highest rate and the Air Force the lowest based on this factor alone. Other critical issues in comparing rates across services include very different recruiting, screening, and discharge policies and practices that influence the level of mental health of recruits, referrals, and outcomes of referrals, including medical discharges, which may or may not be a part of formal suicide prevention programs (Knox et al., 2010; Warner, Appenzeller, Parker, Warner, & Hoge, 2011).

Risk and Protective Factors in the Military

Risk Factors

One of the most important functions of epidemiology is the study of risk factors. To prevent a condition, in this case suicide, it is important to understand the factors that lead to it. General principles focus on targeting risks for which intervention would be expected to have the greatest impact. Some risks are more modifiable than others that are fixed (e.g., alcohol abuse vs. pay grade). Addressing risk factors that are not common in nonsuicidal individuals would have a strong rather than weak effect on the incidence of suicide, as would reducing risk factors characterizing a large proportion of suicides. Among the most frequently associated risk factors for active-duty personnel are relationship problems; unexplained mood change or depression; alcohol involvement; feelings of disgrace, isolation, hopelessness, or worthlessness; financial and legal problems; previous suicide attempts; job/ performance problems; medical/physical evaluation board/administrative discharge processing (Fragala & McCaughey, 1991); work in military security and law enforcement specialties in the Army (Helmkamp, 1996); and apprentice/recruit and blue-collar occupations in the Navy and Air Force (Gaines & Richmond, 1980; Kawahara & Palinkas, 1991). In a Marine Corps population study—of 23 completed suicides, 172 attempters, and 384 nonpsychiatric controls—a history of abuse, neglect, or rejection; lower performance evaluation; symptoms of depression; younger age; history of alcohol abuse; and hopelessness were risk factors that differentiated suicide completers and attempters from controls (Holmes, Mateczun, Lall, & Wilcove, 1998). Additional studies have found that Vietnam veterans with symptoms of posttraumatic stress disorder (PTSD) were significantly more likely to die by suicide than those without such symptoms (Bullman & Kang, 1994; Faberow, Kang, & Bullman, 1990). In a 2009 study of young adults, Wilcox, Storr, and Breslau showed that it was PTSD rather than the trauma itself that increased suicide risk. In an uncontrolled study of 723 Air Force suicides between 1983 and 1993, more than half of the victims were judged to have been depressed and just under a quarter had received mental health care; 40% of the victims had abused alcohol or substances, 66% had difficulties in intimate relationships, 43% had work-related problems, and 16% had legal difficulties (Shaffer, 1997).

Protective Factors

Protective factors are characteristics that are associated with a low risk of suicide. These factors are quite varied and include attitudinal and behavioral characteristics as well as attributes of the environment and culture (Plutchik & Van Praag, 1994). Among the protective factors identified and cited on military suicide prevention websites are social support; belonging and caring; leadership responsibilities; effective coping and problem-solving skills; policies and culture that approve or encourage help-seeking behavior and protect those who seek help; unit cohesion, camaraderie, and support; optimistic outlook; access to assistance services; healthy lifestyle promotion; and spiritual support (e.g., U.S. Marine Corps, 2011). Because positive resistance to suicide is not permanent, programs that support and maintain protection against suicide should be ongoing. All military branches have health promotion-oriented websites that include guidelines and recommendations for building resiliency and hardiness, and the newly created Defense Centers of Excellence for Psychological Health and Traumatic Brain Injury (Defense Centers of Excellence, 2011) evaluate and oversee the military's psychological health programs. Although little research has been conducted that directly links resiliency with reduced suicide risk, there is some evidence that resiliency factors, including family closeness and religiosity, are related to a lower risk of suicidal ideation (O'Donnell, O'Donnell, Warlow, & Steuve, 2004). Promoted as skills that can be used to counter the negative effects of stress, resiliency-building components include such practices as developing stress management skills, viewing setbacks as temporary and/or opportunities for self-discovery, accepting change, and maintaining a sense of humor. Further research is needed on the extent to which such factors can modify suicide risk and be taught as part of a potential intervention program in high-risk individuals.

Suicide Clusters

A suicide cluster is defined as an unexpectedly higher number of suicides occurring within a specified and reasonably small geographical location during a reasonably short time period (Hourani, Warrack, & Coben, 1999a). To determine whether the number is higher than expected, it is necessary first to establish the usual rate in that location for that time. This is particularly difficult in the military because location-specific rates would need to be maintained, and it is not always clear what the geographical unit of investigation should be—for example, command unit, base, temporarily assigned duty site, or departing or receiving command when changing a permanent duty station. Therefore, few military studies have been conducted. There is limited evidence, however, that clusters do occur in the military. For example, an Air Force study concluded that as many as 20% of suicides occurred in a cluster (Rothberg & McDowell, 1988). Navy studies found evidence for time and space clustering within 2 weeks (Hourani et al., 1999a) as well as an imitative phenomenon in a Naval "A" School (an entry-level training school; Grigg, 1988). However, two Marine Corps studies found little or no evidence of clustering (Holmes et al., 1998; Hourani, Warrack, & Cohen, 1999b). Overall, there is more evidence for clustering in civilian than in military populations. Indeed, the CDC (1988) has issued recommendations for the prevention and containment of clusters of suicides, and the AAS has guidelines for the media to discourage imitative suicides (McIntosh, 2012). The civilian literature suggests the following: (1) Both suicide and suicide attempts cluster (Gould & Shaffer, 1986), (2) clustering occurs among psychologically disturbed individuals, (3) cluster victims knew about the suicide but did not personally know the other victims, and (4) clustering is most common in the young (ages 15–24).

Suicide Attempts, Gestures, and Ideation

Until 2005, there were no data on DoD-wide suicide attempts or gestures, although some individual service and command data had been collected and examined (see review in Ritchie, Keppler, & Rothberg, 2003). In the first population-based study to identify and analyze nonfatal suicide attempts (parasuicides) in the U.S. Navy and Marine Corps, hospital and personnel records of 4,578 Navy and Marine Corps hospitalized parasuicides from 1989 to 1995 were examined. The ratios of hospitalized parasuicides to completed suicides were an estimated 7:1 in the Navy and 5:1 in the Marine Corps (Trent, 1999). Parasuicide rates for women were two to three times higher than for men. A psychological disorder was diagnosed in 95% of the cases; the leading diagnosis was personality disorder (53%), followed by substance abuse (36%). The aggregate profile of a parasuicide in this study was as follows: a young (18–21 years) female Navy E1–E2 with a low level of education and a diagnosable mental disorder, who was hospitalized for 1 week after a self-inflicted drug overdose and then returned to duty (Trent, 1999). In a subsequent record review, of 100 consecutive suicidal cases admitted to the Walter Reed Army Medical Center, 94% were admitted with a depressed mood, 67% had a history of attempts or gestures, and 49% had been treated with psychiatric medications prior to admission (Ritchie et al., 2003). Almost half were returned to full-duty status. The following summarizes additional research findings on military suicidal behavior up through the 1990s.

1. During a 6-month period in 1968, 179 instances of suicidal behavior were seen in Army and Air Force personnel psychiatry services. Ninety-seven percent of these individuals were diagnosed with personality disorders or acute situational maladjustment; 88% were returned to duty without hospitalization (Sawyer, 1969).
2. The Army's hospitalized self-inflicted injury rates ranged from 49–94 per 100,000 during 1975–1985. No correlation was observed with death rate or troop strength (Rock, 1988).
3. In a 16-month period between 1989–1991 54 active-duty Army

trainees were seen for parasuicidal behavior; 100% had a principal diagnosis of adjustment disorder (Koshes & Rothberg, 1992).

4. A cluster of 21 Recruit Temperament Survey items (e.g., "Do you feel you will have trouble making good in the service?", "Do you think you have gotten a 'raw deal' from life?") predicted suicide gestures among recruits at the Naval Training Center (Hoiberg & Garfein, 1976).

5. Unlike for active-duty personnel, the primary characteristics among older suicidal veterans utilizing a crisis intervention hotline were loneliness, alcoholism, and unemployment (Porter, Astacio, & Sobong, 1997).

Fortunately, population-based estimates of suicidal ideation and attempts (respondents were asked if they had seriously considered suicide/attempted suicide in the past year) have became available from the anonymous DoD surveys of health-related behaviors (HRB) administered approximately every 3 years to a representative sample of active-duty military personnel worldwide (Bray et al., 2003). In the 2002 survey, the estimated prevalence of the preceding year's suicidal ideation was 5.1% compared with 3.8% in 1998 (Vincus et al., 1999). The difference was statistically significant ($t = 2.5$, $p < .05$) and was primarily accounted for by a large increase in the Navy estimate (1.9% in 1998 to 6.4% in 2002). The other services were about the same and/or not significantly increased (Bray et al., 2003). Overall prevalence rates of self-reported suicidal ideation from the 2005 and 2008 surveys were 4.9% and 4.6%, respectively. Rates in the Air Force of 3.5% in 2005 and 3.1% in 2008 were significantly lower than in the other services (Bray et al, 2009). Major risk factors included screening positive for depression symptoms, PTSD symptoms, and serious psychological distress and receipt of mental health counseling. High risk-taking scores and avoidance coping behaviors also increased risk while active coping behaviors, such as talking to a friend, thinking of a plan, exercising, engaging in a hobby, or saying a prayer when stressed or pressured, were protective. Self-reported suicide attempt rates more than doubled from 0.8% in 2005 to 2.16% in 2008 (Bray et al., 2009). In a 2006 representative study of National Guard and Reservists patterned after the HRB surveys of active-duty personnel, suicidal ideation was significantly higher among Guardsmen and Reservists who had been deployed than their active-duty counterparts (Hourani et al., 2007).

Suicide Assessment and Surveillance

In recent years, suicide surveillance has become an important focus of the DoD. The Suicide Prevention and Risk Reduction Committee (SPARRC) was created to formalize suicide prevention education and to improve the identification of and access to care for high-risk individuals. Representatives of all service branches meet to coordinate suicide prevention and surveillance activities. Up until 2008, each service branch conducted its own suicide surveillance program and collected a varied range of suicide data with its own instruments from varied sources. The exception was the U.S. Department of the Navy (DON), which developed a joint Navy and Marine Corps suicide surveillance system in 1999. This reporting system, based on the DON Suicide Incident Report (DONSIR; Jones, Hawkes, Gelles, Hourani, & Kennedy, 1999), fed a comprehensive database (Jones et al., 2001), providing quantifiable, standardized, and psychological autopsy-related information on all completed active-duty DON suicides. In addition to the demographic, military, incidental, medical, psychological, support service utilization, and command-specific data covered with the DONSIR, this system also collected valuable narratives on circumstances, risk factors, and victims' emotional status. Sources for this reporting system included DD Form 1300 (Report of Casualty), death certificates, autopsy reports, medical records, mental health records, family advocacy and other helping services records, local criminal records, financial and credit reports, personnel records, personnel information files, national criminal databases, and Servicemembers' Group Life Insurance paperwork (Hourani, Hilton, Kennedy, & Robbins, 2001).

Also in 1999, the Air Force instituted the Suicide Event Surveillance System (SESS). This reporting system required agents from the Office of Special Investigations to enter completed suicide data and the mental health staff to enter records of suicide attempts. The SESS was a web-based tool that allowed for direct reporting from any authorized Air Force site in the world. Data sources included all those listed for DONSIR as well as interviews with military members and their families. The U.S. Army tracked suicide data with psychological autopsy reports (Rothberg, 1998) and used a data-gathering surveillance worksheet for suicides based on the SESS model. Information from death records was also obtained.

Given these varied programs, SPARRC recommended that each service maintain separate suicide surveillance databases and that program managers provide the DoD with a required combined report. Such a model would improve DoD population health and prevention efforts by allowing each service to collect and analyze pooled demographics and potential risk factors across the DoD. Differences as well as similarities between personnel of the various services could also be established. As a result, targeted education and risk reduction could be implemented to decrease future suicide events.

In January 2008, the DoD Suicide Event Report (DoDSER) was launched as the first standardized tri-service suicide data registry, replacing the DONSIR that had served to inform its development (Defense Centers of Excellence, 2010). DoDSER collects data on suicide attempts as well as completions and applies not only to active-duty DON personnel but Army, Air Force, and Coast Guard personnel as well. With a major software revision deployed in August 2009 by the National Center for Telehealth & Technology (T2), the secure log-in site allows T2 to:

- Describe the current status
- Track trends and identify patterns
  - Within suicides
  - Between those with suicide behaviors and the population
  - Between the military and civilian cases
- Examine risk factors unique to service members
- Identify possible solutions or interventions
- Evaluate the effectiveness of programs and policies
- Provide senior leaders quality data

The combined suicide database of the DoDSER is an important movement in the development of comparable base population data across services. This joint suicide surveillance program and database now have standardized data collection procedures and enable comparisons across services on some key risk factors. Having access to these comparable data across all services will help researchers, suicide prevention program evaluators, and policymakers to mitigate the issues and limitations of the low base rate of suicide in the military and better inform the development and improvement of suicide prevention efforts.

RESOURCE ISSUES IN SUICIDE PREVENTION AND TREATMENT

Resources

Suicide prevention is a top priority for all mental health providers. This is especially true for the military mental health community, considering the unique stressors placed on the men and women of the armed forces. A large cadre of military and civilian mental health providers from varying backgrounds (e.g., psychologists, psychiatrists, clinical social workers) serve members of the armed forces both in and outside of military treatment facilities across the globe. However, the need for mental health professionals often exceeds the available resources. Additionally, while some service members prefer to see only uniformed mental health providers, others do not feel comfortable receiving mental health treatment within the military. In an effort to ensure that a range of mental health intervention and treatment options are available to members of the military, three initiatives have been implemented by the DoD to complement military healthcare: Military OneSource (2011), Defense Centers of Excellence for Psychological Health and Traumatic Brain Injury (2011), and the National Suicide Prevention Lifeline (2011); all three resources can be reached on a 24-hour basis by phone, e-mail, and live chat.

Military OneSource has evolved from discrete branch-focused websites with separate telephone numbers for accessing services to a comprehensive benefit focusing on the military as a whole. Military OneSource strives to provide a one-stop shop for all members of the military—active, reserve, and guard, as well as family members. Service members and their families can visit *www.militaryonesource.com* or use the toll-free referral and information service (1-800-342-9647), available 24 hours per day, every day of the year. Military OneSource offers a range of services, from relocation assistance to parenting support, and includes mental health resources. Of direct relevance to the DoD's suicide prevention efforts, Military OneSource counselors are available at all hours to guide service members in need of help to appropriate resources. In addition, service members can be connected to civilian mental health providers for 12 free counseling sessions, 11 of which are face to face. This is a critical service when military members and their families do not have access to a military treatment facility or prefer civilian care.

The Defense Centers of Excellence for Psychological Health and Traumatic Brain Injury was established in 2007 by the DoD with the primary mission of serving military members and their families regarding psychological health and traumatic brain injury. Their strategy is to coordinate with a number of military and civilian agencies to facilitate the establishment of policies, procedures, research initiatives, and clinical practices that are in the best interests of military members and their families. Their efforts have had a positive impact in a number of domains, including increased consistency in mental health and traumatic brain injury care across the nation within military and civilian institutions that serve members of the military. Readers can learn more about Defense Centers of Excellence efforts to help service members and their families and available resources at *www.dcoe.health.mil* or at their 24-hour Outreach Center (1-866-966-1020).

The National Suicide Prevention Lifeline, at 1-800-273-TALK (8255), is a free 24-hour confidential crisis hotline service for individuals who are thinking about suicide or are in emotional distress. Callers will be automatically connected to the nearest crisis facility to receive telephonic counseling and appropriate referrals within their local area. Veterans and active-duty military members may also "press 1" to be connected to a military-specific call center located at the Veteran's Affairs Center of Excellence in Canandaigua, New York; this service has been formally endorsed by the DoD.

Service Collaborative Efforts

Leadership Guides for Managing Service Members in Distress

One particular benefit of SPARRC is the sharing of successful resources. The Air Force led the services in their effort to develop a leadership guide for managing service members in distress. In short, this guide helped leaders learn about crises, available resources, how to apply specific kinds of assistance for particular situations, techniques to enhance peer support and self-care strategies, and effective ways to enhance mission readiness. The Air Force leadership guide was a highly successful and popular aspect of their overall suicide prevention effort. The Navy and Marine Corps soon followed suit and developed their own leadership guides based on the Air Force model. The Marine Corps modified the format to more closely match the culture of the Marine Corps and developed a more dynamic website. Demonstrating the benefit of collaboration through the SPARRC and continuous improvement, the Navy recently recrafted their site using a hybrid of the Air Force and Marine Corps models, more effectively leveraging Navy culture. The Army decided not to develop a complete leaders' guide, but did modify the Marine Corps section on suicide prevention to be an Army leaders' guide. Regardless of any service's specific differences, the message remained the same: Once a leader is informed or notices a problem with a service member, he or she needs to get involved and offer help. Links to each service's leadership guide can be found in the reference section: U.S. Air Force (2011a, 2011b), U.S. Army (2011), U.S. Marine Corps (2011), and U.S. Navy (2011).

Frontline Supervisor's Training: PRESS Model

In 2006, the four military branches joined together along with civilian subject matter experts in San Antonio, Texas, at the invitation of the Air Force. The intent was to develop a joint training course to address service member distress and prevent suicides. The eventual course Frontline Supervisors Training, was designed with midmanagement enlisted troops in mind (e.g., noncommissioned officers, petty officers). As most suicides occur among young, enlisted troops, midmanagement enlisted leaders are more likely than other echelons of leadership to notice service members in distress. However, they are typically the least trained within management to handle such personnel-related problems. The PRESS model for suicide gatekeeper training is Prepare (know your subordinates), Recognize (the signs of distress), Engage (your subordinate to find out about their distress), Send (them for help) and Sustain (stay involved during and after treatment). Unlike the Leadership Guides, this resource was developed from inception as a collaborative effort. The services' desire to remain true to their unique cultures and best educate their service members resulted in each branch modifying the training to varying degrees, and implementing it through different procedures. The Air Force's training manual is available online (U.S. Air Force, 2011a, 2011b).

Nomenclature

Suicide nomenclature has been a challenge for decades, as outlined in the Tower of Babel articles (O'Carroll et al., 1996; Silverman, Berman, Sanddal, O'Carroll, & Joiner, 2007). The 2009 DoD and VA Health Executive Council's joint strategic plan mandated that the DoD and VA decide upon a standardized nomenclature system for the reporting of suicides (VA/DoD, 2009). SPARRC, the VA National Suicide Prevention Office, the Mortality Surveillance Division of the Armed Forces Medical Examiner, and CDC took up the task. Ultimately, it was decided to adopt the self-directed violence classification system (Brenner, 2010; U.S. Department of Defense Task Force, 2010). Agreement on the following terms has the potential to increase consistency dramatically within and across the DoD, VA, and CDC: nonsuicidal self-directed violence ideation, suicidal ideation, self-directed violence, nonsuicidal self-directed violence, undetermined self-directed violence, suicidal self-directed violence, suicide attempt, suicide, suicidal intent, preparatory behavior, physical injury, interrupted self-directed violence—by another, interrupted self-directed violence—by self, and fatal.

Service-Level Policy

Army

The Army has launched the most involved and wide-reaching analysis of risk and resilience ever conducted. This Army Study to Assess Risk and Resilience of Suicide (STARRS) began in fall 2010 and will run through 2014, releasing results as they become available. Historically, the Army's suicide rate was lower than that of the civilian population. However, beginning in 2002 its suicide rate began to climb, reaching all-time highs in 2007, 2008, and 2009 (Army STARRS, 2010). The Army responded to this alarming trend by contacting the National Institute of Mental Health for help to better understand psychological resilience, mental health, and risk for self-harm among soldiers. The result was the creation of a multidisciplinary research team from various military and civilian institutions that designed a study with four components: Historical Data Study, New Soldier Study, All Army Study, and the Soldier Health Outcomes Study. Each study seeks to determine risk and protective factors among soldiers at varying points in their military service in an effort to "identify character-istics, events, experiences, and exposures that predict negative or positive health and behavior outcomes" (Army STARRS, 2010).

In 2009, the Army addressed the immediate need for answers to the increasing rate of suicide via the creation of the Army Task Force on Suicide Prevention. This temporary multidisciplinary team, answerable directly to the Secretary of the Army, produced the New Campaign Plan, which syn-chronizes and integrates Army efforts for health promotion, risk reduction, and suicide prevention.

One specific new initiative the Army released for soldiers is an interac-tive video called "Beyond the Front" (WILL Interactive, 2011). This train-ing tool provides an interactive experience in which soldiers have to make decisions based on situational circumstances. The objective is to help sol-diers make the right choices to save a life, reduce stigma, and promote resiliency.

Marine Corps

The Marine Corps has designed and implemented a program known as Never Leave a Marine Behind (2011), a series of suicide prevention train-ings tailored according to rank. The first course was released in 2009, tar-geted to noncommissioned officers. Early results showed a reduction in sui-cides among this targeted population. Intended to be evocative, interactive, engaging courses, more are scheduled for release in 2010 (E1–E3 Marines) and 2011 (staff noncommissioned officers, officers, and family members).

In addition to contacting Military OneSource, Marines also have the option of contacting the newly created D-Stress hotline. The hotline was developed to provide a safety net around a those Marines who may not call OneSource or the National Lifeline because of their perception that these resources do not understand Marine Corps culture. The hotline is manned by former Marines, who provide an immediate experience of comfort and familiarity for Marine callers in distress. This program was launched as a pilot study in the western United States and will be phased in across the world after demonstrating success with supporting Marines.

The Operational Stress Control & Readiness (OSCAR, 2006) pro-gram was initiated in 1999 at Camp Lejeune, North Carolina; in 2003, it was broadened to include all three Marine Corps divisions. The program imbeds psychologists and psychiatrists at the level of an infantry regiment, air wing, or logistics group. The constant presence of mental health assets as organic to a unit prior to, during, and after deployments has helped to reduce stigma and increase mental health awareness and access to care. The practice model is quite different for mental health professionals as OSCAR providers spend much of their time involved with outreach as opposed to the traditional role of clinic-based care. The general guiding principle for an OSCAR mental health provider is to be as close to the fighting force as possible from start to finish of a deployment cycle.

Navy

The Navy launched a modified Frontline Supervisors Training program in April 2010, which includes a comprehensive suicide prevention kit. The training walks attendees through a case study, and the kit includes a new prevention video entitled "Suicide Prevention: A Message from Survivors." This video is a collection of documentary interviews with survivors of suicide attempts or sailors who helped a peer through a suicide crisis. It is designed to be used with small group discussions during training.

The Navy has also developed and delivered Suicide Awareness and Prevention (2012) Workshops, intended to provide fleet leadership with information on all available resources. In addition, these workshops act to institutionalize Navy requirements regarding both the implementation and execution of suicide prevention and awareness policies. Initiatives such as this ensure that policies developed at a central headquarters are, in fact, effectively disseminated throughout the organization.

The Naval Center for Combat & Operational Stress Control (NCCOSC; 2011) is a relatively new initiative of the U.S. Navy Bureau of Medicine and Surgery, which seeks to promote resilience and to put in place best practices for accurate diagnosis and treatment of posttraumatic stress disorder and traumatic brain injury (NCCOSC). One of their primary goals is to teach sailors, Marines, and their family members ways to recognize and treat signs of stress before more severe problems develop.

Air Force

The Air Force has an extensive and successful history of suicide prevention efforts and programs and has often led the services in this domain (Jones et al., 2006). After many successful years of suicide reduction after the implementation of their 1996 suicide prevention program (Knox et al., 2003), the Air Force responded to recent increases in suicide rates with an all-hands half-day "Wingman Stand-Down 2010" for all units that featured leader-led training in suicide prevention to reemphasize the importance of adherence to their program elements. After the stand-down, the Air Force implemented a tiered-training approach to prevent suicide and increase resilience. All personnel complete annual suicide prevention training using computer-based training, but certain career fields, such as military security forces and law enforcement with double the risk for suicide (Helmkamp, 1996), are required to engage in face-to-face training. Supervisors in those fields must complete the jointly developed Frontline Supervisor Training course (U.S. Air Force, 2011b). The Air Force is also developing a series of interactive videos that depict risk factors for suicide in a variety of Air Force work environments (e.g., security forces, aircraft maintenance, and intelligence) and family situations (in the home and relationship problems).

CLINICAL MANAGEMENT OF SUICIDAL PATIENTS

In the mental health arena, suicidal patients are the most common emergency cases seen by clinicians. Caring for suicidal patients consistently ranks as the most stressful occupational challenge faced by mental health professionals (see discussion in Berman & Jobes, 1991). Summarizing recent research, Bongar (2002) indicates that trainees had a 1 in 7 chance of losing a patient to suicide, whereas over the course of their careers psychologists had a 1 in 3 chance and psychiatrists a 1 in 2 chance of experiencing such a loss. He concludes that training programs need to convey that patient suicide is a "real occupational hazard for those clinicians involved in direct patient care" (p. xxi). If the public health threat of suicide is so real that clinicians need to soberly consider the possibility of losing a patient to suicide, then military providers must heed this warning even more, given the unique challenges they face in conducting their clinical activities in difficult environments such as hostile fire zones, remote duty stations, shipboard operations, and overseas settings (Johnson & Kennedy, 2010). To support the fighting force, military mental health professionals must be expert at integrating clinical care and risk management strategies. For an example of a training initiative to enhance the confidence of Air Force clinicians in dealing with suicidal patients, see Oordt et al. (2005).

Service members identified as an increased or imminent risk, but who might be unwilling to seek mental health services on a voluntary basis can be command referred for a routine or emergency evaluation (DoD, 1997a, 1997b). During this process, the clinician is responsible for consulting with the command to ensure the service member's safety, conduct and document a thorough assessment, determine whether outpatient treatment or inpatient hospitalization is clinically indicated, and make recommendations regarding appropriateness of continued service. Both self- and command-referred suicidal service members often present to or are escorted to a military treatment facility for evaluation by any number of personnel (e.g., chain of command, colleague, chaplain). Particularly in deployed settings where immediate access to clinicians can be greatly limited, early identification and management of a suicidal service member may originate with a "battle buddy," combat corpsman or medic, physician's assistant, medical officer, or chaplain from the unit until a mental health provider can travel to the service member or the patient can be evacuated to a higher level of care, such as an area combat stress control team or hospital mental health staff.

In the discussion that follows, we examine the referral processes, safety procedures, and intervention strategies that commanders and helping professionals can use to reduce suicide risk and promote healthy resolution of psychiatric emergencies. Specific attention is given here to identifying cases and referrals, gathering critical assessment data through interviews and consultations, formulating a diagnostic picture, estimating risk, and determining the appropriate level of care. This section concludes with a discussion of dispositional considerations in consulting with commanders about fitness for duty and suitability for military service.

Case Identification and Referral

The cornerstone of military suicide prevention efforts is training leaders (e.g., supervisors), community gatekeepers (e.g., school leaders and agency personnel), coworkers, and family members to act as first responders. A first responder is someone who recognizes the threat or risk of suicide and acts to decrease the risk by linking the suicidal person to an appropriate source of help. Typically, first responders are people in the family, military unit, or work center who have occasion to observe or interact with someone at risk for suicide. The problem is that when someone is in crisis, no one person has all the pieces of the puzzle at his or her disposal to immediately identify the level of risk. For example, a coworker may know about a colleague's dissatisfaction with her job but may not know that she had a previous suicide attempt or has a family history of depression and suicide. Given that more than 80% of those who attempt suicide provide verbal and behavioral clues prior to the incident (Berman & Jobes, 1991), the key to a proactive response is taking seriously anyone who talks about suicide. The questions asked by first responders and the actions they take play an indispensable role in keeping suicidal people safe. For military populations, several tools to educate first responders have been developed. For example, as a metaphor for actions to support individuals deemed at risk for suicide, the Air Force created the acronym LINK: Look for possible concerns, Inquire about those concerns, Note the level of risk, and Know your referral sources and strategies (Staal, 2001; U.S. Department of the Air Force, 2003b). An at-risk person needs immediate attention from professional caregivers. The Army uses the acronym ACE (Act, Care, and Escort) to outline action steps in caring for fellow soldiers (U.S. Army Public Health Command, 2009).

At their heart, the LINK and ACE training strategies emphasize the critical role of first responders in observing problem behaviors and initiating referrals for further assessment to determine the level of risk and intervention options. Another significant aspect of these strategies is to destigmatize help-seeking behaviors for personnel and their families. Once a case is identified, the referral process begins. What may vary is the immediacy of access to specialty consultations and inpatient care for those needing to be in a safe environment. Across a variety of military settings (e.g., hospitals, shipboard operations, field training, combat operations), the essential features of the referral process are similar: (1) Identify the person at risk, (2) link the person to professional support (e.g., chaplains or medical personnel) and inform the chain of command, (3) obtain medical assessment (e.g., triage, emergency room visit, specialty consults, and laboratory panels when indicated), and (4) pursue mental health consultation and evaluation (e.g., safety assessment, determination of treatment level, liaison with the command about findings).

Gathering Critical Assessment Data

The military provides a unique environment in which clinically rich and relevant information is readily available from sources often nonexistent in a civilian setting that patients may not provide themselves. Given the close quarters, accountability, and visibility by peers and command, particularly on deployment, interview and consultation with such sources can often provide critical information and behavioral observations to complement a risk assessment (Payne, Hill, & Johnson, 2008). Also invaluable in terms of assessing psychiatric and medical history is the military's current electronic medical records system for service members and their dependents, the Armed Forces Health Longitudinal Technology Application (AHLTA), which can be accessed from most military treatment facilities stateside and overseas. Even in the deployed environment, clinicians are gaining ever-increasing access to relevant databases, including multiple versions of AHLTA and the Theater Medical Data Store, now allowing for review of medical records generated in theater.

Given that an at-risk person has been appropriately identified and referred, what is the most critical information that helping professionals need to determine diagnosis, level of risk, and intervention options (e.g., outpatient management vs. inpatient treatment)? Efforts directed toward answering this question have produced a large, diverse, and sometimes confusing literature on the assessment of suicide risk, including that for military populations. Indeed, Shaffer (1997) criticized military training materials from the 1980s and early 1990s for the use of unweighted lists of risk factors and warning signs that tend to combine without distinction highly predictive risk factors (e.g., suicide statements and previous attempts) with warning signs common for both suicidal and nonsuicidal populations that have relatively low predictive value (e.g., financial and relationship problems). The net effect was to create long lists of difficult-to-remember warning signs that reduced the visibility and significance of critical factors such as a history of attempts, current suicidal ideation, and a history of depression.

Even with knowledge of the most critical risk factors, it is important to note that "hard and fast actuarial data on the long-term prediction of attempted or completed suicide—predictions that can be directly translated to the emergent clinical moment—do not currently exist" (Bongar, 2002, p. 88). To rephrase the question posed earlier in this section, how do we obtain critical information for risk assessment? The answer, simply put, is to conduct a good diagnostic interview (Rosenberg, 1999; Shea, 1998). The components of such an interview include (1) obtaining identifying information and relevant facts about the presenting problem; (2) gathering information about the history of the problem and other pertinent history (e.g., medical, psychiatric, medication, social, and family data); (3) conducting a mental health screening to assess depression, anxiety, substance use, and psychosis; (4) eliciting specific information about key risk and protective factors; (5) conducting a suicide-specific inquiry about past behavior, present ideation, and intent and access to means for self-harm; (6) formulating a diagnosis and attempting to engage in a safety contract; and (7) estimating the level of risk and making recommendations about the level of care and follow-up (e.g., outpatient vs. inpatient support).

In recent years, input from leading suicidologists has improved education on suicide assessment in the DoD through consultation, training symposia, and research. With respect to policy guidance on risk assessment, military mental health providers follow the accepted canons of professional governing bodies (e.g., American Psychiatric Association and American Psychological Association) regarding the ethical and legal obligations of clinicians to give reasonable care to patients deemed at risk for harm to themselves or others. DoD policy places mental health evaluations related to imminent danger under the purview of credentialed DoD psychologists, psychiatrists, and doctoral-level social workers. However, in practice, initial assessments are often conducted by a variety of professionals, including general medical officers, alcohol counselors, chaplains, psychiatric technicians, and emergency room personnel. According to DoD Instruction 6490.4 (DoD, 1997a), mental health evaluations should include a record review, clinical history, mental status examination, assessments for suicide and homicide potential, psychological testing (if applicable), physical examination (if applicable), diagnosis, and recommendations for treatment and administrative management. Specific questions in the DoD instruction related to suicide assessment are discussed later in this section.

With respect to the methodology of risk assessment, the preponderance of literature focuses on guidelines for data to be gathered, risk factor information, and the clinical decision-making process. Relatively little attention has been given to conducting suicide-focused clinical interviews. The task of obtaining interview data requires both compassionate concern and a tenacious pursuit of critical information from the patient and/or collateral sources (e.g., family members, coworkers, and command representatives). Indeed, the first objective in managing a suicidal emergency is establishing a sound working alliance with the patient (Kleespies, Deleppo, Gallagher, & Niles, 1999). Shea (1998) noted that "if ever there were a moment of critical importance in interviewing, it is the moment when one listens for the harbingers of death" (p. 444). Interviewers who are comfortable talking about a subject as difficult as suicide can offer a basis of hope and set the groundwork for patients to make life-affirming choices in dealing with their pain and despair. One practical methodology for eliciting information from patients on the presence and extent of suicidal ideation is the chronological assessment of suicide events (CASE). The CASE approach (Shea, 1998) offers clinicians an easily learned structure for gathering critical information in four specific regions of inquiry: (1) the presenting concern or suicidal event, (2) recent ideation and incidents over the past 2 months, (3) past suicidal events (2+ months and beyond), and (4) immediate ideation and plans for the future. What is useful for the present discussion is the ease with which questions specified in DoD policy related to suicidal ideation, intent, plan, behaviors, and attempts can be adapted in the CASE approach. The following structured interview links assessment questions from DoD to the natural flow of topics from the CASE approach.

Presenting Ideation or Event

Questions for patients who present with potential suicidal ideation

- "Do you have any thoughts about suicide or hurting yourself?"
- "How long have you had these thoughts?"
- "Do you wish to die?"
- "Do you have a specific plan or intent to kill yourself? Will you hurt yourself or allow yourself to be hurt 'accidentally' or on purpose?"
- "Do you have access to a weapon or other ways to kill yourself?"

Questions for patients who present after a suicide gesture or attempt

- "What did you do to try to kill/hurt yourself?" (Obtain specific information, e.g., the number of pills, amount of alcohol consumed, type of cuts made).
- "Was there a particular stressor or set of stressors that prompted your suicide attempt?"
- "Did you intend to die?"
- "How long had you been planning to do this?"

- "How were you found? How did you get to the hospital?"
- "What are your thoughts about being alive now?"

Recent Suicidal Events (Past 1–2 Months)

- "During this past couple of months, did you think about any ways to commit suicide?"
- "During this time, did you take any action with the intent of killing yourself, but not go through with it?"
- "Over the past month, how much time daily did you think about killing yourself?"
- "As you thought about suicide, was there something you thought would happen or you would achieve through your death?"

Past Suicidal Events (More Than 2 Months Past)

- "Have you ever tried to kill yourself in the past, including when you were a teenager or a child?"
- "If so, what did you do? How many times did this happen? How serious were your injuries? Were you hospitalized? Did you want to die?"
- "What about vague suicidal thoughts/feelings in the past? What were the circumstances?"
- "Has a family member or a friend ever made a suicide attempt or died by suicide? If so, who and when?"

Immediate Concerns

- "Right now, are you having thoughts of killing yourself?"
- "If you had suicidal thoughts later today or tomorrow, what would you do?"
- "Are you willing to make a safety contract so you agree not to kill or hurt yourself?" If yes, write the patient's statement (see Bongar, 2002, for a discussion on the risks and benefits of "no suicide" safety contracts). If no, determine the level of risk and, if warranted, seek consultation regarding psychiatric hospitalization. With answers to these questions in hand, clinicians can move to the next steps in suicide assessment: formulating diagnoses, estimating risk, and determining level of intervention.

Diagnoses, Risk Estimation, and Level of Intervention

When working in a military setting, there are several salient risk factors to take into consideration that may not generalize to a civilian clinical population. For example, Army Suicide Event Report data (2007) suggested that only one-quarter of soldiers who completed suicide had been diagnosed with a psychiatric condition. Furthermore, many military members do not seek out mental health services or demonstrate acute stress or suicidality prior to the suicide act (Hill, Johnson, & Barton, 2006; Payne et al., 2008). Of course, these findings regarding a lack of both formal psychiatric diagnoses or expressed suicidal intent must be interpreted with caution. Relationship and marital stressors are frequently cited stressors among service members who complete suicide. Chart reviews also highlight a possible relationship between disciplinary measures and suicidal thoughts and behavior (Hill et al., 2006). Whereas unit cohesion is cited as a key protective factor in resiliency to combat stress (U.S. Department of the Army, 2006), pressures to conform, fit in, and adhere to the standard can also contribute to maladjustment and increased risk in military populations (Hill et al., 2006). These factors, especially when coupled with a deployed environment where nearly anyone may exhibit some degree of stress or unhappiness at one point or another, can make it particularly challenging to accurately determine and predict those who may go on to attempt or complete suicide.

As in the civilian sector, the fourth edition (text revision) of the American Psychiatric Association's (2000) *Diagnostic and Statistical Manual of Mental Disorders* (DSM-IV-TR) provides the diagnostic framework for mental health decisions in the military. According to DSM-IV-TR, psychiatric diagnoses fall into two broad categories: clinical disorders and other conditions that may be a focus of clinical attention (Axis I) and personality disorders (Axis II). Axis I disorders commonly seen in the military population are V codes (e.g., partner relationship problems), adjustment disorders, anxiety disorders (including posttraumatic stress disorder), substance-related disorders (primarily alcohol abuse/dependence), mood disorders, and psychotic disorders. Personality disorders are enduring patterns of thinking and behaving that result in significant distress or impairment in social and/or occupational functioning. Following from the finding that more than 90% of adults who died by suicide had a diagnosable mental disorder at the time of death, a number of authors have advocated the use of diagnoses associated with high suicide risk in community-based studies as guides for risk assessment in acute cases. Kleespies et al. (1999), summarized findings from studies of completed suicides in which depression was estimated to be a factor in 50% of suicides, alcohol and drug abuse in approximately 20–25%, and schizophrenia in 10%. Duberstein and Conwell (1997) reviewed a number of studies and concluded that 30–40% of all suicides are completed by individuals with Axis II disorders. Of the various types of Axis II disorders, borderline personality disorder and antisocial personality disorder have been most associated with increased suicide risk.

Taken together, these risk estimates suggest that a significant overlap exists between high-risk Axis I and Axis II disorders (Kleespies et al., 1999).

Based on current symptoms, history of suicidal behavior, other risk factors, and the relative presence or absence of protective factors, Joiner, Walker, Rudd, and Jobes (1999), proposed a graduated 5-point continuum for determining suicide risk, ranging from nonexistent to extreme. This continuum offers differential considerations for patients who present with suicidal ideation (SI), no history of suicide attempts (nonmultiple attempters, or NMA), and histories of multiple attempts (MA). Additionally, this framework gives weight to the presence of suicidal desire and plans or preparation for suicide. As this framework has practical value for clinicians in not only estimating risk but also suggesting intervention options, it bears some discussion here. Points on the risk continuum include (1) nonexistent—no current symptoms, no history of suicidal behavior, and few risk factors present; (2) mild—NMA with suicidal ideation of low intensity and short duration or MA with no other risk factors; (3) moderate—MA with current risk factors, NMA with moderate to severe symptoms related to suicidal plans or preparation, or NMA with moderate to severe symptoms of SI but no or limited plans; (4) severe—NMA with moderate to severe symptoms regarding suicide plans and at least one other significant risk factor or MA with two or more risk factors or notable findings; (5) extreme—MA with severe symptoms and specific plans or NMA with plans or preparation for suicide and two or more other risk factors. As an aid in clinical decision making, these risk estimates are linked to intervention options recommended by Joiner et al. (1999) and are integrated with concerns for military providers (see Table 9.1).

Dispositional Considerations of Fitness and Suitability

In the military, diagnostic decisions, estimates of risk, and intervention options are closely linked to dispositional considerations of fitness for duty (for further information, see Chapter 2, this volume). Although the concept of fitness implies a dichotomous decision (fit vs. unfit), in practice there are gradations that permit some flexibility in making personnel decisions. For example, after a course of treatment (outpatient and/or inpatient), a service member whose suicidal ideation was deemed resolved or who made a suicide gesture without serious intent to die may be returned to his or her unit as fit for duty. If the severity of the presenting problem requires more extensive treatment with a specialty provider, a service member can be placed on limited-duty status for a set period of time, usually 6 or 8 months. In cases in which an individual's diagnosis reflects a severe mental illness (e.g., severe mood disorders and psychotic disorders) and the person has a limited probability of returning to full-duty status, then he or she

TABLE 9.1. Risk Estimates and Intervention Options

Level of risk	Intervention considerations and options
Nonexistent/ minimal	• Affirm present coping skills. • Encourage use of social support and seeking help. • Reiterate availability of support and access to emergency services; provide phone contact numbers.
Mild	• Bolster coping skills through individual/group counseling/treatment. • Encourage increased social support at home and/or within the unit. • Liaison with command regarding service member's status. • Reiterate contract for safety and options for crisis intervention (e.g., availability of phone contact, walk-in visits, access to emergency services).
Moderate	• Increase frequency/duration of outpatient follow-up (set plans to address current stressors and reduce symptoms). • Encourage active involvement of family and/or supportive friends/coworkers; engage command support; seek input regarding risk factors. • Reevaluate treatment goals and target suicide-specific concerns (e.g., reduce clinical symptoms and reduce suicidal ideation, reduce feelings of hopelessness, improve problem solving and adaptive coping, and mobilize support system and ensure accessibility to such support). • Consider medication evaluation, if not already in use. • Seek consultation for risk assessment and treatment planning, including indications for psychiatric hospitalization. • Encourage telephone contacts for monitoring purposes. • Reiterate contract for safety and provide business card/phone contacts regarding availability of emergency services. • Modify environment to support safety (e.g., patient turns in pills, weapons). • Advise command regarding deployment suitability and availability for assignment to special duty (e.g., shipboard or overseas duty).
Severe/ extreme	• Provide immediate evaluation for mental health hospitalization. • Initiate protocol for involuntary commitment, if warranted. • Ensure patient is escorted to all medical appointments; monitor patient at all times; engage active involvement of family and command (and police if needed). • Monitor patient at appropriate precaution level (e.g., one to one, line of sight). • As many of the items from the "moderate" level also apply here, make adjustments to the treatment plan as warranted, given changes in symptom/risk level. • Consider aeromedical evacuation to a higher echelon of care, if warranted.

Note. Data from Joiner, Walker, Rudd, and Jobes (1999).

can be processed for a medical discharge. The responsibility for making diagnostic decisions about a military member's psychiatric fitness for duty rests with the local mental health provider. In most cases, the acuity or chronicity of the presenting problem plays a major role in determining a member's duty status. The ultimate determination rests with the Central Physical Evaluation Board in Washington, DC.

Another concept pertinent to military dispositions is suitability. Whereas fitness refers to Axis I, or clinical syndromes, the idea of suitability generally concerns the Axis II, or personality disorder, dimension of diagnoses. Suitability concerns the personality traits, coping skills, and interpersonal capabilities of service members to perform their duties in a safe and harmonious way in their units. Members deemed unsuitable on the basis of a personality disorder may be recommended for administrative separation from the armed services. A personality disorder diagnosis in and of itself, however, does not mean that a person is unsuitable for the military. Typically, a recommendation for separation is made only if the service member's personality problems have been documented to show interference with his or her performance of duty.

Given the weight accorded mental health recommendations in most military settings, providers can often exercise considerable influence on the lives of service members. This is particularly true in dispositional decisions (e.g., evaluations of fitness for duty and determinations of eligibility for security clearances or special assignments), where concerns about suicide or homicide risk may affect a service member's capacity for retention in the military and/or ability to deploy to operational environments. Clinical management in the military thus requires a decision framework in which three separate but related perspectives must be considered: individual status, command mission, and clinical resources; Table 9.2 summarizes key considerations from each perspective. Clinicians and command leaders must weigh the prior factors in deciding to treat members by using local

TABLE 9.2. Case Management Considerations

Individual status	Command mission	Clinical resources
• Diagnostic concerns (acute vs. chronic symptoms/effect on work performance) • Quality of relational support • Legal/administrative concerns • Responsiveness to treatment	• Operational status (type/intensity of work) • Theater of service • Manning requirements • Likelihood of hazardous duty and/or combat deployment	• Treatment availability (outpatient vs. inpatient) Healthcare requirements • Access to specialty care • Aeromedical capabilities

assets or to move them to other echelons of care. Ultimately, diagnostic concerns, mission requirements, and clinical capabilities must be factored into decisions about the return of patients to duty or in making recommendations for administrative separation or medical discharge.

If, after weighing diagnostic and risk-level considerations, a clinician decides to manage a patient on an outpatient basis, then the clinician, patient, and command need to arrange follow-up appointments, discuss level of day-to-day monitoring or establish a predetermined call-in plan, encourage social support (e.g., ensure the person is included in activities or unit functions), and develop a safety plan for emergency contacts if suicidal ideation or behavior recurs. In the past, recommendations typically focused on suggestions on "how not to get sued" and emphasized clinical failures derived from litigation scenarios (Bongar, 2002). While such legal concerns are real, some clinical suicidologists are seeking to develop practice recommendations based on clinical and empirical findings. Although only a few conclusions can be drawn to date, some recommendations do appear to have adequate support (Rudd, Joiner, Jobes, & King, 1999) and merit consideration by military clinicians: (1) intensive follow-up is most effective for patients with a high risk (e.g., history of multiple attempts, mental health history, and/or diagnostic comorbidity); (2) short-term cognitive-behavioral therapy methods that focus on problem solving have been shown to be effective at reducing suicidal ideation and hopelessness for periods of up to 1 year; (3) efforts to reduce suicide attempts require longer treatments that target skill deficits in regulating emotion, tolerating distress, managing anger, and enhancing interpersonal effectiveness; and (4) suicidal patients deemed high risk can be treated on an outpatient basis if psychiatric hospitalization is available for acute situations.

In regard to inpatient treatment, Bongar (2002) summarized the goals of psychiatric hospitalization as (1) protecting the life and safety of suicidal patients; (2) reducing or eliminating suicidal ideation by treating underlying mental disorders; and (3) improving the capacities, skills, and psychosocial resources that foster improved coping by patients after discharge. In the military, service members' chain of command often places them on a safety watch as the most common alternative to or step-down from inpatient psychiatric hospitalization for suicidal ideation and gestures as well as homicidal ideation, self-injurious behavior, and excessive alcohol use (Hassinger, 2003). Safety watches involve close observation (monitoring) and unit assistance (mentoring) by the individual's unit at the direction of a mental health clinician (Hassinger, 2003) and should be considered a temporary level of intervention, as it provides recommendations and restrictions to the command in ensuring the service member's safety and well-being (Payne et al., 2008). The tool is most commonly employed with young, junior enlisted service members who have not been diagnosed with a significant psychiatric condition (Hassinger, 2003) and requires patient reassessment and watch every 2 to 3 days or sooner should the service member demonstrate a decline in functioning or increase in risk (Hassinger, 2003; Hill et al., 2006; Payne et al., 2008).

Depending on the stipulations, safety watches can be delineated as "Buddy Watch" with direct observation from first formation until lights out for lower risk service members (e.g., military-specific suicidal ideation, self-injurious behavior while intoxicated the night prior, or step-down from inpatient hospitalization) or 24-hour watch, where the service member is observed at all times when deemed to be of low to moderate risk (Payne et al., 2008). Related recommendations can range from search and removal of weapons (including firing bolt or pin) and prohibited use of alcohol to ordering a move into the barracks, limiting contact with individuals having a negative impact on the service member's functioning, or facilitating the service members attendance at scheduled appointments (Hassinger, 2003; Hill et al., 2006; Payne et al., 2008). The recommending clinician typically provides verbal consultation and written instructions to the identified escort and command, documenting a description of the service member's safety concerns, warning signs of and actions to take in case of deterioration or decompensation, restrictions to be placed upon the service member, and contact information for the provider (Hassinger, 2003; see Payne et al., 2008, for sample memorandums and operating procedures).

Particularly in contrast to psychiatric hospitalization, safety watches are considered to be less stigmatizing, costly, and resource intensive (Hassinger, 2003). When properly employed, they can also increase social support and interaction between service members, command, and mental health clinicians while avoiding the documented regression, alienation, and reduced retention rates that can occur with inpatient treatment. The available literature suggests that safety watches are most beneficial in cases of what is considered to be "conditional" or "military-specific" suicidal ideation, in which the service member's primary motivation to report or engage in the behavior is driven by a specific, desired outcome, such as avoidance of duty, transfer to another unit, or separation from service (Hassinger, 2003; Payne et al., 2008). Particularly in deployed military settings, weapons and ammunition can be readily accessible, mental health resources limited, and operational demands restrictive. Under such conditions, use of a safety watch can not only prove invaluable in helping conserve the fighting force, but also help mitigate the potential for "evacuation syndrome," wherein clusters of service members present to mental health with symptoms known to increase their chances of medical evacuation from theater (Hill et al., 2006; Payne et al., 2008).

One of the greatest shortcomings of safety watches is the lack of empirical support demonstrating their efficacy (Hassinger, 2003; Payne et al., 2008). Furthermore, by itself, a safety watch cannot be considered treatment and may still result in some degree of stigmatization of the identified service member as well as decreased morale of the unit in relation to personnel demands associated with providing the supervision and oversight. Those who have been shown to do poorly on safety watches may have unresolved psychiatric concerns, negative or hostile reaction from the unit, or an ulterior motive for their behavior (Hill et al., 2006). Overall, available anecdotal and retrospective chart reviews suggest a preponderance of adverse outcomes during watch while in garrison (Hassinger, 2003) and recovery with full return to duty within 2 weeks for most service members receiving psychiatric treatment while under watch in theater (Hill et al., 2006). Important factors for clinicians to consider when recommending a safety watch include the usefulness and relevance of the increased supervision, severity of the service member's psychiatric presentation and diagnosis, estimated level of risk and prognosis, and availability of unit resources (Hassinger, 2003).

Across the DoD, a large network of professionals is involved in providing outpatient and inpatient care on a daily basis to military members and their families. When treatments go well, patients get on with their lives and little attention is drawn to the services provided. When bad outcomes such as suicide occur, however, intense scrutiny can be brought to bear on the services and systems in place. In some cases, this scrutiny can engender a culture of fear, and little can be learned from the situation. In other cases, a process can unfold that brings to light service delivery problems that can be improved to prevent future incidents. An example of the latter in a military treatment facility is the Suicide Prevention Advisory Group, which met at Tripler Medical Center in Hawaii after a series of seven suicides in a 15-month span by patients recently evaluated by hospital staff or in active treatment (Hough, 2000). Each case was analyzed, and a series of 11 recommendations was ultimately presented to the hospital for implementation. Among the key recommendations were the following: (1) Provide ongoing education to mental health providers on the assessment and treatment of suicidal patients; (2) increase awareness in the local community about depression and risk factors for depression as well as awareness about the availability of treatment resources; (3) educate staff on the criteria to be used in making decisions about whether or not to admit patients to the psychiatry ward, including involuntary admissions; and (4) improve communication between the hospital and outlying clinics regarding suicidal patients. Implementation of these recommendations increased awareness of staff and residents about assessment and treatment of suicidal patients. Such awareness contributed to the ending of the suicide cluster, as no suicides occurred in the ensuing 22 months.

Several considerations are important concerning the return of service members to their units after psychiatric hospitalization (F. C. Budd, personal communication, March 2004): (1) clear communication by attending mental health providers to senior command leaders about patients' diagnosis and disposition, including a considered opinion about the prognosis; (2) documentation of a clear follow-up plan, including face-to-face appointments with a mental health provider on at least a weekly basis until patients' risk level is significantly reduced; and (3) advising patients of their responsibilities for treatment compliance and positive behavioral choices (e.g., commanders cannot overlook misconduct or irresponsible choices such as drinking and driving). Also, mental health providers need to recognize that commanders have an array of nonmedical options to support their troops, such as reassignment of service members to new work centers or supervisors for a "fresh start"; designation of a buddy or mentor to facilitate positive adjustment; and involvement of service members in social activities, educational pursuits, and special projects to promote competence and skill building. Patients recommended for separation from the service because of personality disorders or chronic adjustment problems need to be informed about the status of their cases. These patients sometimes generate animosity from others for not fulfilling their contracts or "not pulling their weight," but interest in their well-being can prevent an escalation of distress that could create an additional administrative burden or contribute to readmission for suicidal ideation or behavior.

SUMMARY

This chapter emphasized epidemiological concerns, suicide prevention resources, and clinical practices in assessment and treatment. Specific attention was given to four areas: cross-service comparisons, risks and protective factors, population-based research on suicides, and suicidal gestures and attempts. Multidisciplinary and community-based suicide prevention programs have been noted for each service. Also, practical strategies for clinical assessment and intervention were discussed with an eye to the issues and concerns of troop leaders. As the military has been at the forefront of national efforts in suicide prevention, continued collaboration among the services should spur further innovation in addressing suicide as a serious public health problem in the United States.

REFERENCES

American Association of Suicidology. (2012). U.S.A. suicide: 2007 official final data. Retrieved from *suicidology.org/e/document_library/get_file?folderId= 254&name-DLFE-441.pdf*. Accessed March 16, 2012.
American Association of Suicidology & U.S. Army Center for Health Promotion

and Preventive Medicine. (2000). *Suicide prevention: A resource manual for the United States Army.* Aberdeen Proving Ground, MD: Author.

American Psychiatric Association. (2000). *Diagnostic and statistical manual of mental disorders* (4th ed., text rev.). Washington, DC: Author.

Army Chief of Public Affairs. (2000, Spring). Hot topics: Suicide prevention. *Soldiers,* pp. 1–15.

Army STARRS. (2010). *Army Study to Assess Risk and Resilience in Servicemen.* Retrieved from *www.armystarrs.org.*

Army Suicide Event Report. (2007). Retrieved March 9, 2012, from *media. mcclatchydc.com/smedia/2009/05/29/19/Army-Suicide.source.prod_affiliate.91.pdf.*

Associated Press. (2008, February 12). *Most vet suicides among Guard, Reserve troops.* Retrieved February 5, 2011, from *www.msnbc.msn.com/id/23132421.*

Association of the United States Navy (AUSN). (2011). *Suicide rates among servicemembers and veterans alarm lawmakers.* Retrieved February 5, 2011, from *www.ausn.org/Advocacy/LegislativeUpdates/tabid/270/ArticleType/ArticleView/ArticleID/1784/Default.aspx.*

Berman, A. L., & Jobes, D. A. (1991). *Adolescent suicide assessment and intervention.* Washington, DC: American Psychological Association.

Black, S. A., Gallaway, M. S., Bell, M. R., & Ritchie, E. C. (2011). Prevalence and risk factors associated with suicides of Army soldiers 2001–2009. *Military Psychology, 23,* 433–451.

Bongar, B. (2002). *The suicidal patient: Clinical and legal standards of care* (2nd ed.). Washington, DC: American Psychological Association.

Bray, R. M., Hourani, L. L., Rae, K. L., Dever, J. A., Brown, J. M., Vincus, A. A., et al. (2003, November). *Department of Defense survey of health related behaviors among military personnel.* Raleigh, NC: Research Triangle Institute International.

Bray, R. M., Pemberton, M. R., Hourani, L. L., Witt, M., Rae Olmstead, K. L., Brown, J. M., et al. (2009, September). *2008 Department of Defense Survey of Health Related Behaviors among Active Duty Military Personnel.* Raleigh, NC: RTI International.

Brenner, L. A. (2010). *Self-directed violence classification system.* Retrieved January 30, 2011, from *www.mirecc.va.gov/visn19/docs/SDVCS.pdf.*

Bullman, T. A., & Kang, H. K. (1994). Posttraumatic stress disorder and the risk of traumatic deaths among Vietnam veterans. *Journal of Nervous and Mental Disease, 182,* 604–610.

Carr, J. R., Hoge, C. W., Gardner, J., & Potter, R. (2004). Suicide surveillance in the U.S. military—reporting and classification biases in rate calculations. *Suicide and Life-Threatening Behavior, 34*(3), 233–241.

Centers for Disease Control and Prevention. (1988). CDC recommendations for a community plan for the prevention and containment of suicide clusters. *Morbidity and Mortality Weekly Reports, 37*(S6), 1–12.

Centers for Disease Control and Prevention. (1997). Regional variations in suicide rates—United States, 1990–1994. *Morbidity and Mortality Weekly Reports, 46*(34), 789–793.

Centers for Disease Control and Prevention. (1998). Suicide among black youths—

United States, 1980–1995. *Morbidity and Mortality Weekly Reports, 47*(10), 193–196.

Centers for Disease Control and Prevention, National Center for Injury Prevention and Control. (2010). *WISQARS leading causes of death reports, 1999–2009)*. Retrieved from *webappa.cdc.gov/sasweb/ncipc/leadcaus10. html.*

Christenson, S. (2010, May 14). Army still plagued by suicides. *San Antonio Express-News.* Retrieved from *www.mysanantonia.com/news/military/article/Army-still-plagued-by-suicides-793814.php.*

Defense Centers of Excellence. (2010). *National Center for Telehealth and Technology.* Retrieved February 5, 2011, from *t2health.org/programs-surveillance. html.*

Defense Centers of Excellence. (2011). *What we do, who we are, how we do it.* Retrieved January 30, 2011, from *www.dcoe.health.mil.*

Defense Manpower Data Center. (2011). U.S.ctive dutymilitary deaths—1980 through 2011. Retrieved from *siadapp.dmdc.osd.mil/personnel/CASUALTY/ death_Rates1.pdf.*

Donnelly, J. M. (2011, January 24). Understanding suicides in the U.S. military. *CQ Weekly—Vantage Point,* p. 188.

Duberstein, P. R., & Conwell, Y. (1997). Personality disorders and completed suicide: A methodological and conceptual review. *Clinical Psychology: Science and Practice, 4*(4), 359–376.

Faberow, N. L., Kang, H. K., & Bullman, T. A. (1990). Combat experience and postservice psychosocial status as predictors of suicide in Vietnam veterans. *Journal of Nervous and Mental Disease, 178,* 32–37.

Fragala, M. R., & McCaughey, B. G. (1991). Suicide following medical/physical evaluation boards: A complication unique to military psychiatry. *Military Medicine, 156,* 206–209.

Gaines, T., & Richmond, L. H. (1980). Assessing suicidal behavior in basic military trainees. *Military Medicine, 145,* 263–266.

Gould, M. S., & Shaffer, D. (1986). The impact of suicide in television movies: Evidence of imitation. *New England Journal of Medicine, 315,* 690–694.

Grigg, J. R. (1988). Imitative suicides in an active duty military population. *Military Medicine, 153,* 79–81.

Harvard Mental Health Letter. (2003, May). *Confronting suicide* (Part I). Cambridge, MA: Harvard Medical School.

Hassinger, A. D. (2003). Mentoring and monitoring: The use of unit watch in the 4th Infantry Division. *Military Medicine, 168*(3), 234–238.

Helmkamp, J. C. (1995). Suicides in the military: 1980–1992. *Military Medicine, 160,* 45–50.

Helmkamp, J. C. (1996). Occupation and suicide among males in the U.S. armed forces. *Annals of Epidemiology, 6,* 83–88.

Hill, J. V., Johnson, R. C., & Barton, R. A. (2006). Suicidal and homicidal soldiers in deployment environments. *Military Medicine, 171*(3), 228–232.

Hoiberg, A., & Garfein, A. D. (1976). Predicting suicide gestures in a naval recruit population. *Military Medicine, 412,* 327–331.

Holmes, E. K., Mateczun, J. M., Lall, R., & Wilcove, G. L. (1998). Pilot study of suicide risk factors among personnel in the United States Marine Corps (Pacific forces). *Psychological Reports, 83,* 3–11.

Hough, D. (2000). A suicide prevention advisory group at an academic medical center. *Military Medicine, 165,* 97–100.

Hourani, L. L., Bray, R. M., Marsden, M. E., Witt, M., Peeler, R., Scheffler, S., et al. (2007). *2006 Department of Defense Survey of Health Related Behaviors in the Reserve Component* (Report RTI/9842/001/201-FR). Raleigh, NC: RTI International.

Hourani, L. L., Hilton, S., Kennedy, K., & Robbins, D. (2001). *Department of the Navy suicide incident report (DONSIR): Summary of 1999–2000 findings* (Report No. 01-22). San Diego, CA: Naval Health Research Center.

Hourani, L. L., Warrack, A. G., & Coben, P. A. (1999a). A demographic analysis of suicide among U.S. Navy personnel. *Suicide and Life-Threatening Behavior, 29,* 365–375.

Hourani, L. L., Warrack, A. G., & Coben, P. A. (1999b). Suicide in the U.S. Marine Corps: 1990–1996. *Military Medicine, 164,* 551–555.

Hu, G., Wilcox, H. C., Wissow, L., & Baker, S. P. (2008). Mid-life suicide: An increasing problem in U.S. whites, 1999–2005. *American Journal of Preventive Medicine, 36,* 589–593.

Johnson, W. B., & Kennedy, C. H. (2010). Preparing psychologists for high-risk jobs: Key ethical considerations for military clinical supervisors. *Professional Psychology: Research and Practice, 41,* 298–304.

Joiner, T. E., Walker, R. L., Rudd, M. D., & Jobes, D. A. (1999). Scientizing and routinizing the assessment of suicidality in outpatient practice. *Professional Psychology: Research and Practice, 30,* 447–453.

Joint Service Committee. (2000). Military rules of evidence 513. In *Manual for courts-martial.* Washington, DC: U.S. Government Printing Office.

Jones, D. E., Hawkes, C., Gelles, M., Hourani, L., & Kennedy, K. R. (1999). *Department of the Navy suicide incident report* (NAVMC 11410). Washington, DC: U.S. Department of the Navy.

Jones, D. E., Kennedy, K. R., Hawkes, C., Hourani, L. L., Long, M. A., & Robbins, N. L. (2001). Suicide prevention in the Navy and Marine Corps: Applying the public health model. *Navy Medicine, 92*(6), 31–36.

Jones, D. E., Kennedy, K. R., & Hourani, L. L. (2006). Suicide prevention in the military. In C. H. Kennedy & E. A. Zillmer (Eds.), *Military psychology: Clinical and operational applications* (pp. 130–162). New York: Guilford Press.

Kawahara, Y., & Palinkas, L. A. (1991). Suicides in active-duty enlisted Navy personnel. *Suicide and Life-Threatening Behavior, 21,* 279–291.

Kessler, R. C., Berglund, P., Borges, G., Nock, M., & Wang, P. S. (2005). Trends in suicide idedation, plans, gestures, and attempts in the United States, 1990–1992 to 2001–2003. *Journal of the American Medical Association, 293*(20), 2487–2495.

Kleespies, P. M., Deleppo, J. D., Gallagher, P. L., & Niles, B. L. (1999). Managing suicidal emergencies recommendations for the practitioner. *Professional Psychology: Research and Practice, 30,* 454–463.

Knox, K. L., Litts, D. A., Talcott, G. W., Feig, J. C., & Caine, E. D. (2003). Risk of suicide and related adverse outcomes after exposure to a suicide prevention programme in the U.S. Air Force: Cohort study. *British Medical Journal, 327,* 1376–1378.

Knox, K. L., Pflanz, S., Talcott, G.W., Campise, R.L., Lavigne, J.E., Bajorska, A., et al. (2010). The US Air Force suicide prevention program: Implication for public health policy. *American Journal of Public Health, 100,* 2457–2463.

Koshes, R. J., & Rothberg, J. M. (1992). Parasuicidal behavior on an active duty Army training post. *Military Medicine, 157,* 350–353.

Kovach, G. C. (2010, May 2). Suicide: The unseen enemy for marines. *San Diego Union-Tribune.* Retrieved *ebird.osd.mil/ebfiles/e20100503749372.html.*

Kruzel, J. J. (2009, July 30). Uncertainty about military suicides frustrates services. *Armed Forces Press Services.* Retrieved *www.af.mil/news/story.asp?id=123161224.*

Kuehn, B.M. (2009). Soldier suicide rates continue to rise. *Journal of the American Medical Association, 201,* 1111–1113.

Litts, D. A., Moe, K., Roadman, C. H., Janke, R., & Miller, J. (1999, November 26). Suicide prevention among active duty Air Force personnel: United States, 1990–1999. *Morbidity and Mortality Weekly Report, 48*(46), 1053–1057.

Loeb, V. (2004, January 15). Military cites elevated rate of suicides in Iraq. *Washington Post,* p. A14.

McIntosh, J. L. (2012). *U.S.A. suicide: 2009 official final data.* Washington, DC: American Association of Suicidology.

Military OneSource. (2011). *A 24/7 resource for military members, spouses and families.* Retrieved January 30, 2011, from *www.militaryonesource.com.*

National Institute of Mental Health. (2009). *Evidence-based prevention is goal of largest ever study of suicide in the military.* Retrieved July 16, 2009, from *www.nimh.nih.gov/science-news/2009/evidence-based-prevention-is-goal-of-largest-ever-study-of-suicide-in-the-military.shtml.*

National Suicide Prevention Lifeline. (2011). *With help comes hope.* Retrieved January 30, 2011, from *www.suicidepreventionlifeline.org.*

Naval Center for Combat and Operational Stress Control. (2011). Retrieved February 5, 2011, from *www.med.navy.mil/sites/nmcsd/nccosc/Pages/welcome.aspx?slider2=1.*

O'Carroll, P. W., Berman, A. L., Maris, R. W., Moscicki, E. K., Tanney, B. L., & Silverman, M. M. (1996). Beyond the Tower of Babel: A nomenclature for suicidology. *Suicide and Life-Threatening Behavior, 26*(3), 237–252.

O'Donnell, L., O'Donnell, C., Warlow, D. M., & Steuve, A. (2004). Risk and resiliency factors influencing suicidality among urban African American and Latino youth. *American Journal of Community Psychology, 33,* 37–49.

Oordt, M. S., Jobes, D. A., Rudd, M. D., Fonseca, V. P., Runyan, C. N., Stea, J. B., et al. (2005). Development of a clinical guide to enhance care for suicidal patients. *Professional Psychology: Research and Practice, 36*(2), 208–218.

Operational Stress Control & Readiness. (2006). *Operational Stress Control and Readiness (OSCAR): The U.S. Marine Corps initiative to deliver mental health swervice to operating forces.* Retrieved March 9, 2012, from *www.dtic.mil/cgi-bin/GetTRDoc?AD=ADA472703.*

Operational Stress Control & Readiness. (2008). *2008 USMC Combat Operational*

Stress Control Conference. Retrieved February 3, 2011, from *www.usmc-mccs.org/cosc/conference/index.cfm.*

Payne, S. E., Hill, J. V., & Johnson, D. E. (2008). The use of unit watch or command interest profile in the management of suicide and homicide risk: Rationale and guidelines for the military mental health professional. *Military Medicine, 173*(1), 25–35.

Plutchik, R., & Van Praag, H. M. (1994). Suicide risk: Amplifiers and attenuators. In M. Hillbrand & N. J. Pollone (Eds.), *The psychobiology of aggression* (pp. 173–186). Binghamton, NY: Haworth.

Porter, L. S, Astacio, M., & Sobong, L. C. (1997). Telephone hotline assessment and counseling of suicidal military service veterans in the USA. *Journal of Advanced Nursing, 26,* 716–722.

Ritchie, E. C., Keppler, W. C., & Rothberg, J. M. (2003). Suicidal admissions in the United States military. *Military Medicine, 168,* 177–181.

Rock, N. L. (1988). Suicide and suicide attempts in the Army: A 10-year review. *Military Medicine, 153,* 67–69.

Rosenberg, J. I. (1999). Suicide prevention: An integrated training model using affective and action-based interventions. *Professional Psychology: Research and Practice, 30,* 83–87.

Rothberg, J. M. (1998). The Army psychological autopsy: Then and now. *Military Medicine, 163,* 427–433.

Rothberg, J. M., & McDowell, C. P. (1988). Suicide in United States Air Force personnel, 1981–1985. *Military Medicine, 153,* 645–648.

Rudd, M. D., Joiner, T. E., Jobes, D. A., & King, C. A. (1999). The outpatient treatment of suicidality: An integration of science and recognition of its limitations. *Professional Psychology: Research and Practice, 30,* 437–446.

Sawyer, J. B. (1969). An incidence study of military personnel engaging in suicidal behavior. *Military Medicine, 134,* 1440–1444.

Secretary of Veterans Affairs. (2008). *VA secretary appoints panel of national suicide experts.* Retrieved February 1, 2012, from *www.va.gov/opa/pressrel/pressrelease.cfm?id=1506.*

Shaffer, D. (1997). *Suicide and suicide prevention in the military forces: Report of a consultation.* New York: Columbia University.

Shea, S. C. (1998). *Psychiatric interviewing: The art of understanding* (2nd ed.). Philadelphia: Saunders.

Silverman, M. M., Berman, A. L., Sanddal, N. D., O'Carroll, P. W., & Joiner, T. E. (2007). Rebuilding the Tower of Babel: A revised nomenclature for the study of suicide and suicidal behaviors. *Suicide and Life-Threatening Behavior, 37*(3), 264–277.

Staal, M. A. (2001). The assessment and prevention of suicide for the 21st century: The Air Force's community awareness training model. *Military Medicine, 166,* 195–198.

Stander, V. A., Hilton, S. M., Kennedy, K. R., & Robbins, D. L. (2004). Surveillance of completed suicide in the Department of the Navy. *Military Medicine, 169,* 301–306.

Suicide Awareness and Prevention Workshops. (2011). Retrieved February 3, 2011, from *www.npc.navy.mil/CommandSupport/SuicidePrevention.*

Suicide Awareness and Prevention Workshops. (2012). Retrieved March 9, 2012, from *www.public.navy.mil/bupers-npc/support/suicide_prevention/Pages/default.aspx*.

Tornberg, D. N. (2004, April 15). *DoD health officials concerned over military suicides*. Retrieved March 9, 2012, from *www.defense.gov/news/newsarticle.aspx?id=26856*.

Trent, L. K. (1999). *Parasuicides in the Navy and Marine Corps: Hospital admissions, 1989–1995* (Technical Document 99-4D). San Diego, CA: Naval Health Research Center.

U.S. Air Force. (2011a). *Frontline supervisors training: Manual for instructors and students*. Retrieved January 30, 2011, from *airforcemedicine.afms.mil/idc/groups/public/documents/afms/ctb_091855.pdf*.

U.S. Air Force. (2011b). *Leader's guide for managing personnel in distress*. Retrieved January 30, 2011, from *airforcemedicine.afms.mil/idc/groups/public/documents/webcontent/ knowledgejunction.hcst?functionalarea=Le adersGuideDistress&doctype=subpage&docname=CTB_030121&incbann er=0*.

U.S. Army. (2011). *Combat and operational stress control manual for leaders and soldiers*. Retrieved January 30, 2011, from *rdl.train.army.mil/soldierPortal/atia/adlsc/view/public/9509-1/fm/6-22.5/toc.htm*.

U.S. Army Public Health Command. (2009). *Suicide prevention*. Retrieved February 5, 2011, from *phc.amedd.army.mil/topics/healthyliving/bh/Pages/SuicidePreventionEducation.aspx*.

U.S. Department of the Air Force. (2003, January). *Suicide and violence prevention, education, and training* (Air Force Instruction AFI 44-154). Washington, DC: Author.

U.S. Department of the Army. (2006, July). *Combat and operational stress control* (Field Manual 4-02.51 [FM 8-51]). Washington, DC: Author.

U.S. Department of Defense. (1997a, August 28). *Requirements for mental health evaluations of members of the armed forces* (DoDI 6490.4). Washington, DC: Author.

U.S. Department of Defense. (1997b, October 1). *Mental health evaluations of members of the armed forces* (DoDD 6490.1). Washington, DC: Author.

U.S. Department of Defense. (1999). *Community approach to suicide prevention program expanded* (Report No. 283-99). Washington, DC: U.S. Department of Defense, Office of Assistant Secretary of Defense, Public Affairs.

U.S. Department of Defense Task Force. (2010). *The challenge and the promise: Strengthening the force, preventing suicide and saving lives: Final report of the Department of Defense Task Force on the prevention of suicide by members of the armed forces*. Retrieved January 30, 2011, from *www.health.mil/dhb/downloads/Suicide%20Prevention%20Task%20Force%20 final%20 report%208-23-10.pdf*.

U.S. Department of Veterans Affairs, U.S. Department of Defense. (2009). *FY 2009 annual report joint strategic plan FY 2010–2012*. Retrieved January 30, 2011, from *www.va.gov/OP3/docs/StrategicPlanning/va_DoD_AR_JSP.pdf*.

U.S. Marine Corps. (2007). *Protective factors*. Retrieved February 5, 2011, from *www.usmc-mccs.org/suicideprevent/protective.cfm*.

U.S. Marine Corps. (2011). *Leaders' guide for managing marines in distress.* Retrieved January 30, 2011, from *www.usmc-mccs.org/leadersguide.*

U.S. Marines. (2011). *Never leave a marine behind: Suicide prevention training.* Retrieved February 3, 2011, from *www.marines.mil/news/messages/Pages/MARADMIN52011.aspx..*

U.S. Navy. (2010). *Front line supervisors training: Suicide prevention: A message from survivors* [video]. Retrieved February 3, 2011, from *www.npc.navy.mil/NR/rdonlyres/89B577E4-A747-4074-A0BE-191EFE580290/0/NAV10189.txt.*

U.S. Navy. (2011). *Navy leader's guide for managing sailors in distress.* Retrieved January 30, 2011, from *www-nehc.med.navy.mil/LGuide/index.aspx.*

U.S. Public Health Service. (1999). *The surgeon general's call to action to prevent suicide.* Washington, DC: U.S. Government Printing Office.

Viebeck, E. (2010). *Panel recommends new DoD office for suicide prevention.* Retrieved March 19, 2012, from *thehill.com/blogs/blog-briefing-room/news/115689-panel-recommends-new-dod-office-for-suicide-prevention.*

Vincus, A. A., Ornstein, M. L., Lentine, D. A., Baird, T. U., Chen, J. C., Walker, J. A., et al. (1999, October). *Health status of military females and males in all segments of the U.S. military.* Raleigh, NC: RTI International.

Warner, C. H., Appenzeller, G. N., Parker, J. R., Warner, C. M., & Hoge, C. W. (2011). Effectiveness of mental health screening and coordination of in-theater care prior to deployment to Iraq: A cohort study. *American Journal of Psychiatry in Advance, 168,* 378–385.

Wilcox, H. C., Storr, C. L., & Breslau, N. (2009). Posttraumatic stress disorder and suicide attempts in a community sample of urban young adults. *Archives of General Psychiatry, 66*(3), 605–611.

WILL Interactive. (2011). Beyond the front: Beyond the front: An interactive life preservation training program. Retrieved on February 3, 2011, from *willinteractive.com/products/beyond-the-front.*

CHAPTER 10

Substance Abuse Services and Gambling Treatment in the Military

Ingrid B. Pauli
Carrie H. Kennedy
David E. Jones
William A. McDonald
Revonda Grayson

In 1770, Admiral Edward Vernon of the Royal Navy directed that sailors in the West Indies fleet be given a daily ration of grog, rum, or whiskey diluted with water (Mateczun, 1995). The Admiral's intent was to minimize the harmful effects of drinking straight liquor on the health of sailors under his charge. The American Navy, patterned after its British predecessors, continued the practice and even formalized it through congressional legislation in 1794, marking the first documented formal substance abuse prevention effort in the U.S. military. The rationing of grog remained in effect until 1862, when it was abolished by a general order, although alcohol on U.S. Navy vessels was not banned entirely until 1914 (Sobocinski, 2004).

Substance use patterns in the military have typically been monitored during periods of conflict. During the Civil War, for example, alcohol abuse and opium use were common (Jones, 1995). In a sample of Civil War veterans from Indiana, 22.4% admitted to alcohol abuse and 5.2% noted abuse

of chloral hydrate, cocaine, morphine, or opium (Dean, 1997). Historically, however, the worst substance problems were evident in the Vietnam
War: In 1971, 34% of soldiers admitted to marijuana use and 50% to the
use of heroin (Jones, 1995). Toward the end of the war, more service members were medically evacuated for drug use than for war wounds (Reinstein, 1972; Stanton, 1976; Watanabe, Harig, Rock, & Koshes, 1994). In
contrast, U.S. forces' exposure to alcohol during the first Persian Gulf War
was minimal, in part because of the relatively short duration of the war,
but mainly because Muslim tradition forbids the consumption of alcohol
and Saudi Arabia prohibited its importation. Under these environmental
conditions, alcohol was more difficult to acquire, and many alcohol-related
problems were reduced substantially during this conflict (Watanabe et al.,
1994). The same prohibitions against alcohol have been present for the
more recent and current wars in Iraq and Afghanistan. However, there
have been numerous journalistic reports on the ease of obtaining drugs and
alcohol in theater (McCanna, 2007; Schlesing 2005; Weaver, 2005; Von
Zielbauer, 2007). According to Von Zielbauer (2007), alcohol- and drug-
related charges were involved in more than one-third of all Army criminal prosecutions of soldiers in the two war zones in 2007. An inspection
was conducted by the Army for the 2007 fiscal year, which revealed that
alcohol, illicit drugs, and controlled medications are widely available in
the contemporary operating environment from various sources to include
contractors, third-country nationals, local nationals, coalition forces from
other nations, and mail from home (Kaner et al., 2007). Despite the apparent availability of illicit drugs in theater, the Army reports that it maintains
an in-theater urinalysis "clean" rate of 98% (McCannna, 2007).

In 1980, the U.S. Department of Defense (DoD) began the first in a
series of systematic studies on health-related behaviors of military personnel across periods of peace and war (Bray et al., 1983, 1995, 2003, 2005,
2009). These studies included surveillance of substance use trends and their
impact on military readiness. Overall, the most recent survey results reveal
that the military has made a noteworthy improvement in combating illegal
drug use. Prevalence rates declined from 27.6% in 1980 to 3.4% in 2002.
Beginning with the 2005 survey, participants were asked about misuse of
prescription drugs in addition to use of illegal drugs, which may account
for a recent trending upward of reported drug use. In 2005, the prevalence
of drug use was 5% and in 2008 it was 12% (Bray et al., 2009). The overall
decline in drug use by military members since the 1980s is largely attributable to the military's zero-tolerance policy for illicit drug use (Mehay &
Pacula, 1999). However, the most recent findings suggest that as illegal
drug use has declined substantially since the 1980s, the misuse of prescription drugs has increased, more than doubling across all DoD services since
2005 (Bray et al., 2009). While alcohol abuse levels have proven somewhat

variable over the course of this longitudinal survey, they have not shown the same overall decline as did drug use. Data from these surveys indicate declining abuse rates from 1980 to 1998, but reveal a significant increase from 1998 to 2008. The abuse rate for 2008 (20%) is not significantly different from when the survey began in 1980 (21%) (Bray et al., 2009). These surveys also looked at the serious consequences associated with alcohol abuse and considered serious consequences to include time away from work as a result of alcohol use, arrest for driving under the influence, fighting, causing an accident, illness, and low performance ratings, among others. Nearly one-quarter of all heavy drinkers, defined by consumption of five or more drinks on the same occasion at least once a week, had one or more serious consequences, with productivity loss as the most prevalent of the consequences endorsed (Bray et al., 2009).

The costs associated with alcohol misuse are numerous and varied. A study of the TRICARE Prime (the military healthcare) program of high alcohol consumption among beneficiaries conservatively estimated the annual cost to the program to be approximately $1.2 billion (Dall et al., 2007), with a breakdown of $425 million in increased medical costs and $745 million in reduced readiness (Harwood, Zhang, Dall, Olaiya, & Fagan, 2009). Alcohol problems affect mission readiness in a variety of ways. Service members who are heavy drinkers (five or more drinks at least once per week) are more likely than nondrinkers and light drinkers to be late to work, to leave work early, to exhibit decreased job performance, and to suffer on-the-job injuries (Fisher, Hoffman, Austin-Lane, & Kao, 2000). An estimated 10,400 active-duty service members are unable to deploy each year because of drinking, and another 2,200 are separated from service each year because of alcohol problems. These early separations cost the DoD about $108 million annually, and missed deployments resulting from alcohol problems costs the DoD $510 million per year (Harwood et al., 2009). A recent Air Force report indicated that 33% of suicides, 57% of sexual assaults, 29% of domestic violence incidents, and 44% of motor vehicle accidents are alcohol related (U.S. Air Force, 2006). Taking into consideration the ultimate cost of substance misuse, a review of more than 14,000 casualty records maintained by the Defense Manpower Data Center reveals that between 2001 and 2009 at least 430 military members have died from drug or alcohol use, with an overall increasing trend, up nearly threefold from 2001 to 2009 (Tilghman & McGarry, 2010). Whereas quantifying the negative impact of substance abuse on the military is relatively simple, addressing the problem is complicated.

Military members face a great deal of stress not typically encountered by the civilian population (e.g., loss of personal freedom, deployment to dangerous areas, frequent moves and/or absences from family). The military lifestyle itself is considered a contributing factor to abusive levels of alcohol use (Watanabe et al., 1994; Bray et al., 2007). This high level of stress is associated with increased high-risk behaviors such as heavy episodic drinking during off-duty hours, particularly after combat or on return home from a deployment (Ames, Cunradi, Moore, & Stern, 2007; Spera et al., 2010). A study of health outcomes of U.K. soldiers found significantly heavier alcohol consumption among those deployed to Bosnia for a peacekeeping mission compared with personnel who had not deployed (Hotoph et al., 2006). Some authors suggest that certain subgroups of military personnel are at increased risk of significant alcohol problems, including U.S. Marines (Schuckit et al., 2001) and U.S. Army Rangers (Sridhar et al., 2003). From a demographic perspective, the military faces particular challenges because a majority of personnel are young adult males, a population considered at heightened risk for substance abuse problems. One 5-year longitudinal study found that 75% of U.S. Navy recruits used alcohol prior to enlistment and 31% had used illegal drugs (Ames, Cunradi, & Moore, 2002). In fact, a study following high school students into adulthood found that those who enter the military were more likely than other young adults to have been heavy drinkers in high school (Bachman, Freedman-Doan, O'Malley, Johnston, & Segal, 1999).

Although substance-related problems continue among uniformed personnel, significant attention has been given to reducing their impact across the military community. This chapter addresses the widespread prevention efforts under way throughout the military (e.g., zero tolerance, deglamorization campaigns, random urinalysis, and mandatory education), early intervention services (e.g., alcohol screenings and intense education), the components of a comprehensive evaluation of a possible substance or gambling disorder, and the comorbidity of substance use disorders (SUDs) and posttraumatic stress disorder (PTSD). The final section examines treatment options available for active-duty service members who experience problems with alcohol, drugs, and/or gambling (e.g., outpatient, intensive outpatient, and residential treatment).

PREVENTION AND EDUCATIONAL SERVICES

Many early prevention efforts in the military focused on punishment for offenses. Alcohol-related incidents were the primary cause for 80% of U.S. Navy floggings until the practice was abolished in 1850 (Mateczun, 1995). Before 1970, chronic alcohol and drug problems were generally met with legal punishment and discharge from the service. In 1970, Congress stipulated that efforts be directed toward treatment and rehabilitation rather than automatic punishment and discharge (Watanabe et al., 1994). Another significant event in the 1970s was the development of an office to focus on the prevention of drug abuse, which was created in response to significant increases in drug- and alcohol-dependent military personnel in Vietnam. The earliest prevention efforts emphasized education and the detection of drug use (Watanabe et al., 1994). In 1971, the U.S. Army began urine testing for opiates upon the completion of Vietnam tours and quickly added routine, unannounced testing for opiates, barbiturates, and amphetamines. In the 1980s and later, programs were developed that have become increasingly standardized. Military policy mandates prevention training for 100% of new military members, and annual training is required for all troops, in addition to random urine drug testing. Whereas each service manages its own prevention programs, they all retain the same basic objectives of promoting mission readiness and the health and wellness of troops through the prevention of substance abuse. Each branch of the military maintains a comprehensive prevention program. These prevention services include direct contact with all recruits and service members as well as specialized training for members of the chain of command and prevention specialists, who are assigned to various units.

The Navy's program is an excellent example of using a public website to disseminate best-practice information on alcohol abuse prevention to support local commands (*www.npc.navy.mil/commandsupport/nadap*). Suggestions include first identifying the target population, followed by the evaluation of environmental risk and protective factors inherent in different locales and situations. "Three R's" (relationship, relevance, and responsibility) are identified to form a core program: a positive mentoring relationship; the relevance of everyone's role in the overall success of the mission; and the responsibility of individuals to learn and integrate expectations and policies as well as leadership's responsibility to provide information and facilitate the prevention program. The website contains recommendations specific to the Navy's environment and lifestyle, including planning ahead for port calls, the most effective use of drug and alcohol program advisors (DAPA), and preparing sailors for liberty in both U.S. and foreign ports.

In the military system, prevention services and substance abuse counseling fall under the purview of certified prevention specialists, drug demand reduction coordinators, and drug and alcohol abuse counselors. In most situations, the provision of prevention services is not a primary responsibility of military psychologists. Psychologists and psychiatrists across the military, however, are often assigned to oversee substance abuse treatment programs as licensed independent practitioners (LIP). In the role of LIP, the psychologist or psychiatrist can interact with literally thousands of military members and is often called upon to help develop local command-sponsored prevention programs. The LIP is also encouraged to work in conjunction with prevention specialists and drug demand reduction coordinators to accomplish such preventive interventions as:

1. Taking full advantage of opportunities to allow substance abuse counselors to provide prevention education and on-site substance abuse screenings to service members.
2. Utilizing local television (e.g., Armed Forces Network), radio, and newspapers (e.g., *Stars and Stripes*) to disseminate prevention information and program availability.
3. Providing prevention briefs to commands about availability of illegal and/or addictive substances specific to the local area or, in the case of deployed ships and units, to locations being visited. For example, such briefings in Japan commonly provide warnings to troops about the consequences of testing positive for opiates that are available in over-the-counter cough medicines from Japanese pharmacies and warnings about hallucinogenic mushroom use on Okinawa. Also, service members are warned that alcoholic beverages in Japanese bars catering to the military can include as many as five shots of liquor per drink.

As with prevention services, each branch of the military offers alcohol education aimed at promoting responsible drinking. These early intervention programs are geared toward personnel at risk for developing more serious problems such as alcohol abuse or dependence. Educational programs are typically recommended at the first sign that an individual is making unwise decisions about alcohol use. The trigger for a referral to an early intervention program is usually an alcohol-related incident (ARI), for example, an arrest for drunk and disorderly conduct, underage drinking, or drunk driving. Generally, a single alcohol-related incident or concerns of the command about an individual's pattern of alcohol use will result in referral to an early intervention program. Courses usually involve 15 to 20 hours of training and discussion related to improving awareness about the effects of alcohol on the body and brain, identifying risky situations, and making positive choices for responsible drinking. The primary goals are to promote responsible drinking, prevent further alcohol-related incidents, and prevent the development of clinical and psychosocial substance abuse problems.

The DoD continues to pursue inventive ways to prevent and address problem drinking. In 2007, the DoD launched the "That Guy" deglamorization campaign specifically to address the rising rate of binge drinking among junior enlisted personnel highlighted in the Bray et al. 2005 survey results. DoD's "That Guy" campaign is based on a social marketing theory about behavior, using a unique peer-to-peer, rather than a top-down, approach. The campaign utilizes humor to increase awareness of the often humiliating problems associated with binge drinking. The campaign's innovative website, *www.thatguy.com*, won a 2007 Webby Award and offers resources for members who think they may have a problem with alcohol and for commands who wish to align with this campaign. In a similar vein, the military is addressing use of other problematic substances, including tobacco and caffeine, with Internet and other media-based resources. In 2007 the military launched a "Make Everyone Proud" campaign called Train2Quit. The program, which can be accessed at *www.ucanquit2. org/train2quit.aspx*, offers step-by-step processes for quitting smoking; an online message board that allows participants to ask questions, share opinions, and get support from others who are attempting to quit smoking; educational information; live chat; games to play to distract one from smoking; and self-assessment tools (Fortin, 2010). While there is currently no equivalent online resource to address caffeine misuse, a series of articles ran in the Army, Navy, and Air Force Times addressing caffeine addiction (Anderson, 2009a, 2009b, 2009c).

REFERRAL AND ASSESSMENT SERVICES

Diagnostic evaluations to determine the presence of substance use disorders generally occur in several stages: referral, screening, and comprehensive evaluation. Although service members are encouraged to self-refer if they think they may have an alcohol problem, the most common referral route for a screening is an ARI or concern on the part of command leadership. Given that various levels of the chain of command are involved in processing documentation related to an ARI, there is limited confidentiality in drug and alcohol abuse referrals. For the most part, alcohol screening and intervention services are considered "commander's programs," or resources that senior leaders can use to ensure that their troops get needed help. Command-level advisors on drug and alcohol issues across the services include DAPA (Navy), Substance Abuse Control Officers (SACO; Marine Corps), Army Substance Abuse Program (ASAP; Army), and the Air Force Alcohol and Drug Abuse Prevention and Treatment program (ADAPT). Table 10.1 provides the various regulations for substance abuse evaluations for each branch of the military.

Primary-care physicians play a key role in the screening and diagnosis of alcohol-related problems. Gold and Aronson (2012) identified a four-step screening process: (1) Inquire about current and past alcohol use with all patients, including any family history of substance-related problems; (2) for individuals identified as "drinkers," obtain enough detailed information to differentiate between moderate and heavy drinkers; (3) use standard screening questionnaires such as CAGE (e.g., Have you ever felt the need to <u>c</u>ut down on drinking? Have you ever felt <u>a</u>nnoyed by criticism of your drinking? Have you ever had <u>g</u>uilty feelings about your drinking? Have

TABLE 10.1. Substance-Related Instructions by Branch of Service

Instruction	Air Force	Army	Coast Guard	Marine Corps	Navy
Alcohol rehabilitation failure	AFI 44-121 AFI 36-3207 AFI 36-3208	AR 600-85	COMDTINST M1000.6 Chapters 12 and 20	MCO P1900.16F	MILPERSMAN article 1910-152
Drug abuse	AFI 44-121 AFI 44-120	AR 600-85 Chapter 1	COMDTINST M1000.6 Chapter 20	MCO P1900.16F SECNAVINST 5300.28D	SECNAVINST 5300.28D MILPERSMAN article 1910-146, 1910-150
Aviation personnel	AFI 44-121 AFI 48-123 Attachments 4–7	AR 600-85 Chapter 7	COMDTINST M6410.3 Chapter 9	BUMEDINST 5300.8	BUMEDINST 5300.8
Submarine and nuclear weapon personnel	AFM 10-3902	AR 50-5	No specific instruction.	SECNAVINST 5510.35A	SECNAVINST 5510.35A OPNAVINST 5355.3B
Substance use and security clearances	AFM 10-3902	AR 380-67	COMDTINST M5520.12B	SECNAVINST 5510.30A	SECNAVINST 5510.30A
Substance abuse prevention and control	AFI 44-121 Section 3B	AR 600-85 Chapter 2	COMDTINST M1000.6 Chapter 20	MCO P1700.24B Chapter 3 SECNAVINST 5300.28C OPNAVINST 5350.4D	SECNAVINST 5300.28D OPNAVINST 5350.4D
Standards for provision of substance-related disorder treatment services	AFI 44-121 Section 3F	AR 600-85 Chapters 3 and 4	COMDTINST M1000.6 Chapter 20	MCO P1700.24B Chapter 5 BUMEDINST 5353.4A	BUMEDINST 5353.4A
Use of disulfiram (Antabuse)	AFI 44-121 Section 3.15.9	AR 600-85 Chapter 4	No specific instruction.	BUMEDINST 5353.3	BUMEDINST 5353.3

Note. AFI, Air Force Instruction; AR, Army Regulation; BUMEDINST, Department of the Navy, Bureau of Medicine and Surgery Instruction; COMDTINST, United States Coast Guard, Commandant Instruction; MCO, Marine Corps Order; MILPERSMAN, Navy Military Personnel Manual; OPNAVINST, Chief of Naval Operations Instruction; SECNAVINST, Secretary of the Navy Instruction. Full reference entries for the specific publications noted in this table are listed in the reference list under the "U.S. Department of . . ." entries.

258

you ever taken a morning *e*ye opener?); (4) based on information from steps 1–3, ask more specific questions to determine whether criteria for an alcohol use disorder are met and to assess for evidence of any medical, psychiatric, or behavioral complications associated with excessive drinking and/ or other substance use. In their review of 22 studies, Kaner et al. (2007) found that general practitioners can help patients alter patterns of harmful drinking with brief interventions, including feedback on alcohol use and dangers, identification of high-risk situations for drinking and coping strategies, increased motivation, and the development of a personal plan to reduce drinking.

It is also common for substance problems to be detected by emergency room physicians (e.g., when patients present after fights or accidents while intoxicated), mental health providers (e.g., diagnoses made during outpatient evaluation or while on the inpatient mental health unit), and internists (e.g., patients admitted for detoxification). A strong collaboration with these areas of medical treatment facilities is important and can lead to an increase in referrals and earlier detection of problems. Storer (2003) noted significant benefits to brief inpatient interventions both in preventing second alcohol-related hospitalizations to U.S. Naval Medical Center Portsmouth and in reducing the length of stay of individuals who were readmitted.

Once a referral is made, the active-duty member undergoes an outpatient or inpatient substance abuse screening. Screenings focus mainly on the extent of the alcohol or drug use. Substance-related diagnoses are based on criteria set by the fourth edition of the *Diagnostic and Statistical Manual of Mental Disorders* (DSM-IV; American Psychiatric Association, 1994). If DSM-IV criteria are met for either substance abuse or dependence, a provisional diagnosis is made by the screener and the individual is referred for a more comprehensive evaluation. The majority of referrals are for single ARIs. Many of these one-time incident referrals do not meet diagnostic criteria for a substance use disorder. Although some service members are returned to their commands with recommendations for "no action," many are recommended for early intervention education. For example, from October 2009 to October 2010, a total of 1,078 active-duty patients (primarily Navy personnel) were referred to the Substance Abuse Rehabilitation Program at U.S. Naval Medical Center Portsmouth. Thirty-eight percent of these patients ($n = 408$) did not meet criteria for a substance use disorder but did warrant attendance at the Navy's IMPACT class, a 3-day alcohol education course (E. Pauli, personal communication, November 22, 2010).

A word of caution is offered here about both the overdiagnosis and the underdiagnosis of alcohol abuse among military personnel. Some clinicians strictly adhere to DSM-IV criteria for alcohol abuse and will sometimes make the diagnosis based on two alcohol-related incidents that occur within a 12-month period regardless of their severity. A common example might involve a 19- or 20-year-old service member who is referred for evaluation because he or she has had two underage drinking incidents (involving one or two beers) but no accompanying behavioral problem such as fighting or disorderly conduct. This type of individual might be better served by an early intervention approach rather than alcohol treatment if the infraction is attributable to simple rule breaking rather than a bona fide substance use disorder. On the other hand, too strict an interpretation of the 12-month cluster criterion may mean that service members with recurrent episodes of clinically significant abusive drinking that spans several years could be underdiagnosed because their incidents do not fall within the stipulated 12-month time frame. The text revision of DSM-IV (American Psychiatric Association, 2000) offers clinicians a diagnostic modification: "In order for an Abuse criterion to be met, the substance-related problem must have occurred repeatedly during the same 12-month period or been persistent" (p. 198). Thus, a service member with four ARIs at 18-month intervals across several duty stations could be found to meet the criteria for alcohol abuse even though the incidents did not occur within the same 12-month period. These service members may seek "geographic cures," as the documentation of incidents from one command sometimes does not arrive at the next duty station. Alcohol abuse diagnoses could be made in these cases because maladaptive drinking patterns have been found to have been persistent over significant time periods.

Service members who meet criteria for substance abuse or dependence during a screening then undergo a comprehensive evaluation that typically covers topics addressed in a traditional psychological evaluation as well as an in-depth exploration of the onset of substance use, changes in use over time, current use, triggers to maladaptive use, availability of a support system, current stressors, and coping strategies. Diagnostic information is integrated with treatment placement criteria from the American Society of Addiction Medicine (ASAM; Mee-Lee, 2001) to determine the appropriate level of care (for an evaluation example, see Appendix 10.1). ASAM placement criteria establish guidelines for outpatient treatment, intensive outpatient treatment, residential treatment, and medically managed intensive inpatient treatment (detoxification and/or inpatient mental health). Patient placement decisions are based on assessment of various dimensions, including acute intoxication/withdrawal risk, medical conditions, coexisting psychological diagnoses, treatment acceptance and resistance, relapse potential, and the recovery environment (e.g., see U.S. Department of the Navy, 1999).

Integration of diagnostic and placement criteria in the treatment of substance abuse problems requires a thorough knowledge of withdrawal symptoms (e.g., the revised Clinical Institute Withdrawal Assessment for Alcohol scale, or CIWA-Ar; Sullivan, Sykora, Schneiderman, Naranjo, & Sellers, 1989), evaluation procedures, and comorbidities of substance abuse problems with other mental health and/or medical problems ("dual diagnoses"). Of particular concern in today's military environment is the rate of PTSD in individuals returning from deployments to war zones. Given the significant co-occurrence of PTSD with substance abuse problems, the following section provides related epidemiological, assessment, and treatment information.

PTSD AND SUDS

PTSD and SUDs commonly occur in conjunction with one another (Norman, Tate, Wilkin, Cummins, & Brown, 2010) and individuals with these co-occurring diagnoses are known to require much more intensive addiction services than addicted individuals with no PTSD component (Brown, Stout, & Mueller, 1999). Norman et al. (2010) report that individuals with co-occurring SUDs and PTSD have worse treatment outcomes, experience more psychiatric, medical, legal, and social problems, and tend to relapse sooner than those with just one of these disorders. As many as 25% (Brown, Recupero, & Stout, 1995) to 50% (Brady, Back, & Coffey, 2004) of civilians seeking substance abuse treatment meet diagnostic criteria for PTSD at some point in their lives. Stecker, Fortney, Owen, McGovern, and Williams (2010) report rates of PTSD co-occurring with SUDs to be 34–88%, and distinguish that among men with PTSD substance use is the most prevalent comorbidity, and among women substance use is second only to depression.

Given exposure to combat and traumatic incidents associated with training exercises, peacekeeping missions, and humanitarian relief, the military population as a group is thought to be at a particularly high risk of developing PTSD and other mental health disorders. Two large surveys of veterans of Operation Iraqi Freedom (OIF) and Operation Enduring Freedom (OEF) found rates of PTSD of 14% and 18%, respectively (Tanielian & Jaycox, 2008; Seal et al., 2009). Thomas et al. (2010) report that the incidence of PTSD is 2 to 3 times higher among OIF and OEF veterans exposed to combat compared with those who did not report significant combat exposure. Also, PTSD has been associated with increased alcohol consumption in deployed military personnel (Asmundson, Stein, & McCreary, 2002). Several studies have examined a link between combat exposure and problem drinking. One study looking at Iraq veterans found that nearly 20% of those deployed for 9–12 months reported severe alcohol problems and that this association was partly accounted for by combat exposure (Rona et al., 2007). Veterans report regular use of substances to manage PTSD symptoms (Ruzek, 2003), and 75% of Vietnam veterans who met the criteria for PTSD following their military service also met the criteria for SUDs (Jacobsen, Southwick, & Kosten, 2001). In a study that surveyed 1,120 soldiers returning from Iraq, of the 1,080 soldiers who responded to alcohol-related questions, 25% screened positive for alcohol misuse 3–4 months after returning home, and those who screened positively had significantly more combat experiences than those who screened negatively (Wilk et al., 2010). In a study of 110 deceased veterans with prior diagnoses of PTSD and residential treatment for it between 1990 and 1998, 14.7% of deaths were directly related to chronic substance abuse (e.g., liver disease; Drescher, Rosen, Burling, & Foy, 2003). In addition to increased substance abuse in the PTSD population, suicide risk is also higher. One study of veterans found that almost 70% of those with PTSD also had suicidal thoughts, and 25% had attempted suicide in the preceding 6 months (Butterfield et al., 2005). Drescher et al. (2003) found that 8.3% of veterans' deaths were by suicide, and suicide risk is known to be compounded by substance-related problems (Suominen, Isometsa, Haukka, & Lonnqvist, 2004; Wilcox, Conner, & Caine, 2004).

Individuals with PTSD and SUDs whose PTSD symptoms are not brought into remission demonstrate significantly poorer outcomes concerning their substance use (Ford, Russo, & Mallon, 2007; Hien et al., 2010; Read, Brown, & Kahler, 2004). Conversely, PTSD treatment has been shown to reduce not only immediate but also long-term risk of SUD relapse if provided during the transitional period beginning soon after discharge from inpatient SUD treatment and during the long-term recovery period (Ford et al., 2007). Unfortunately, PTSD screening and treatment are not currently standard parts of all military substance abuse programs.

A recommended screening instrument, the PTSD CheckList—Military Version (PCL-M), can be easily integrated into the existing substance abuse questionnaires that are completed by every military member as a part of the substance use evaluation process. The PCL-M is in the public domain and may be reproduced (Weathers, Litz, Huska, & Keane, 1994; see Figure 10.1). It may be acquired online at the Deployment Health Clinical Center (*www.pdhealth.mil/guidelines/appendices.asp*).

The need not only for PTSD screenings but also for concurrent treatment for both disorders has been recognized by some providers, and some military substance abuse programs include integrated treatment of PTSD within that realm; however, this decision is currently at the discretion of individual treatment facilities and is not standardized throughout the services. Ouimette, Brown, and Najavits (1998) suggested that all substance abuse patients be routinely screened for PTSD, that they receive more intensive substance abuse treatment than individuals without PTSD, and that

Patient's name: _____

Instruction to patient: Below is a list of problems and complaints that veterans sometimes have in response to stressful life experiences. Please read each one carefully; put an X in the box to indicate how much you have been bothered by that problem *in the last month*.

No.	Response	Not at all (1)	A little bit (2)	Moderately (3)	Quite a bit (4)	Extremely (5)
1.	Repeated, disturbing *memories, thoughts, or images* of a stressful military experience from the past?					
2.	Repeated, disturbing *dreams* of a stressful military experience from the past?					
3.	Suddenly *acting* or *feeling* as if a stressful military experience *were happening* again (as if you were reliving it)?					
4.	Feeling *very upset* when *something reminded* you of a stressful military experience from the past?					
5.	Having *physical reactions* (e.g., heart pounding, trouble breathing, or sweating) when *something reminded* you of a stressful military experience from the past?					
6.	Avoid *thinking about* or *talking about* a stressful military experience from the past or avoid *having feelings* related to it?					
7.	Avoid *activities* or *situations* because they *remind you* of a stressful military experience from the past?					
8.	Trouble *remembering important parts* of a stressful military experience from the past?					
9.	Loss of *interest in things that you used to enjoy?*					
10.	Feeling *distant* or *cut* off from other people?					
11.	Feeling *emotionally numb* or being unable to have loving feelings for those close to you?					
12.	Feeling as if your *future* will somehow be *cut short?*					
13.	Trouble *falling* or *staying asleep?*					
14.	Feeling *irritable* or having *angry outbursts?*					
15.	Having *difficulty concentrating?*					
16.	Being *"super alert"* or watchful on guard?					
17.	Feeling *jumpy* or easily startled?					

FIGURE 10.1. PTSD Checklist—Military Version (PCL-M).

they receive concurrent support and treatment for both diagnoses. Given the high rates of traumatic exposure reported by veterans of combat operations in Afghanistan and Iraq, these recommendations should be adopted for today's active-duty population.

LEVELS OF TREATMENT

As noted previously, the military offers admission to treatment for SUDs based on the ASAM patient placement criteria (Mee-Lee, 2001). In general, an alcohol abuse diagnosis warrants outpatient treatment (ASAM Level I), although an individual considered to be at heightened risk (e.g., multiple alcohol-related incidents and severe psychosocial problems) could be placed in a more intensive level of treatment. In the same vein, an alcohol dependence diagnosis generally warrants either intensive outpatient treatment (Level II) or residential treatment (Level III). Exceptions to this rule might include those who previously completed treatment for alcohol dependence and were able to remain sober for a significant period of time but then had a brief relapse. If such individuals want to stay sober and demonstrate singular motivation to follow a recovery plan, they may be best served by a time-limited period of outpatient treatment (OP) or a revision of their after-care plan to include increased attendance in Alcoholics Anonymous (AA) meetings, developing and following a relapse prevention plan, and/or establishing environmental changes that support an abstinence-based lifestyle.

The length of OP treatment differs among the services, ranging from weekly meetings for 2–3 months to daily sessions for about 2 weeks. OP treatment typically focuses on substance education, stress management, and boosting coping strategies. It is considered appropriate for individuals who are exhibiting problematic alcohol or drug use and who may be developing a more serious substance problem, but who have not yet demonstrated signs of dependence. In some ways, OP is an extension of early intervention in that the emphasis is on education, alternative activities to drinking or other substance use, and the development of more adaptive behaviors and stress management techniques. In OP, however, members attend individual therapy, receive an introduction to AA or comparable mutual-support programs, and are integrated into group therapy with individuals with varying levels of severity of substance abuse. Military members attending OP in Ausburg, Germany, reported that the intensive education, stress management, and values clarification components of the program were the most helpful aspects of their treatment (Fisher, Helfrich, Niedzialkowski, Colburn, & Kaiser, 1995).

Intensive outpatient treatment (IOP) is appropriate for those individuals with significant alcohol or drug problems that can be effectively treated in an outpatient environment. Given the level of military structure, this model is the most frequently used because there are significant command supports in place for abstinence and alternative activities. IOP generally lasts 2–3 weeks and focuses on the same areas as OP, but it provides more in-depth education, increased individual and group therapy, and an emphasis on regular attendance at 12-step recovery meetings such as AA. Residential treatment is available for individuals who need that higher level of structure in order to remain abstinent during the treatment program or who have comorbid disorders that require additional medical and/or mental health support.

In some IOP and residential programs, the introduction of amethystic medication such as disulfiram, naltrexone, or acamprosate may serve as an adjunct to behavioral interventions. Disulfiram is a medication that interferes with the body's breakdown of alcohol by blocking the action of the enzyme aldehyde dehydrogenase, causing accumulation of the toxic intermediate metabolite acetaldehyde, with the result that an individual who drinks alcohol while taking the medicine becomes nauseated, hypotensive, and flushed (Garbutt, West, Carey, Lohr, & Crews, 1999). Naltrexone is an opioid antagonist that reduces the reinforcing effects of alcohol and, subsequently, alcohol cravings and the amount of alcohol consumed by individuals in relapse (Carmen, Angeles, Ana, & Maria, 2004). Until 2004, these two were the only medications approved by the U.S. Food and Drug Administration (FDA) for use in the treatment of alcoholism (Petrakis, Leslie, & Rosenheck, 2003; FDA, 2004). In July 2004, a third medication, acamprosate calcium, was approved by the FDA for the treatment of alcohol dependence. The mechanism of action of this medication is not well understood, but it is thought to interact with glutamate and gamma-aminobutyric acid neurotransmitter systems and thus to restore a normal excitatory/inhibitory balance, hypothetically correcting an imbalance caused by heavy drinking (FDA, 2004). Acamprosate is intended for use in individuals who have already undergone physical withdrawal from alcohol, and it assists in the maintenance of abstinence. Decisions to use these medications must be based not only on medical indications and contraindications but also on operational realities such as upcoming deployments or time to be spent in the field. Monitoring of these types of medications generally cannot be done in these environments. It should be noted that individuals who require treatment with any of these amethystic agents are specifically prohibited from reentering certain jobs, particularly in aviation.

TREATMENT OF PATHOLOGICAL GAMBLING IN THE MILITARY

In the United States, rates of problem and pathological gambling vary from 0.42 (Petry, Stinson, & Grant, 2005) to 2.3 (Kessler et al., 2008) to 5.4%

of the population in some areas (Volberg, 1996). Although not reaching the higher of these proportions, pathological gambling is also no stranger to the military. Prevalence of pathological gambling in the military is estimated at 1.2% overall, with the Air Force at 0.7%, the Army and Marine Corps at 1.4% each, and the Navy at 1.5% (Bray et al., 2003).

Despite these rates, which would indicate that thousands of military members meet diagnostic criteria for pathological gambling, there are only three known structured treatment programs. The first is an outpatient program at Nellis Air Force Base in Las Vegas, which treats only local service members because the Las Vegas environment is considered a high risk for gamblers in outpatient treatment. The second is an outpatient program at the U.S. Naval Hospital in Okinawa, Japan, which because of its location also generally treats only local service members as well as their adult family members, retirees, and other eligible beneficiaries. The third is a residential treatment program at the Naval Hospital in Camp Pendleton, California, which treats active-duty members from any service and from any location.

Other disorders often occur in conjunction with a diagnosis of pathological gambling. It is estimated that as many as 50% of pathological gamblers also meet criteria for a substance abuse diagnosis (Petry & Armentano, 1999), 76% meet criteria for a depressive disorder (National Research Council, 1999), 48–70% experience suicidal ideation, and 13–20% attempt suicide (Petry & Armentano, 1999). Suicide is clearly a significant concern in a population with access to firearms and other lethal means of suicide. Military rates of suicidal ideation in compulsive gamblers have been documented to range from 20 (Kennedy, Cook, Poole, Brunson, & Jones, 2005) to 50% (M. Catanzaro, personal communication, October 9, 2003). It should be noted that in a study of all individuals referred for gambling treatment in the first year of the Okinawa program who were experiencing suicidal ideation (i.e., 7/35), none had a recurrence of suicidal thoughts or behavior once treatment had begun (Kennedy et al., 2005).

A profile of the active-duty pathological gambler was offered by Kennedy et al. (2005) after the first year of the Okinawa program, to which 25 active-duty members, seven spouses, and three DoD civilians were referred. The average age was 33.2 years, with the median ranks falling between E4 and E6. The mean reported debt per individual was $11,407.35, with a standard deviation of $17,746.26. The average reported financial losses from gambling per individual were $24,154.41, with a standard deviation of $33,125.22. Of the 25 active-duty members referred for treatment, 21 were retained in the military and four were court-martialed and subsequently discharged for crimes related to their gambling.

Military policy regarding confidentiality in cases of pathological gambling differs from that of substance use disorders. Whereas substance abuse has to be reported to a command, a gambling problem per se does not. Most pathological gambling cases encountered by military psychologists involve addictive behaviors associated with legal activities such as slot machines and casino games. Unless a service member who seeks help for pathological gambling presents with suicidality or another issue that requires mandatory reporting, he or she will enjoy a greater degree of confidentiality than substance patients and can thus self-refer with less fear of stigma, career-damage and similar impediments.

The treatment of pathological gambling has many similarities to that of other addictions as well as some differences. A discussion of appropriate treatment options and the development of a treatment program are unfortunately beyond the scope of this chapter. It is important to note, however, that mental health and/or addiction providers who are considering the introduction of a gambling treatment option into their program must obtain additional, specialized training in order to do so. Besides the tailored individual and group therapy that is provided, treatments must consider the other unique characteristics of this population. For example, the clinic will have to have a consultant available for financial counseling, spousal education, potential marital counseling, and emergent suicide risk assessments. The evaluation of the pathological gambler cannot be a brief screen, as is done for a preliminary substance abuse evaluation. Because of the severity and frequency of suicidality, as well as other comorbid mental health issues and substance use disorders, a full psychological evaluation or, at a minimum, a suicide risk assessment must be provided. For a sample gambling evaluation, see Appendix 10.2.

SUMMARY

Although SUDs continue to be a problem in the military, each service provides a comprehensive range of services, from prevention programs to progressively intensive levels of treatment. Early intervention is provided at the first indication of a possible problem, and excellent treatment options exist and are available to any military member who needs them. The military environment provides significant social support to military members with substance problems and state-of-the-art treatment for all members. Although substance abuse and pathological gambling are very difficult to treat in any arena, military members have an array of educational and treatment options that support readiness and recovery.

REFERENCES

American Psychiatric Association. (1994). *Diagnostic and statistical manual of mental disorders* (4th ed.). Washington, DC: Author.

American Psychiatric Association. (2000). *Diagnostic and statistical manual of mental disorders* (4th ed., text rev.). Washington, DC: Author.

Ames, G. M., Cunradi, C. B., & Moore, R. S. (2002). Alcohol, tobacco, and drug use among young adults prior to entering the military. *Prevention Science, 3,* 135–144.

Ames, G. M., Cunradi, C. B., Moore, R. S., & Stern, R. (2007). Military culture and drinking behavior among U.S. Navy careerists. *Journal of Studies on Alcohol and Drugs, 68,* 336–344.

Anderson, J. R. (2009a, August 7). Caffeine, I wish I could quit you. *Army Times.* Retrieved from *www.armytimes.com/offduty/health/offduty_caffeine_quitting_080609.*

Anderson, J. R. (2009b, August 7). The buzz about caffeine: Healthy kick or addictive drain? Try not to lose sleep over it. *AirForce Times. Retrieved from www. airforcetimes.com/offduty/health/offduty_caffeine_main_080609.*

Anderson, J. R. (2009c, August 7). On the good ship Caffeine Buzz. *Navy Times.* Retrieved November 30, 2010, from *www.navytimes.com/offduty/health/ offduty_caffeine_sailor_080609.*

Asmundson, G. J. G., Stein, M. B., & McCreary, D. R. (2002). Posttraumatic stress disorder symptoms influence health status of deployed peacekeepers and non-deployed military personnel. *Journal of Nervous and Mental Disease, 190,* 807–815.

Bachman, J. G., Freedman-Doan, P., O'Malley, P. M., Johnston, L. D., & Segal, D. R. (1999). Changing patterns of drug use among U.S. military recruits before and after enlistment. *American Journal of Public Health 89,* 672–677.

Brady, K. T., Back, S. E., & Coffey, S. F. (2004). Substance abuse and posttraumatic stress disorder. *Current Directions in Psychological Science, 13,* 206–209.

Bray, R. M., Guess, L. L., Mason, R. E., Hubbard, R. L., Smith, D. G., Marsden, M. E., et al. (1983). *1982 worldwide survey of alcohol and non-medical drug use among military personnel.* Research Triangle Park, NC: RTI International.

Bray, R. M., Hourani, L. L., Rae, K. L., Dever, J. A., Brown, J. M., Vincus, A. A., et al. (2003). *2002 Department of Defense survey of health related behaviors among military personnel.* Research Triangle Park, NC: RTI International.

Bray, R. M., Hourani, L. L., Rae Olmstead, K. L., Witt, M., Brown ,J. M., Pemberton, M. R., et al. (2007). *2005 Department of Defense survey of health related behaviors among military personnel.* Research Triangle Park, NC: RTI International.

Bray, R. M., Kroutil, L. A., Wheeless, S. C., Marsden, M. E., Bailey, S. L., Fairbank, J. A., et al. (1995). *1995 Department of Defense survey of health related behaviors among military personnel.* Research Triangle Park, NC: Research Triangle Park, NC: RTI International.

Bray, R. M., Pemberton, M. R., Hourani, L. L., Witt, M., Rae Olmstead, K. L., Brown, J. N., et al. (2009). *2008 Department of Defense survey of health related behaviors among active duty military personnel,.* Research Triangle Park, NC: RTI International. Retrieved November 22, 2010, from *www.tricare.mil/2008HealthBehaviors.pdf.*

Brown, P. J., Recupero, P. R., & Stout, R. (1995). PTSD substance abuse comorbity and treatment utilization. *Addictive Behaviors, 20,* 251–254.

Brown, P. J., Stout, R. L., & Mueller, T. (1999). Substance use disorder and posttraumatic stress disorder comorbidity: Addiction and psychiatric treatment rates. *Psychology of Addictive Behaviors, 13*, 115–122.

Butterfield, M. I., Stechuchak, K. M., Connor, K. M., Davidson, J., Wang, C., MacKuen, C. L., et al. (2005). Neuroactive steroids and suicidality in posttraumatic stress disorder. *American Journal of Psychiatry, 162*, 380–382.

Carmen, B., Angeles, M., Ana, M., & Maria, A. (2004). Efficacy and safety of naltrexone and acamprosate in the treatment of alcohol dependence: A systematic review. *Addiction, 99*, 811–828.

Dall, T. M., Zhang, Y., Chen, Y. J., Askarinam Wagner, R. C., Hogan, P. F., Fagan, N. K., et al. (2007). Cost associated with being overweight and with obesity, high alcohol consumption, and tobacco use within the military health system's TRICARE Prime-enrolled population. *American Journal of Health Promotion, 22*, 120–139.

Dean, E. T. (1997). *Shook over hell: Post-traumatic stress, Vietnam, and the Civil War*. Cambridge, MA: Harvard University Press.

Drescher, K. D., Rosen, C. S., Burling, T. A., & Foy, D. W. (2003). Causes of death among male veterans who received residential treatment for PTSD. *Journal of Traumatic Stress, 16*, 535–543.

Fisher, C. A., Hoffman, K. J., Austin-Lane, J., & Kao, T. (2000). The relationship between heavy alcohol use and work productivity loss in active duty military personnel: A secondary analysis of the 1995 Department of Defense worldwide survey. *Military Medicine, 165*, 355–361.

Fisher, E. M., Helfrich, J. C., Niedzialkowski, C., Colburn, J., & Kaiser, J. (1995). A single site treatment evaluation study of a military outservice member drug and alcohol program. *Alcoholism Treatment Quarterly, 12*, 89–95.

Ford, J. D., Russo, E. M., & Mallon, S. D. (2007). Integrating treatment of posttraumatic stress disorder and substance use disorder. *Journal of Counseling and Development, 85*, 475–490.

Fortin, C. A. (2010, July 21). New help to quit smoking comes from DoD: Train-2Quit offers tools to kick the habit. *Northwest Military*. Retrieved from *www. northwestmilitary.com/news/focus/2010/07/northwest-military-ranger-airlifter-newspaper-JBLM-quit-smoking-help-train2quit.*

Garbutt, J. C., West, S. L., Carey, T. S., Lohr, K. N., & Crews, F. T. (1999). Pharmacological treatment of alcohol dependence: A review of the evidence. *Journal of the American Medical Association, 281*, 1318–1325.

Gold, M. S., & Aronson, M. D. (2012). *Screening for alcohol misuse*. Retrieved March 12, 2012, from *www.uptodate.com/contents/screening-for-alcohol-misuse.*

Harwood, H. J., Zhang, Y., Dall, T. M., Olaiya, S. T., & Fagan, N. K. (2009). Economic implications of reduced binge drinking among the military health system's TRICARE Prime plan beneficiaries. *Military Medicine, 174*, 728–736.

Hien, D. A., Jiang, H., Campbell, A. N. C., Hu, M. C., Miele, G. M., Cohen, L. R., et al., (2010). Do treatment improvements in PTSD severity affect substance use outcomes?: A secondary analysis from a randomized clinical trial in NIDA's Clinical Trials Network. *American Journal of Psychiatry, 167*(1), 95–101.

Hotoph, M., Hull, L., Fear, N. T., Browne, T., Horn, O., Iversen, A., et al. (May–June, 2006). The health of U.K. military personnel who deployed to the 2003 Iraq War: A cohort study. *The Lancet, 367*(9524), 1731–1741.

Jacobsen, L. K., Southwick, S. M., & Kosten, T. R. (2001). Substance use disorders in patients with posttraumatic stress disorder: A review of the literature. *American Journal of Psychiatry, 158,* 1184–1190.

Jones, F. D. (1995). Disorders of frustration and loneliness. In R. Zajtchuk & R. F. Bellamy (Eds.), *Textbook of military medicine: War psychiatry* (pp. 63–84). Washington, DC: Office of the Surgeon General, U.S. Department of the Army.

Kaner E. F., Dickinson H. O., Beyer F. R., Campbell F., Schlesinger C., Heather N., et al. (2007). Effectiveness of brief alcohol interventions in primary care populations. *Cochrane Database of Systematic Reviews,* Issue 2. Art.

Kennedy, C. H., Cook, J. H., Poole, D. R., Brunson, C. L., & Jones, D. E. (2005). Review of the first year of an overseas military gambling treatment program. *Military Medicine, 170,* 683–687.

Kessler, R. C., Hwang, I., Labrie, R., Petukhova, M., Sampson, N. A., Winters, K. C., et al. (2008). DSM-IV pathological gambling in the National Comorbidity Survey Replication. *Psychological Medicine, 38*(9), 1351–1360.

Mateczun, J. (1995). U.S. Naval combat psychiatry. In R. Zajtchuk & R. F. Bellamy (Eds.), *Textbook of military medicine, war psychiatry: Warfare, weaponry and the casualty* (pp. 211–242). Washington, DC: Office of the Surgeon General, U.S. Department of the Army.

McCanna, S. (2007, August 7). *It's easy for soldiers to score heroin in Afghanistan; simultaneously stressed and bored, U.S. soldiers are turning to the widely available drug for a quick escape.* Retrieved from *www.salon.com/print.html?URL=/news/feature/2007/08/07/afghan_heroin.*

Mee-Lee, D. (2001). *ASAM service member placement criteria for the treatment of substance-related disorders* (2nd ed., rev.). Chevy Chase, MD: American Society of Addiction Medicine.

Mehay, S. L., & Pacula, R. L. (1999). *The effectiveness of workplace drug prevention policies: Does "zero tolerance" work?* (Working paper 7383). Cambridge, MA: National Bureau of Economic Research.

Norman, S. B., Tate, S. R., Wilkins, K. C., Cummins, K., & Brown, S. A. (2010). Posttraumatic stress disorder's role in integrated substance dependence and depression treatment outcomes. *Journal of Substance Abuse Treatment, 38,* 346–355.

Ouimette, P. C., Brown, P. J., & Najavits, L. M. (1998). Course and treatment of service members with both substance use and posttraumatic stress disorders. *Addictive Behaviors, 23,* 785–795.

Petrakis, I. L., Leslie, D., & Rosenheck, R. (2003). Use of naltrexone in the treatment of alcoholism nationally in the Department of Veterans Affairs. *Alcoholism: Clinical and Experimental Research, 27,* 1780–1784.

Petry, N. M., & Armentano, C. (1999). Prevalence, assessment, and treatment of pathological gambling: A review. *Psychiatric Services, 50,* 1021–1027.

Petry, N. M., Stinson, F. S., & Grant B. F. (2005). Comorbidity of DSM-IV pathological gambling and other psychiatric disorders: Results from the National

Epidemiologic Survey on Alcohol and Related Conditions. *Journal of Clinical Psychiatry, 66*(5), 564–574.

Read, J. P., Brown, P. J., & Kahler, C. W. (2004). Substance use and posttraumatic stress disorders: Symptom interplay and effects on outcome. *Addictive Behaviors, 29,* 1665–1672.

Reinstein, M. (1972). Drugs and the military physician. *Military Medicine, 137,* 122–125.

Rona, R. J., Fear, N. T., Hull, L., Hull, L., Greenberg, N., Earnshaw, M., et al. (2007). Mental health consequences of overstretch in the UK armed forces: first phase of a cohort study. *British Medical Journal, 335,* 603.

Ruzek, J. I. (2003). Concurrent posttraumatic stress disorder and substance use disorder among veterans: Evidence and treatment issues. In P. Ouimette & P. J. Brown (Eds.), *Trauma and substance abuse* (pp. 191–207). Washington, DC: American Psychological Association.

Schlesing, A. (2005, January 3). Drugs, booze easy for GIs to get in Iraq. *The Arkansas Democrat-Gazette.* Retrieved from *www.november.org/stayinfo/breaking3/GIDrugs.html.*

Schuckit, M. A., Kraft, H. S., Hurtado, S. L., Tschinkel, S. A., Minagawa, R., & Shaffer, R. A. (2001). A measure of the intensity of response to alcohol in a military population. *American Journal of Drug and Alcohol Abuse, 27,* 749–757.

Seal, K. H., Metzler, T. J., Gima, K. S., Bertenthal, D., Maguen, S., & Marmar, C. R. (2009). Trends and risk factors for mental health diagnoses among Iraq and Afghanistan veterans using Department of Veterans Affairs health care, 2002–2008. *American Journal of Public Health, 99*(9), 1651–1658.

Sobocinski, A. (2004). A few notes on grog. *Navy Medicine, 95,* 9–10.

Spera, C., Franklin, K., Uekawa, K., Kunz, J. F., Szoc, R. Z., Thomas, R. K., et al.. (2010). Reducing drinking among junior enlisted Air Force members in five communities: Early findings of the EUDL program's influence on self-reported drinking behaviors. *Journal of Studies on Alcohol and Drugs, 71*(3), 373–383.

Sridhar, A., Deuster, P. A., Becker, W. J., Coll, R., O'Brien, K. K., & Bathalon, G. (2003). Health assessment of U.S. Army Rangers. *Military Medicine, 168,* 57–62.

Stanton, M. D. (1976). Drugs, Vietnam, and the Vietnam veteran: An overview. *American Journal of Drug and Alcohol Abuse, 3,* 557–570.

Stecker, T., Fortney, J., Owen, R., McGovern, M. P., & Williams, S. (2010). Co-occurring medical, psychiatric, and alcohol-related disorders among veterans returning from Iraq and Afghanistan. *Psychosomatics, 51*(6), 503–507.

Storer, R. M. (2003). A simple cost-benefit analysis of brief interventions on substance abuse at Naval Medical Center Portsmouth. *Military Medicine, 168,* 765–768.

Sullivan, J. T., Sykora, K., Schneiderman, J., Naranjo, C. A., & Sellers, E. M. (1989). Assessment of alcohol withdrawal: The Revised Clinical Institute Withdrawal Assessment for Alcohol Scale (CIWA-Ar). *British Journal of Addiction, 84,* 1353–1357.

Suominen, K., Isometsa, E., Haukka, J., & Lonnqvist, J. (2004). Substance use and male gender as risk factors for deaths and suicide: A 5-year follow-up study after deliberate self-harm. *Social Psychiatry and Psychiatric Epidemiology, 39,* 720–724.

Tanielian, T., & Jaycox, L. H. (2008). *Invisible wounds of war?: Psychological and cognitive industries, their consequences, and services to assist recovery.* Santa Monica, CA: RAND Center for Military Health Policy Research.

Thomas, J. L, Wilk, J. E., Riviere, L. A., McGurk, D., Castro, C. A., & Hoge, C. W. (2010). Prevalence of mental health problems and functional impairment among active component and National Guard soldiers 3 and 12 months following combat in Iraq. *Archives of General Psychiatry, 67*(6), 614–623.

Tilghman, A., & McGarry, B. (2010, September). Troop deaths soar with prescriptions for war wounded. *Army Times.* Retrieved from *www.armytimes.com/news/2010/09/military-wounded-prescriptions-troop-deaths-soar-080910.*

U.S. Department of the Navy. (1999). *Standards for provision of substance related disorder treatment services* (BUMEDINST 5353.4A). Washington, DC: Author.

U.S. Food and Drug Administration. (2004, July 29). *Center for drug evaluation and research approval package for: Application number 21-431.* Retrieved March 20, 2012, from *www.accessdata.fda.gov/drugsatfda_docs/nda/2004/21-431_campral_Pharmr-P1.pdf.*

Volberg, R. A. (1996). Prevalence studies of problem gambling in the United States. *Journal of Gambling Studies, 12,* 111–128.

Von Zielbauer, P. (2007, March 12). In Iraq American military finds it has an alcohol problem. *International Herald Tribune.* Retrieved from *www.times.com/2007/03/12/world/americas/12iht-alcohol.4885466.html?scp=18sq=In%20Iraq%20American%20military%20finds20%20it%20has%20an20%alcohol%20problem&st=cse.*

Watanabe, H. K., Harig, P. T., Rock, N. L., & Koshes, R. J. (1994). Alcohol and drug abuse and dependence. In R. Zajtchuk & R. F. Bellamy (Eds.), *Textbook of military medicine: Military psychiatry: Preparing in peace for war* (pp. 61–90). Washington, DC: Office of the Surgeon General, U.S. Department of the Army.

Weathers, F. W., Litz, B. T., Huska, J. A., & Keane, T. M. (1994). *PCL-M for DSM-IV.* Washington, DC: National Center for PTSD, Behavioral Science Division. Retrieved March 20, 2012, from *www.pdhealth.mil/guidelines/appendicies.asp.*

Weaver, T. (2005, July 21). Drug, alcohol problems sometimes follow troops to Iraq. *Stars and Stripes.* Retrieved from *www.stripes.com/news/drug-alcohol-problems-sometimes-follow-troops-to-Iraq-1.36098.*

Wilcox, H., Conner, K., & Caine, E. D. (2004). Association of alcohol and drug use disorders and completed suicide: An empirical review of cohort studies. *Drug and Alcohol Dependence, 76,* S11–S19.

Wilk, J. E., Bliese, P. D., Kim, P. Y., Thomas, J. L., McGurk, D., & Hoge, C. W. (2010) Relationship of combat experiences to alcohol misuse among U.S. soldiers returning from Iraq war. *Drug and Alcohol Dependence, 108,* 115–121.

APPENDIX 10.1. Substance Abuse Intake Evaluation

NAME: John Doe
SSN: 000-00-1111
RANK/RATE/SERVICE: PO3/USN
DOB: 01 January 1988
DATE OF EVALUATION: 08 May 2010

Introduction: The patient is a 22-year-old single Caucasian male, E-4/AD/USN, with approximately 4 years of continuous active duty. He was referred for treatment following a screening on 29 Apr 10 during which he was diagnosed with alcohol dependence. He has been stationed at White Beach Naval Facility for 7 months of a 24-month tour. He was seen on this date for an evaluation to begin treatment. He was advised of the limits of his confidentiality and rights, and consented to participate.

Chief Complaint: "I have a drinking problem."

History of Present Illness (HPI): The incident leading to the present evaluation occurred on 25 Apr 10 when the patient was involved in an alcohol-related incident (ARI) for being UA (unauthorized absence) to unit physical training. Regarding this event, the patient reported consuming approximately 16 drinks on the previous night and slept through the scheduled training.

The patient reported that his first introduction to alcohol was at age 16, and he began regular drinking when he was 19 years old. During the first year of his regular drinking he consumed eight drinks per occasion two times per week. He stated that he felt the effects of his alcohol use after five drinks, and eight drinks were required before he was intoxicated. He estimated that during the past 12 months he consumed alcohol three times per week. He normally consumed 10 drinks per occasion. He reported that he felt the effects of alcohol after 10 drinks, and 15 drinks were required before he was intoxicated. He endorsed a history of monthly blackouts during the last 7 months. The patient denied withdrawal symptoms. He acknowledged a family history of alcoholism (paternal uncle and grandfather). The patient reported that his last consumption of alcohol was on 02 May 10, when he consumed approximately six drinks. The patient and records indicated no previous ARIs. The patient denied any previous alcohol treatment/education.

The patient reported a prior history of illicit substance use (marijuana), for which he indicates he has a drug waiver. Regarding the use of tobacco products, he reported that he smokes a pack of cigarettes per day and does not desire to quit at this time. He denied use of oral tobacco.

Diagnostic Criteria: The patient's substance abuse file and psychosocial assessment revealed the following information about DSM-IV criteria for alcohol dependence:

a. The patient endorsed a marked tolerance or markedly diminished effect with continued use of the same amount. The patient noted that initially it took 8 drinks for him to become intoxicated and it now takes 15.
b. The patient endorsed substance often taken in larger amounts or over a longer period than intended. The patient reported that he is often late to work due to drinking the night before but that he has been unable to limit his intake.
c. The patient endorsed persistent desire or unsuccessful efforts to cut down or control substance use. The patient reported that he has tried to stop drinking independently on at least four occasions but has been unsuccessful.
d. The patient endorsed continued substance use despite knowledge of having a persistent or recurrent psychological or physical problem that is caused or exacerbated by the use of the substance. The patient noted that he has experienced repetitive alcohol-related blackouts for the past 7 months.

Some symptoms of the disturbance have persisted for at least 1 month or have occurred repeatedly within the past 12-month period.

Results of Brief Screening Instruments: The patient was administered the Alcohol Use Disorders Identification Test (AUDIT) questionnaire on 29 Apr 10 with a raw score of 22 on his AUDIT and 3 out of 4 on the CAGE test. A value of 8 or greater on the AUDIT indicates possible alcohol abuse or dependence.

The patient was administered the PTSD Checklist—Military Version. There was no indication of PTSD symptoms. He received a raw score of 0 on the South Oaks Gambling Screen (SOGS), which is not indicative of problem gambling. The patient was administered a nutrition screening. There were no nutritional problems noted.

Mental Health History: The patient denied the following: suicidal ideation, gestures, or attempts. The patient denied self-mutilation. The patient denied previous hospitalizations for psychiatric treatment. The patient denied having difficulty concentrating, dysphoria, and anxiety. The patient also denied disturbances in sleep and in appetite. In the past year, he acknowledged some work-related difficulties and increased conflict or arguments with significant others. The patient denied anger control problems.

Past Developmental/Social History: The patient reported being the eldest of three siblings. He denied a history of emotional, physical, and sexual abuse. He graduated from high school on time. The patient reported having several friends and typically maintained good relations with his peers. He reported that he is single and has no children. The patient noted no religious affiliation. The patient reported that he enjoys rock climbing. He denied financial problems. His upbringing included middle-class European American cultural/ethnic influences.

Psychological and Social Stressors: The patient denied significant psychosocial stressors. He rated his current ability to cope with stressors as fair. The following characteristic was chosen as being self-descriptive: "active." The patient endorsed "upbeat" as a descriptor of his mood. He was arrested for underage possession of alcohol and DUI (prior to his entering the service) for which he did community service.

Medical History: The patient acknowledged a family history of alcohol problems but denied a family history of illicit substance abuse. He denied a significant medical history and rated his general level of health as good. Currently he is not under the care of a physician or taking any medication. The patient denied experiencing any current pain (0/10) or having a condition that frequently results in pain. He denied use of nutritional supplements.

The patient meets ASAM criteria for <u>admission to</u> IOP. The following dimensional criteria apply:

Dimension 1: Withdrawal Risk

Severity of condition was rated: High   Moderate   Minimal   *<u>None</u>*
Current withdrawal problems: Yes   *<u>No</u>*
Stated goal(s) in this dimension:
Progress toward goal: Worse   No Change   Improved   Resolved   *<u>N/A</u>*
See recommendations below: Pt report his last drink was 02 MAY 10.

Dimension 2: Biomedical Conditions and Complications

Severity of condition was rated: High   Moderate   Minimal   *<u>None</u>*
Current medical conditions: Yes   *<u>No</u>*
Stated goal(s) in this dimension:
Progress toward goal: Worse   No Change   Improved   Resolved   *<u>N/A</u>*
See recommendations below:

Dimension 3: Emotional/Behavioral/Cognitive Conditions and Complications

Severity of condition was rated: High   Moderate   Minimal   *<u>None</u>*
Based on: Stress Mgt   Anger Mgt   Unresolved Grief   Suicide History   PD Dx
Other   Specify:
Stated goal(s) in this dimension:
Progress toward goal: Worse   No Change   Improved   Resolved   *<u>N/A</u>*
See recommendations below:

Dimension 4: Resistance to Change

Severity of condition was rated: High   *<u>Moderate</u>*   Minimal   None
Based on: *<u>Screening Evaluation</u>*   Completion of Goals   Attendance
    Group Behavior   Other   Specify:
Stated goal(s) in this dimension: To educate the patient on the effects of alcohol
    and the disease of alcoholism.
Progress toward goal: Worse   *<u>No Change</u>*   Improved   Resolved   N/A
See recommendations below:

Dimension 5: Relapse/Continued Use/Continued Problem Potential

Severity of condition was rated: *High*   Moderate   Minimal   None
Based on: BAC Group Interaction   *Urge to Use*   Prior Relapse   Other   Specify:
Stated goal(s) in this dimension: To identify and apply coping skills for relapse
    triggers and high-risk situations.
Progress toward goal: Worse   *No Change*   Improved   Resolved   N/A
See recommendations below:

Dimension 6: Recovery Environment

Severity of condition was rated: High   *Moderate*   Minimal   None
Based on: *Barracks Environment*   AA Involvement   Spouse Support
    Other   Specify:
Stated goal(s) in this dimension: To identify a support network, drink refusal
    skills, and alternatives to drinking.
Progress toward goal: Worse   *No Change*   Improved   Resolved   N/A
See recommendations below:

Dimension 7: Operational

Severity of condition was rated: High   Moderate   *Minimal*   None
Based on: Command Support
Stated goal(s) in this dimension:
Progress toward goal: Worse   *No Change*   Improved   Resolved
See recommendations below:

Mental Status Examination (MSE): The patient arrived for the present evaluation
appropriately groomed and properly dressed in the uniform of the day. Rapport
was easily established and maintained. The patient did not appear defensive or
anxious. The patient did not demonstrate psychomotor abnormalities. Attention
and concentration were adequate during the present evaluation. Observation of the
patient did not reveal evidence of memory, thought, or speech difficulties. Affect
was broad and mood congruent. The patient denied hallucinations and delusions.
The patient denied current suicidal or homicidal ideation, plan, or intent. He convincingly contracted for safety.

Diagnostic Impressions:
    Axis I: 303.90 Alcohol Dependence, with Physiological Dependence
    Axis II: 799.90 Diagnosis Deferred on Axis II
    Axis III: No Diagnosis as per Physical Examination
    Axis IV: Routine Military Duties

Stage of Change: Contemplation

Recommendations:

1. Attend IOP classes Monday through Friday 0730–1130.
2. Attend at least two AA meetings per week.

3. Attend individual and group counseling sessions as scheduled.
4. Write in your journal daily.
5. Follow your treatment plan.
6. Abstain from alcohol.
7. Abstain from all establishments whose primary purpose is to sell alcohol.
8. The patient understands that he may page the Duty Counselor at 555-1000 if he is at risk of relapse.
9. Patient was assessed not to have any learning needs or barriers. The patient was educated about the diagnosis and rationale for treatment, and the patient expressed understanding.

J. A. Smith, GSM2 USN
Navy Drug & Alcohol Counselor
(*Intern*)

D. E. Jones, PhD, ABPP
CAPT, MSC, USN
Clinical Psychologist

APPENDIX 10.2. Psychological Evaluation

NAME: A. B. Jones
SSN: 123-45-6789
RANK/RATE/SERVICE: LCPL/USMC
DOB: 01 January 1988
DATE OF EVALUATION: 24 February 2010

Identifying Data: The service member is a 22-year-old married male with 1 year, 5 months CADU. He was encouraged to self-refer for gambling problems by an individual in his chain of command who is also a gambler in treatment.

History: The history of the present problem was taken from the service member and was considered reliable. He noted that he started gambling approximately 3 years ago and immediately developed a problem. He reported that at first he was betting on dogs, horses, and slot machines, but when transferring overseas he began gambling solely on slot machines. He reported that in the past 9 months he has gambled $14,000, some of which was family savings, and that he is $3,800 in debt. The service member reported preoccupation with gambling, chasing his losses, gambling more than he intended to, felt that he was unable to stop, lied to his wife about his gambling, and that this weekend she notified him that she wanted to file for marital separation after discovering loans that she was unaware of. The service member reported that after his wife told him about the separation he started drinking. He reported that he drank three to four beers and eight mixed drinks. He noted that he became suicidal and attempted to hang himself in his bathroom with a belt. He reported that his roommate heard the shower bar crash in the bathroom, forced his way in, and stopped him from trying again. Despite the suicide attempt this weekend, the service member denied symptoms of a mood, anxiety, psychotic, eating, and/or somatization disorder.

Psychological History: The service member noted that he sought help for his gambling in October 2009 and was prescribed Zoloft to address the problem. He noted that he took the Zoloft for a week and did not return to treatment. He denied a history of suicidal ideation or suicide attempts prior to this weekend.

Medical History: The service member denied a significant medical or surgical history. He denied current pain (0/10). He denied a history of head injuries and seizures.

Substance History: The service member denied a history of substance abuse and illegal drug use. He noted that he drinks three to four caffeinated sodas per day and smokes a pack of cigarettes daily.

Family Mental Health/Substance Abuse History: The service member denied a family history of mental health problems, pathological gambling, or substance abuse.

Personal History: The service member is the oldest of two siblings raised in an intact Arizona home. He denied a childhood history of emotional, physical, and sexual abuse. He noted some discipline/behavioral problems in grade school, but he graduated on time with a C average.

The service member noted that he has been married for 1 year 8 months and they have one child. The service member reported serious marital conflict related to the lies that he has been telling about finances and gambling. He noted that if he cannot successfully get treatment for his gambling problem he will lose his wife and child.

Psychological Testing: The service member was administered the South Oaks Gambling Screen. He scored a 15, which is considered indicative of a significant gambling problem. He was also administered the Beck Depression Inventory–II, on which he received a 6. This was not considered indicative of a clinical depression.

Mental Status Examination: Mental status examination at the time of the evaluation revealed an appropriately groomed male dressed in the uniform of the day. He was alert and oriented to person, place, time, and situation. He was cooperative, and eye contact was direct. There were no atypical behaviors or psychomotor disturbances noted. Speech was normal in range, rate, and intensity, though he often paused when answering questions or answered minimally when embarrassed. Cognitive functioning, judgment, insight, and impulse control appeared intact in the clinical interview. Thought processes appeared clear and goal-directed. Auditory and visual hallucinations were denied. His affect was restricted and congruent with his nervous mood. He adamantly denied current suicidal/homicidal ideation, plan, and intent and convincingly contracted for safety.

Diagnostic Impressions (DSM-IV):
    Axis I: 312.31 Pathological Gambling
                  V61.10 Partner Relational Problem
    Axis II: No Diagnosis
    Axis III: No Diagnosis
    Axis IV: Routine Military Duties, Economic Problems

Plan:

1. The service member is recommended to attend the Gambling Treatment Program at the Substance Abuse Rehabilitation Program. His first group therapy appointment is at 1730 on 25 Feb 10.
2. The service member was referred to a financial counselor. He was accepted as a walk-in appointment as soon as he leaves SARP today.
3. The service member was instructed not to drink until this crisis stage has passed. He noted that he understood this rationale and would not have a problem abstaining from alcohol indefinitely.
4. The service member was encouraged to attend the weekly Gambler's Anonymous meeting (Thursdays at 1800).
5. The service member understands that he may call for an earlier appointment at

any time (555-1234) or call the after-hours counselor at 555-0000 if at risk for relapse.

6. The service member adamantly denied suicidal ideation and readily and convincingly contracted for safety. He was able to articulate a thorough plan for safety.

7. These findings were discussed with the service member, who agreed with the results of the evaluation and the current plan.

8. Clinic POC is SSGT Smith or Dr. Watson at 555-1234.

C. H. Watson
CDR/MSC/USN
Head, Substance Abuse
Rehabilitation Program

J. A. Smith
SSGT/USMC
Substance Abuse Counselor

★ CHAPTER 11 ★

Crisis and Hostage Negotiation

Russell E. Palarea
Michael G. Gelles
Kirk L. Rowe

On September 5, 1972, at the Olympics in Munich, Germany, 13 members of the Palestinian terrorist organization Black September invaded the Olympic village and took 11 Israeli athletes and coaches hostage. The terrorists demanded that they be flown to Egypt and that 200 Palestinian prisoners being held in Israeli jails be released. The terrorists stated that (1) if actions to meet their demands were not taken immediately, two athletes would be killed and (2) if they were not given transportation to Egypt, all the athletes would be killed. In the end, when authorities demanded surrender at the airport, the result was the death of all 11 Israeli athletes, one police officer, and 10 attackers (McMains & Mullins, 1996).

Because of the concern about the loss of life in hostage situations and the close scrutiny of police practices that grew out of the 1960s and the Munich terrorist incident, the New York City Police Department evaluated the effectiveness of tactical confrontations in the 1970s (McMains & Mullins, 2001). At that time, Harvey Schlossberg (1979), a detective with a PhD in psychology, noted the lack of literature about negotiation techniques in law enforcement, and he and Lieutenant Frank Boltz from the New York City Police Department developed new tactics for crisis negotiation. They viewed crisis negotiation principles from the perspective that the incident was a crisis for the hostage taker; emphasized the importance of containing and negotiating with the hostage taker and understanding his or her motivation and personality; and stressed the importance of slowing down an incident so time could work for the negotiator. Schlossberg noted four alternatives to an incident similar to the one in Munich: (1) assault, (2) selected sniper fire, (3) chemical agents, and (4) contain and negotiate. The first three options were originally the norm for police departments and included a high probability for violence, injury, and death. Although a primary goal was to limit loss of life, the first three options most often resulted in injury and death to the hostage, hostage taker, or police officers, and sometimes all three. With the development of negotiation strategies, law enforcement now had another option, one that often led to a peaceful outcome. Minimizing and eliminating loss of life is a guiding principle for negotiations today (McMains & Mullins, 2001).

PSYCHOLOGICAL APPLICATIONS TO CRISIS NEGOTIATIONS

Crisis negotiation is closely linked to the behavioral sciences and, more specifically, to psychology. Changes and developments in the field of psychology have inevitably influenced hostage negotiations. For decades, the negotiator has been confronted with many situations that require establishing a dialogue with an individual who may or may not have hostages but who has been found to be mentally ill. The need for understanding what "crazy" or "erratic behavior" might represent led the field of hostage negotiations to develop a relationship with psychology and psychiatry communities in order to better understand different types of aberrant behavior. As a result, negotiators became closely aligned with mental health professionals, who taught negotiators about mental illness and consulted with them on difficult or challenging cases. Thus, psychologists and psychiatrists became active members of negotiating teams and frequently became negotiators on the frontline. Today, psychologists and psychiatrists with operational training and experience are active consultants to negotiators, but they no longer typically become primary negotiators.

The 1972 incident in Munich brought to light the need to develop responses other than tactical maneuvers. The hostage negotiation option originated in Munich to address traditional hostage-taking incidents; however, Gist and Perry (1985) found that negotiators were primarily called out for domestic, barricaded, and suicidal incidents. Ninety percent included domestic incidents, jilted lovers, and individuals with mood disorders, psychosis, or suicidal intent. McMains (1988) found that over a 5-year period in the 15 largest U.S. cities fewer than 18% of negotiated incidents involved hostages. Fifty percent of the calls involved barricaded subjects without hostages, and 17% involved high-risk suicide attempts in which others were at risk of injury. Hatcher, Mohandie, Turner, and Gelles (1998) noted a change in that negotiators worked more with emotionally disturbed individuals, trapped criminals, and domestic incidents and less with terrorists and prisoners.

Communications Skills

The second generation of negotiations involves more use of active-listening and crisis intervention skills in order to reach a peaceful resolution, and it transformed what was once hostage negotiation into a comprehensive field of crisis negotiation. Active listening (i.e., paraphrasing, reflecting feelings, reflecting meaning, and summing up reflections; Bolton, 1984) involves basic skills for effective psychologists, which are taught to negotiators. These techniques are used by negotiators to engage in effective communication in order to build trust and rapport, help the individual feel understood, and enable that person to resume more adaptive levels of coping, thus defusing the crisis state (Vecchi, Van Hasselt, & Romano, 2005).

In effective communication, the negotiators must focus beyond the spoken words and on the style, intensity, and context of the communication of the individual and then apply that effectively to themselves and their approach to the situation (Taylor, 2002; Taylor & Donald, 2004). Considerable emphasis has been placed on active listening in the training of negotiators to gain insight into a subject's motivation and intention (Van Hasselt, Baker, et al., 2005). For example, if a hostage taker in a barricade situation asks for a relative (e.g., a mother or spouse) to be brought to the scene, the negotiator must ask, "Why does he want this relative at the scene?" Many negotiators initially focus on a request as an opportunity to gain leverage or provide the hostage taker with something that will lead to some gain for the police. What negotiators are now learning is to consider the communication within the larger context: understanding the nature of the relationship with the relative and the relative's role in this crisis or recognizing that the relative may, in fact, increase the possibility of violence. In many cases, the relative's presence facilitates a witnessed suicide or, worse, a homicide–suicide.

In the case of suicidal individuals, negotiators may be drawn into a debate with a barricaded suspect over the benefits of suicide. It is common for negotiators, when focused solely on the content of the communication, to become increasingly frustrated. What negotiators are taught instead is to listen for the *idea* that the barricaded individual might be trying to engage the negotiator in his or her suicide. A failure to see that the subject is attempting to reenact with others his or her frustration from being misunderstood, for example, significantly raises the possibility of suicide.

Active-listening skills have been well articulated in the literature. However, the previous examples highlight the need to listen to the information provided by a subject and understand its relevance to the context in which the crisis has arisen. What is currently motivating the subject at a particular time? How does this reflect other behaviors that suggest movement toward violence? The negotiator must adapt to the speaker, listen for ideas rather than facts, not be distracted by emotional statements, and respond to any situation that may arise (e.g., withdrawal, intoxication, suicide; McMains & Mullins, 1996).

Another communication skills issue involves the use of linguistic style matching in negotiations. Taylor and Thomas (2008) reviewed 18 categories of linguistic style in four successful and five unsuccessful negotiations. They found that at the conversational level successful negotiations involved more coordination of linguistic styles between the hostage taker and negotiator, including problem-solving style, interpersonal thoughts, and expressions of emotion. When negotiators communicated in short, positive bursts and used low sentence complexity and concrete thinking, hostage takers would often match this style. This allowed for more synchronization between the hostage taker and negotiator, which facilitated additional psychological constructs that resulted in successful negotiations, such as establishing a common framing of the problem, developing interdependence, and using adaptive problem-solving techniques. Overall, the driving factor that determined linguistic style-matching behavior depended on the dominant party in the negotiation: Successful cases were marked by the negotiator taking the dominant role, implementing a positive dialogue, and dictating the hostage taker's response.

Persuasion and Compliance

Another key psychological contribution to crisis negotiation was Cialdini's (1993) six psychological strategies for negotiators: reciprocity, commitment, social proof, liking, authority, and scarcity. The first principle, reciprocity, simply means that when people are provided with something from someone else (e.g., goods, favors, or compliments), they feel compelled to respond in kind (Webster, 2003). In negotiations, the crisis negotiator can provide a small concession and later ask for something larger in return. Reciprocity is so effective that people often give more than they receive; they may comply even though what they received was something they did not ask for and it came from someone they disliked. In a hostage situation, the simple act of listening places the subject in a position of reciprocity.

Two compliance techniques that fall under reciprocity are the "door in your face" effect and the "that's not all" effect. These are basic social psychology concepts that are often used as sales techniques. When a person asks for a large favor and is refused (door in your face), compliance with a smaller favor is much more likely than if the person had initially asked only for the small favor (Webster, 2003). This technique is commonly seen in negotiations when the negotiators ask for the release of the hostages and then reduce their request to some or just one of the hostages. The "that's not all" technique involves requesting something negotiators know the subject will reject. While the subject is contemplating the request, the negotiator reduces it, which then appears to be a concession and is likely to result in the acceptance of the second offer.

The second principle is commitment. Once people commit themselves, their desire to remain consistent is strong and they may agree to something that may not be in their best interest (Webster, 2003). In negotiations, just talking to the negotiator implies a commitment. The longer individuals communicate with the negotiator, the more committed they become to a peaceful resolution.

The third principle, social proof, describes how individuals look to others to determine how they should think or behave in certain situations. This principle suggests that people behave within the context of the others around them. In crisis negotiations, the negotiators may explain to a barricaded subject how others have dealt with similar predicaments, hoping that the subject will follow this lead. The negotiators mirror the gestures and language style of the hostage taker, and when they sense that they are matching the subject, they attempt to influence his or her thoughts, feelings, and behavior.

Liking, the fourth principle, applies to the aforementioned negotiation technique of active listening. In general, people tend to like others who are nonthreatening, who listen, understand, and are worthy of respect. If a person describes another in these terms, he or she is more likely to comply with that person's requests, and the negotiator attempts to achieve this status with the hostage taker. Active listening goes far in achieving this goal and, combined with the impression that the negotiator is attempting to assist the hostage taker, significantly helps in peaceful resolutions by enhancing positive feelings of the hostage taker toward the negotiator.

The fifth principle, authority, is based on the notion that people with authority have significant influence. In crisis negotiations, the negotiator is the lifeline for the subject and is viewed as the authority figure. Whatever the subject wants or needs will come through the negotiator. Authority figures are also often seen as trustworthy and credible experts, and people have been socialized to obey authority even when this may be contraindicated. The crisis negotiator leverages all of these attributes in an effort to gain compliance and eventually a peaceful surrender.

The sixth principle, scarcity, helps to determine something's value. In negotiating, the more the subject's independence is limited, the more

attractive self-sufficiency and freedom become. When discussing conces-
sions or providing the subject with something requested, it is most effective
to grant reasonable requests slowly. Overall, these six compliance strategies
help shift the focus of crisis negotiation from outcome to the negotiation
process.

In addition to Cialdini's (1993) principles, recent research on compliance has focused on gaining the hostage taker's cooperation through
the content of the negotiation, specifically by using low- versus high-
probability requests. Hughes (2009) assessed hostage taker compliance
to naturally occurring requests by reviewing the audio content of three
different hostage negotiations. Negotiator requests were defined as high
probability (e.g., answering clarification questions, discussing thoughts and
feelings, and performing simple behaviors) and low probability (e.g., for-
feiting a negotiating item, such as releasing hostages, giving up a weapon,
or surrendering to police). Findings indicated that during the negotiation,
the hostage taker's compliance with a series of naturally occurring high-
probability requests increased the probability of compliance with a subsequent low-probability request. However, Hughes cautioned that while
low-probability request compliance was achieved during the negotiation
process, this is not indicative of a successful outcome, as two of the three
incidents ended violently.

Interpersonal Dynamics

In addition to the negotiator–hostage taker relationship, the crisis response
team also focuses on the relationship that develops between the hostage
taker and the hostages. The most powerful depiction of this is in a phenomenon known as Stockholm Syndrome, and its promotion is a vital strategy
of negotiators during an incident.

In August 1973, two individuals attempted to rob a bank in Stockholm, Sweden. Police responded before their escape, and the robbers took
four employees hostage for 5 days. Following a peaceful resolution, authorities were surprised when the former hostages showed great sympathy for
their captors and animosity toward the police. The former hostages refused
to testify at their trial and spoke on behalf of the hostage takers, and some
tried to raise money to help pay for their defense (McMains & Mullins,
2001).

The Stockholm Syndrome consists of one or more of the following conditions (Ochberg, 1980): (1) Hostages begin to have positive feelings toward
their captors, (2) the captors begin to have positive feelings for the hostages,
and (3) the hostages begin to have negative feelings toward authorities. If
the hostages are kept together, the interaction between the hostages and

hostage taker is positive, and the hostages are not abused, the Stockholm Syndrome usually develops, often within a few hours (Strentz, 1979).

A more recent study called these conditions into question. In a review of five hostage cases from the FBI's Hostage Barricade Database System, de Fabrique, Van Hasselt, Vecchi, and Romano (2007) identified anomalies to the Stockholm Syndrome conditions. Their results scrutinized Strentz's (1979) finding that a passage of time is needed to take place for the hostage–hostage taker relationship to build. They argue that the length of time needed for the syndrome to develop must be better defined, as the time in their incidents ranged between 40 minutes to 7 hours. The condition of being treated kindly by the hostage takers was also contradicted in their case studies, as one of their cases involved the physical and verbal abuse of a hostage who later developed Stockholm Syndrome. Their one consistent finding with the previous literature was that the hostages and hostage takers maintain a reasonable level of interpersonal contact. Another contradictory view was provided by Giebels, Noelanders, and Vervaeke (2005), who cautioned using a psychiatric label to describe the positive bond between hostages and hostage takers.

Given the Stockholm Syndrome's positive impact on the safety of the hostages, crisis negotiators are trained to encourage its development. This is achieved by trying to get the hostage taker to use the names of the hostages, by inquiring about any medical needs, and by not using the term "hostage." The crisis negotiator may also request that the hostage taker pass on personal messages to the hostages from their family members (McMains & Mullins, 1996).

A more recent incident in Atlanta, Georgia, in March 2005 clearly illustrates the transference that develops between a hostage taker and a hostage. Brian Nichols held Ashley Smith hostage for approximately 7 hours in her own apartment. She was able to remain calm throughout the ordeal and early on began talking about herself, her daughter, and the death of her husband 4 years before. As they continued to talk, Nichols became calmer and untied Smith; she followed him in her car so he could get rid of his stolen vehicle. Nichols was surprised when Smith did not drive off. After returning to her apartment, Smith made him pancakes, and he let her go to see her daughter at church. Illustrating the bond they developed, he asked Smith as she was leaving if there was anything he could do, such as hang curtains, while she was gone. He was apprehended after she called 911 (Metz, 2005). In this case the hostage taker allied with the hostage, though there was no reciprocation by the hostage. Rather, she displayed an intelligent tactical strategy, using a basic tenet of Stockholm Syndrome, in gaining the hostage taker's trust as a means to escape the situation and alert authorities.

Problem-Solving Approaches

Along with communications skills, interpersonal dynamics, and compliance strategies, crisis negotiators are trained to help subjects in crisis use problem-solving techniques. Negotiators help them focus on solutions as opposed to problems, successes instead of failures, and the future rather than the past (Webster, 2003). For example, in cases involving hostage takers who are depressed, it is critical for the psychologist to give the negotiator insight into the subjects' level of information processing as well as their degree of helplessness and hopelessness. Frequently, depressed individuals have difficulty with attention and concentration. Therefore, speaking slowly and more concretely and offering simple solutions not only help subjects engaged in negotiations to problem solve but also increase the probability that they will be able to reliably process what is communicated to them. In cases where the negotiator communicates too abstractly, with little consideration for the complexity of the ideas or the speed in which information is communicated, the hostage takers can become confused and frustrated and misinterpret what is being said, leading them to action that could be lethal.

THE ROLE OF THE PSYCHOLOGIST
IN CRISIS NEGOTIATIONS

The process of crisis negotiation is dynamic and ever changing. Just as psychotherapy requires constant reassessment of goals and objectives to increase the likelihood of success, so too does crisis negotiation. Because of their ability to work in high-stress settings, their understanding of the strategies of crisis negotiations, and their frequent service in remote and embedded environments, U.S. Department of Defense psychologists may become vital members of a crisis negotiation team.

As this field has developed, the importance of the role of a psychological consultant as part of the negotiation team has become increasingly clear. Research suggests an upward trend in the use of such consultants. Butler, Leitenberg, and Fuselier (1993) reported that 39% of 300 police departments surveyed used mental health consultants. McMains and Mullins (2001) noted that departments using psychological consultants reported a higher incidence of negotiated surrenders and fewer incidents of death or injury to the hostages, hostage takers, or the tactical team.

A psychologist with appropriate training is well equipped to work as a consultant during crisis negotiation. The people with whom the law enforcement teams are negotiating for a peaceful resolution are those individuals for whom psychologists in many cases provide assessment and treatment.

Psychologists not only have extensive knowledge about human behavior but, more important, are experts in addressing active suicidality as well as the types of mental illness or altered mental states that may result in an individual becoming a barricaded subject or taking hostages.

Preincident Roles of the Operational Psychologist

Psychologists play a major role prior to a negotiation. They participate actively in the screening and selection of negotiators. In addition, they provide training for negotiators on a wide range of topics—including active-listening skills, persuasion techniques, crisis intervention, interpersonal relationships, psychiatric disorders and pharmacological treatment, assessment of personality types, threat assessment, and aggression potential—as well as participate in training exercises (Fuselier, 1981b; Galyean, Wherry, & Young, 2009).

Intraincident Roles of the Operational Psychologist

The psychologist has several functions as a consultant to a negotiation team during incidents (Fuselier, 1988). As an on-scene participant-observer, the psychologist monitors negotiations, translating relative information and behavior of the hostage taker, with an emphasis on the assessment of potential violence. Also, the psychologist manages the stress level of the negotiator and liaisons with collateral sources and other professionals to support the ongoing assessment of the subject in crisis. The psychologist must help negotiators in not only assessment but also management of the different behaviors that are presented during a negotiation. The differing patterns of behavior and clinical syndromes presented in negotiation scenarios call for a variety of approaches in managing the hostage taker. Given the complexity of hostage situations, there is a high risk that events will agitate the subject. The psychologist assists the negotiator in moving beyond any misperceptions or problems and helps to prevent escalation of the incident.

Because all behavior occurs within a context, the psychologist is in a position to assess the critical interface between the mental state of the hostage taker and the situation that is unfolding. The key to initial assessment in a negotiation scenario is to evaluate the motivation for the hostage taker to engage in negotiation, and it is critical to understand the events that led to a barricaded situation and interaction with law enforcement. An assessment of the context allows the psychologist to evaluate more clearly the motivation of the hostage taker. For example, is the situation based on a terrorist group's attempt to promote a political or religious cause and gain publicity? Are the individuals going to use violence as the punctuation to their communication, as was seen in Iraq? Is the situation the result of a botched robbery, with the hostage taker motivated to negotiate an escape? Is the subject suicidal and barricaded, with or without hostages, over a failed relationship and a sense of helplessness? Is the individual delusional or hallucinating? Are hallucinations the result of drugs or mental illness?

Assessing the situation also includes evaluating whether the hostage taker has engaged in predatory or affective violence (Meloy, 1992). In cases of predatory violence, the hostage taker demonstrates minimal levels of arousal, does not demonstrate emotion, acts in a purposeful and planned manner, and demonstrates behavioral responses that are not time limited. Generally, these individuals demonstrate a level of heightened awareness, often the case in criminal escapes, botched robberies, or terrorist acts. When the hostage taker demonstrates indicators consistent with affective violence, the goal is threat reduction (Van Hasselt, Flood, et al., 2005). These individuals show an intense level of arousal and considerable emotion in the form of anger and fear; they are often reactive, and there is a heightened but diffuse level of awareness. This phenomenon is generally observed in domestic violence situations, with the serving of warrants, and with individuals who are either under the influence of a substance or mentally ill.

In any context in which a negotiation is initiated and an assessment pursued, it is critical to evaluate the hostage taker's motivation for negotiation. For example, an individual who has been interrupted during a homicide–suicide may have little interest in negotiating if he has already made a decision. The approach will be more solution oriented, geared toward buying time and offering alternatives. In situations in which the individuals are reactive and emotional, the preferred strategy is to create some sense of containment, using time to allow them to utilize their available resources and reduce the tendency to act impulsively.

The art and science of psychological consultation in crisis negotiations has evolved over the years. The concept of psychological profiles has become increasingly outdated and of little use to negotiators. Traditional psychiatric diagnosis is also of limited relevance. Rather, demonstrated critical variables include behavioral indicators or behavioral constellations and their associated personality styles, which are assessed by accounting for the contexts in which they occur.

Psychological consultants to the negotiator engage in behavioral assessment that is ongoing and continuous, as well as situational and context specific, and it generates inferences and hypotheses that they want to corroborate. However, most critically, psychologists assess the motivation behind each communication and try to determine throughout the negotiation whether the hostage taker is *making* or *posing* a threat (Fein & Vossekuil, 1998, 1999). As consultants, psychologists are interested in what a person says and does, giving insight into whether the negotiation process is increasing or decreasing the potential for violence and/or peaceful resolution.

Turner and Gelles (2003) discuss five variables that help to assess any communication for potential violence: the degree to which the communication is organized, fixated on a theme, or blaming; whether it is focused on a specific person or target; and whether an action plan or time imperative is articulated. Today, as a result of considerable work in the area of targeted violence (Fein & Vossekuil, 1998, 1999), psychologists can help assess the potential for violence in the behavior and communication of a hostage taker. Also, with current developments in indirect assessment, psychologists contribute significantly to the analysis of gathered intelligence through interviews with family members, assessing the hostage taker's mental status, recognizing potential mental illness, and utilizing data about his or her actions and patterns of behavior. However, given ethical dilemmas regarding the boundaries between "health provider" and "operational psychology consultant," consultations with other mental health professionals should be approached with caution (Gelles & Palarea, 2011).

Psychologists function as an adjunct resource to the team, offering expertise in understanding behavior (Bahn & Louden, 1999) and helping to translate behavior for the on-scene commander and the negotiator. As a mental health professional, the psychologist thinks and interprets behavior differently than a tactical commander, who serves as a strategic decision maker. Because negotiation is a law enforcement function, psychologists *do not, and should not,* function as a negotiator. It is uncommon for psychologists to know about the process of negotiations, the resources of law enforcement, or the public safety responsibility of law enforcement (McMains & Mullins, 2001). Using a psychologist as a negotiator may also escalate a situation by implying that an individual is mentally ill or by dredging up previous negative experiences with the mental health system (Hatcher et al., 1998). Psychologists function as consultants, and their expertise is used by the negotiation team to plan its strategy. One difficulty for psychologists is that, after hours and possibly days of negotiations, the final resolution may require tactical operations to capture or kill the hostage taker (Fuselier, 1981b). This may also cause serious injury and/or the death of the hostages, security force members, and other bystanders.

In addition to focusing on the hostage taker, monitoring the stress of the negotiators is a key role of the psychological consultant. Crisis negotiators are highly trained, have superior verbal skills, and are able to think quickly and perform effectively under tremendous stress. But even these superior performers experience a high level of stress both during and after negotiations. The negotiators are under significant pressure to successfully conclude negotiations and prevent harm to innocent people. Although time is a great ally for the negotiators, increasing the chances of a positive resolution, the more time that passes, the more impatient the tactical arm of the crisis response team becomes. This creates added pressure for the negotiators, who must remain collected and rational. Psychologists should monitor the negotiators and provide feedback. If they believe that a negotiator is losing objectivity, they can recommend a new negotiator. The internal and external pressures on negotiators ebb and flow throughout the process, and psychologists are a great asset in monitoring these stressors. To the extent possible, they can also monitor and promote the well-being of hostages (Giebels et al., 2005).

Postincident Roles of the Operational Psychologist

Following an incident, psychologists provide stress management education, particularly when incidents have an adverse outcome, as well as team debriefings and counseling to team members. Unsuccessful negotiations that result in death and injury are a significant cause of stress for the hostage negotiator. One recent example occurred in September 2004 in Beslan, Russia, where Chechen terrorists were holding children and teachers. After authorities stormed the school, more than 300 children and teachers were killed. When there are adverse outcomes like this, negotiators commonly feel guilty, angry, and depressed (Bohl, 1992). Although initially these feelings are considered normal, a psychological consultant can help restructure the perception of the event, showing the negotiator and the team how to use the experience to learn and move forward. When negotiators fail to manage symptoms appropriately after a poor outcome, long-term problems may occur, such as mood disturbance, occupational or marital problems, and substance abuse. Negotiators are also at risk of developing posttraumatic stress disorder (Bohl, 1992). A psychologist's expertise is invaluable when helping negotiators in this capacity.

Research on the Use of Mental Health Professionals on Negotiation Teams

One key area that has received recent research attention is the attitudes about mental health professionals participating on crisis negotiation teams. In one study, Galyean et al. (2009) surveyed 20 Lubbock, Texas, SWAT team members' views on mental health professionals' consultation. They found that SWAT team members valued having mental health professionals serve both as a consultant to the negotiation and as the actual negotiator, as well as in providing other psychological support to the team. However, the SWAT team members reported they did not value training assistance and postincident counseling or debriefing as highly as other contributions to the mission.

A second study by Hickman (2010) assessed the opinions of 73 team members about the involvement of mental health professionals on hostage negotiations teams. The assessed items included the usefulness of mental health professionals in various roles, their perceived benefit, and their quality of relationship with team members. Results indicated that 74% of hostage negotiation team members found that mental health professionals are valuable assets to the team. Team members reported that mental health professionals were most useful in specific, peripheral roles, such as providing intraincident consultation to the negotiator, conducting postincident critiques, and performing counseling for victims. However, team members least favored scenarios in which mental health professionals served in the role of negotiator. Overall, team members agreed that psychological knowledge is important in this mission and were willing to receive more training in this area.

CHARACTERISTICS OF INDIVIDUALS WHO TAKE HOSTAGES

During the 1980s and mid-1990s, it became common for negotiators to describe the hostage taker in terms of diagnoses and psychological profiles. This was a direct reflection of the influence and input of mental health professionals on the evolution of crisis negotiation. Although diagnostic labels were helpful, they proved to be more of an impediment than an asset in understanding the complexities of the hostage taker, especially in assessing the potential for violence.

Over the past decade, psychologists have begun to revise their positions on mental illness and dangerousness. It would be fair to conclude, with some degree of confidence, that mental illness does not often translate into violent behavior, nor do violent individuals generally suffer from mental illness (Monahan, 1992). "Mental illness" has become a misnomer for dangerousness, and diagnostic labels have become less useful in describing behavior and developing interventions in crises.

There continue to be certain behavioral clusters that are associated with a high potential for violence, such as suicidal, paranoid, and homicidal behaviors. These behaviors can be associated with delusions or hallucinations but are not mutually inclusive to any psychiatric disorder. However, they are critical to the resolution of any crisis. Although suicidal and paranoid behavior may be evident to law enforcement personnel, antisocial or inadequate personality types who exhibit these behaviors provide a very different challenge for the negotiator.

Nomenclature will continue to be revised and redefined to reflect behavioral patterns and personality styles that are useful in operations and place less emphasis on clinical diagnoses. For example, suicidal and paranoid behaviors are considered very risky in a crisis. They are also two behavioral dimensions that cross several diagnostic categories. Evaluating them is important, not in the diagnosis, but in paying specific attention to the content and process of the behavior in the crisis. Hallucinations and delusions as components of a psychotic or schizophrenic disorder are unimportant. Examining and assessing what the voices are saying and how fears of persecution increase or decrease the risk of violence is critical.

Similarly, determining the type of personality disorder is less relevant than attending to the subject's style. Unfortunately, personality disorders—as listed in the fourth edition of the *Diagnostic and Statistical Manual of Mental Disorders* (DSM-IV; American Psychiatric Association [APA], 1994) are associated with certain criteria that tend to be overly categorical when interacting with and assessing an individual in a crisis. Although the label may be helpful in orienting negotiators to patterns of behavior, the degree of stress inherent in the situation is likely to distort the discernable behavioral constellation of the disorder. Whereas the presence or absence of behaviors is useful in developing approaches, adjusting communications, and negotiating parameters, their intensity offers a certain degree of insight into the progress made in negotiations, the degree of deception by the subject, and the assessment of his or her potential for violence.

Finally, beyond the diagnostic label, insight has been gained into behaviors that suggest a person is moving from idea to action. There are markers people display that suggest they are seriously contemplating action. Communications that reflect the projection of responsibility, egocentricity, organization, and a focus on specific individuals, along with an action plan and time imperative, indicate a considerable risk of violence (Turner & Gelles, 2003). Similarly, barricaded subjects with hostages but no demands to be met by a third party are probably intent on killing the hostages and then committing suicide (Fuselier, Lanceley, & Van Zandt, 1991).

Negotiators will continue to be confronted with different challenges, and it is critical that they assess and manage the potential for violence. The communications and behavior demonstrated by a hostage taker must be evaluated in the context in which they are occurring. Whereas the presence or absence of a mental illness may or may not shed light on how to approach or negotiate with a perpetrator, attention to communications and the ongoing assessment of behavior are the keys to defusing or mitigating the potential for a violent outcome (Gelles, 2001).

Terrorists

Terrorists are dramatically different from other types of hostage takers, are generally not mentally disturbed, and may only be taking captives for the express purpose of killing them. Terrorist behavior is generally very highly structured, well planned, and rational (Wilson, 2000), and taking hostages is usually done to obtain as much publicity as possible to draw attention to a cause or plight. The likelihood of hostages being killed is high because many terrorists are ready to be "martyrs." Negotiators try to convince the hostage takers that they have been successful in spreading their message and that by killing hostages they will be discredited in the public eye, thus also discrediting the message. As the war on terror has shown, this method has been far from successful; not only have terrorists killed their hostages, but they have publicly displayed their executions. In these cases, the captives were never truly hostages but, from the start, were a graphic way to threaten and intimidate. Negotiation may be best used to give the tactical team time to locate the captives and formulate a plan for rescue or assault on the hostage takers.

Psychotic Individuals

When a hostage taker has either auditory hallucinations or delusional thought processes, it is best that the negotiator not confront these symptoms. In stark contrast to an individual who may be floridly psychotic, strictly delusional individuals may easily sustain rational conversation, outside of the delusional topic. The best approach to negotiation with these individuals is to discuss other topics while developing rapport and exploring other resolutions to demands (Fuselier, 1981a) before or instead of focusing on any delusional content. When necessary, it is critical to differentiate delusions that reflect grandiosity (e.g., the belief that one is Jesus Christ or a supreme being) from those reflecting paranoia and persecution. When a persecutory delusion is present, the hostage taker's communications concern actions that are in the service of self-preservation. When communications shift in theme from self-defensiveness (e.g., blaming) to self-preservation (e.g., threat of being destroyed), the potential for violence is increased.

In cases of command hallucinations, it is useful to have hostage takers describe what the voices are suggesting. For example, if they tell the negotiator that the voices are telling them to kill the hostages, put bags over their heads, or treat them as inanimate objects, the potential for violence will be assessed as high. It would be assessed lower if the voices are bothersome or frightening and hostage takers do not want to hurt anyone. This provides an opportunity for the negotiator to offer some solutions.

In negotiating with a psychotic individual, the negotiators should never confront the hallucination or delusion. Instead, they can actively listen and demonstrate interest in the subject's world, asking what the voices are saying, but they must not criticize or challenge his or her view of reality. The negotiators can reinforce the idea that the voices are asking the individual to do things he or she does not want to do and offer some solutions to mediate the influence of the hallucinations, but they should never suggest that they seek the help of a mental health provider.

Depressive Symptomatology

Suicide is a significant concern in individuals with depressive symptoms, and negotiators are advised to be attentive to suicidal ideation. After establishing contact, the negotiator initiates communications and develops rapport in an effort to establish a working alliance. As rapport, credibility, and trust increase, it is easier to help steer individuals with a mood disorder toward a peaceful surrender. Negotiators should provide reflective, nonjudgmental statements that offer specific solutions and recommendations while remaining empathic and focusing on the short term. Continuously monitoring plans for suicide is imperative, as suicidal ideation may wax and wane throughout negotiations.

When consulting on cases involving individuals who are suicidal, psychologists should be sensitive to sudden improvements in mood or a carefree attitude that reflects a resolution of ambivalence about committing suicide. A depressive disorder with psychotic features significantly increases the risk for harm to the hostage taker and possible hostages or victims, typically family members (Fuselier, 1981a). In addition, there are instances when an individual chooses not to commit suicide but rather force police officers to carry out the act (accomplishing a police-assisted suicide), and consultants must consider this as a possibility when assessing an individual's behavior (Mohandie, Meloy, & Collins, 2009).

Maladaptive Personality Traits

When the hostage taker has, by clinical standards, an antisocial personality disorder or malignant narcissism, it is helpful if the psychologist can metabolize the clinical formulation into a more operationally relevant description. When the negotiator has to negotiate with a criminal personality, it is more useful for the psychologist to define that personality as a behavioral style. In this case, the hostage taker's personality would be described as an exploitative behavioral style, which generally exhibits the following features: entitlement, grandiosity, immediate gratification, defensive and reactive to criticism, focused on the present, not future oriented, and limited ability to form attachments, make commitments, and demonstrate loyalty. These people tend to be manipulative, impulsive, blaming, predatory, and lacking in remorse.

When these persons present themselves as hostage takers, it is most important to first assess their motivation and determine whether it is instrumental (achieve a recognizable goal), expressive (demonstrate power), or stimulus seeking. Does the situation reflect the potential for affective or predatory violence? What could increase or decrease the potential for violence? What themes or ideas should the negotiator avoid? When initiating negotiations, the negotiator must choose words carefully to avoid threatening the ego of the hostage taker. The negotiator must control the level of stimulation and avoid the appearance of being indecisive or ambivalent. In almost all cases, negotiators should try to help the hostage taker save face. Negotiators are advised not to parent or direct the hostage taker, avoid discussions of jail sentences and "help," avoid focusing on the hostages (Zakrzewski, 2003), recognize the need to blame others, and recognize the need for immediate gratification. During the course of the negotiation, there will be much give and take, and negotiators should be prepared to give small things (e.g., cigarettes, candy, and soda) but never alcohol or other dangerous substances.

Those classified as avoidant or dependent personality types can be more appropriately labeled operationally as demonstrating an inadequate behavioral style. These individuals are generally quite bright but have not had much experience in applying their intellect. They may have a history of succeeding only with the help of others, have had difficulty persevering, and have probably been self-defeating. Overall, they are constantly trying to prove themselves. During the course of a negotiation, they tend to make excessive demands, to change their demands on impulse, to refuse to negotiate with police, and to have a hostage speak for them. The general approach in negotiations is supportive, and negotiators should try to avoid bringing up past failures (Zakrzewski, 2003), to offer simple solutions, and to reinforce what is offered as explanations for the predicament. Negotiators are advised to always be sensitive to suicide as a possible solution to another failure.

MAKING CONTACT

The first 15 to 45 minutes are the most dangerous time during a hostage crisis and can have a significant impact on the eventual outcome (Dolan & Fuselier, 1989). During this time, emotions are at their peak for the hostages, hostage taker, and the first responders. Upon arriving at the scene of the incident, the crisis negotiators try to make contact with the hostage taker as soon as possible in order to begin gathering intelligence. The first request is usually for surrender, and occasionally the individual will comply. Given this possibility, a surrender plan should already be in place to help allay the subject's anxiety and to ensure a peaceful conclusion. If there is not a quick resolution, the negotiator must immediately begin to assess the subject's behavior and motivation, whether there are hostages, and the nature of the demands (Zakrzewski, 2003). The negotiator should attempt to have the hostage taker talk about what led up to the incident and provide the opportunity to vent about his or her challenges in life, which may include relationships with friends and family, occupation, health concerns, mental health issues, and substance use. The psychological consultant has a clear role in the indirect assessment of the hostage taker, whose motivation is then considered. The team may better understand motivation by learning whether the hostage taker is psychotic, delusional, depressed, suicidal, or homicidal. Does he or she have a specific personality style? Who are the hostages? Does the hostage taker know the hostages, or were they simply in the wrong place at the wrong time? What are the hostage taker's demands? In negotiations, there are usually material demands, for example, money or the release of select individuals from prison. However, emotional needs and frustrations are often at the base of the material demands.

Demands can be either instrumental or expressive (Miron & Goldstein, 1979). Instrumental demands are concrete and specific and benefit the hostage taker. They may include money, food, a car, or the retreat of the police (McMains & Mullins, 2001). Expressive demands are less tangible and involve the hostage taker's emotional goals, which often revolve around frustration with some area of life. The expressive demands are what drive the instrumental demands (McMains & Mullins, 2001). The skill of the negotiator is critical in managing both sets of demands. It is a balancing act, using bargaining skills to manage the instrumental needs and crisis negotiation skills to manage the expressive needs. As evident by news reports of hostage-taking situations, the expressive demands are at the forefront for the hostage taker, suicidal person, or barricaded subject, and vary greatly, and they have at times included a request for an apology for some real or imagined wrong by a specific person, business, or government agency.

As the primary negotiator continues to talk to the hostage taker, the extension of time is a vital goal. Time decreases emotions and anxiety and increases rational thinking. As time passes, a relationship will develop between the hostage taker and the negotiator, which will allow the hostage taker to take the suggestions of the negotiator more seriously. Time also increases the opportunity for a hostage to escape and for the hostage taker to consider alternatives. As time passes, hostage takers decrease their expectations, and basic human needs (sleep, food, water, and waste elimination) come into play. Experience in the field shows that many stalled negotiations begin to progress after the hostage taker has missed a meal (Zakrzewski, 2003). Time permits improved intelligence and better decision making for the crisis response team. Finally, time allows for tactical planning and rehearsing if the need arises.

Zakrzewski (2003) cautions that, although mostly positive, there are some negative elements in having an incident continue. As negotiations become extended, people become tired and more apt to make mistakes. The longer the incident, the more likely people will become bored and irritable, thus losing objectivity. This can lead to pressure to move toward a tactical response. The pressure from the media can also be a negative factor in the management of a protracted event. The cost of maintaining an incident can be very expensive, both monetarily and in human resources.

During negotiations, the hostage taker often sets deadlines for meeting demands. The Special Operations and Research Unit at the Federal Bureau of Investigation Academy found only one U.S. incident in which a hostage was killed because a deadline was not met (Fuselier, 1981b). However, this has not been the case in the war on terror. Many hostages have been killed as the terrorists threatened. The difference between terrorist and other hostage situations are vast.

When dealing with hostage takers in more traditional situations, meeting their deadlines is often manageable; at times, they even forget the deadlines they have set (Fuselier, 1981b). However, deadlines set by the crisis response team are often more difficult to handle. A deadline from the on-scene commander for a tactical response at a set time is the one that is most difficult for the crisis negotiator. These are the types of pressures negotiators attempt to deal with during each negotiation. More often today than in the past, both tactical and negotiation teams work better together, knowing that the negotiation team needs ample time to work and that the tactical option is usually used when all attempts to negotiate have failed.

An extreme example of problems related to the differences between the tactical and negotiation teams occurred in 1993 in Waco, Texas. This incident is ripe with lessons for military negotiation teams. The Bureau of Alcohol, Tobacco, and Firearms (ATF) raided Mt. Carmel, the home of the sect known as the Branch Davidians, in February 1993. They were there to serve a weapons warrant, but the Davidians were ready when the ATF arrived and a firefight broke out, leaving four ATF agents dead and 16 wounded. The operation was then turned over to the FBI. Throughout the long standoff, the negotiators were able to secure the release of 23 children (McMains & Mullins, 2001). However, the compound went up in flames on April 19, 1993, when the FBI's tactical team attempted to insert tear gas in an effort to bring the Davidians out. It is believed that the Davidians set the fires while the gas was entering. One of the significant lessons learned from the standoff is the essential need for communication between the negotiation and tactical teams. On at least three occasions, the negotiators learned what the tactical team was doing (destroying cars, playing loud music, and running over their guard house) from David Koresh, the Branch Davidian leader. As the negotiators tried to gain the trust of Koresh, the tactical team's actions quickly eroded any leverage the negotiators were building in attempts to secure the release of the Davidians, or at least their children. A fascinating turning point toward the end of the siege occurred when the Davidians released seven more hostages. While the negotiation team was celebrating the release of the hostages, the tactical team immediately began destroying the Davidians' cars with their tanks (McMains & Mullins, 2001). This devastating incident should not be seen as a failure of the negotiation process but rather a failure of the tactical and negotiation teams to work as one unit.

USE OF NON-NEGOTIATORS

During a negotiable event, the question about the use of nonnegotiators will undoubtedly arise. Family members, friends, coworkers, mental health professionals, members of the clergy, and on-scene commanders may want to negotiate. For example, a man suffering from paranoid schizophrenia barricaded himself in his home. His mental illness was well known to his family and neighbors, but recently he had become agitated about his perception that the government was controlling citizens' lives, and he posted numerous signs on his front yard, alerting the community to the local government's attempts to control them. The neighbors complained, and the police responded. The man asked to speak to his father, and the request was facilitated by the police. Upon the arrival of his father, the man promptly committed suicide. Experience in crisis negotiations shows that permitting nonnegotiators to speak to a hostage taker has a high probability of further agitation. It may also be the case that the subject is planning to commit suicide, and a particular family member, friend, coworker, or commander is exactly the person he or she wants to hear or see this occur. The military crisis response team should do everything possible to prevent an audience.

ETHICAL ISSUES IN CRISIS NEGOTIATIONS

Crisis negotiation consultations present numerous situations in which psychologists are faced with ethical dilemmas. Despite this situation, the topic of psychological ethics in crisis negotiations has not been addressed in the literature; the extent of the discussion involved justifying psychologists' role in this mission (Call, 2008). However, in response to recent controversies in operational psychology consultation, Kennedy and Williams (2011; see also Chapter 14, this volume) brought together experts to discuss ethical conflicts in specific operational mission areas, including crisis negotiations (Gelles & Palarea, 2011).

Gelles and Palarea (2011) reviewed the various roles psychologists provide in crisis negotiations and identified typical ethical dilemmas that arise from these roles. They noted that ethical conflicts naturally arise between the needs of the law enforcement agency (the client), the needs of any persons taken hostage (society), and the needs of the subject in crisis. In order to anticipate and proactively address these role conflicts and mixed agency issues, the consulting psychologist is advised to identify the different roles in the consultation process, to draw boundaries between these roles, and not to violate these boundaries (see also Kennedy, 2012). For example, the psychologist should remain in the objective role as consultant to the negotiation process and not serve as the actual negotiator or as the on-scene strategic decision maker. The psychologist is also mindful of keeping operational and clinical roles separate, and does not provide clinical mental health services to the negotiation team when functioning as an operational member of the same team. Instead, a separate clinical psychologist is brought in to provide mental health support and debrief the negotiation team members, including the operational psychologist serving on the team.

Additionally, Gelles and Palarea (2011) conducted an analysis of the APA Code of Ethics (APA, 2002) on specific applications to crisis negotiations, indirect assessment issues, training and competency issues, and other considerations in consulting with law enforcement. One common argument against psychologists serving on negotiation teams is that it violates the "Do No Harm" code (Principle A, APA, 2002, p. 3; Ethics Code 3.04, APA, 2002, p. 6), as the psychologist may participate in a negotiation that ultimately ends with a tactical intervention in which the subject is killed by the police (Call, 2008). However, Gelles and Palarea point out that the purpose of the psychological consultation is to preserve life, and thus avoid harm. They argue that the psychologist's role is to assist the negotiation team with gaining insight into the subject's mental health, motivations, and risk for violence in order to ensure the safety of the subject in crisis, any hostages taken, the police, and bystanders and assist with bringing the situation to a peaceful resolution. Furthermore, they differentiate between the negotiation phase and the tactical phase, and advise that the psychologist is not involved with the scene commander's decision to use a tactical intervention; once the scene commander has decided to shift from negotiation to tactical resolution, the psychologist's intraincident consultation has ended. Other key elements of the APA ethics code addressed by Gelles and Palarea include identifying and avoiding multiple relationships (Ethics Code 3.05, APA, 2002, p. 6), establishing and maintaining competence (Ethics Codes 2.01 and 2.03, APA, 2002, pp. 5–6), and conducting an indirect assessment of the subject in crisis (Ethics Code 9.01, APA, 2002, p. 13).

Finally, Gelles and Palarea (2011) provided the following guidelines in order to more clearly define roles and boundaries in psychological consultation for crisis negotiations:

• *Identify the client, the psychologist's role, and the roles of other team members.* The client is the law enforcement organization, not the hostage taker, hostages, or other involved parties. The psychologist's role is to consult with the law enforcement team as they conduct the negotiation.

• *Remain in the role of an expert psychologist consultant.* The psychologist should remain in the objective role as subject matter expert consultant and should never become the negotiator.

• *Remain autonomous in consultation and free from external influence and pressure.* The psychologist should be mindful of not letting the high-energy environment, the scene commander's agenda, or the political agendas of senior leadership influence the consultation.

• *Identify the boundaries of the psychologist's role.* The psychologist only serves as a consultant and never as the on-site strategic decision maker. The psychologist consults with the negotiator and scene commander on the negotiation process, but never makes operational decisions, such as shifting from negotiation to tactical resolution.

• *Appreciate the uniqueness of each crisis situation.* The psychologist gives careful thought and consideration to each negotiation and subject in crisis, understands the limitations of models and templates, and keeps his or her biases and prejudices in check.

• *Clearly delineate the boundaries between operational consultants and healthcare providers.* The psychologist must keep the clinical healthcare provider and operational consultation roles separate. Before entering into an operational consultation role, the psychologist must first receive appropriate training and supervision.

• *Establish and maintain professional competence.* Psychologists conducting consultation on this mission should receive crisis negotiation training and supervision, join their local crisis negotiation association and conduct liaison with other crisis negotiation professionals, and establish a network of psychologists consulting on this mission in order to discuss and resolve ethical dilemmas.

CONCLUSIONS

In closing, military psychologists can provide valuable consultation to the crisis negotiation team. Across the nation, law enforcement agencies report a steady increase in the use of mental health consultants in crisis negotiations and thus a significantly higher incidence of negotiated surrenders and fewer deaths and injuries (McMains & Mullins, 2001). With the change in the world since September 11, 2001, and subsequent wars in Iraq and Afghanistan, hostages have frequently been on the forefront of media reports. Trained military consultants are in a position to provide significant assistance in both foreign and domestic situations. Psychologists can serve a fundamental role in this area and contribute directly to the optimal resolution of crises. Overall, negotiation is a means of significantly increasing the chances of peaceful resolution, and the psychological consultant provides vital assistance in the formulation of the approach to a given individual and situation.

REFERENCES

American Psychiatric Association. (1994). *Diagnostic and statistical manual of mental disorders* (4th ed.). Washington DC: Author.

American Psychological Association. (2002). Ethical principles of psychologists and code of conduct. *American Psychologist, 57,* 1060–1073.

Bahn, C., & Louden, R. J. (1999). Hostage negotiation as a team enterprise. *Group, 23,* 77–85.

Bohl, N. K. (1992). Hostage negotiator stress. *FBI Law Enforcement Bulletin, 61,* 24–26.

Bolton, R. (1984). *People skills.* Upper Saddle River, NJ: Prentice Hall.

Butler, W. M., Leitenberg, H., & Fuselier, G. D. (1993). The use of mental health professional consultants to hostage negotiations teams. *Behavioral Science and the Law, 1,* 213–221.

Call, J. A. (2008). Psychological consultation in hostage/barricade crisis negotiations. In H. Hall (Ed.), *Forensic psychology and neuropsychology for criminal and civil cases* (pp. 263–288). Boca Raton, FL: CRC Press.

Cialdini, R. B. (1993). *Influence: Science and practice* (3rd ed.). Glenview, IL: Scott, Foresman.

de Fabrique, N., Van Hasselt, V. B., Vecchi, G. M., & Romano, S. J. (2007). Common variables associated with the development of Stockholm Syndrome: Some case examples. *Victims and Offenders, 2,* 91–98.

Dolan, J. T., & Fuselier, G. D. (1989). A guide for first responders to hostage situations. *FBI Law Enforcement Bulletin, 58,* 9–13.

Fein, R. A., & Vossekuil, B. (1998). *Protective intelligence and threat assessment investigations* (NCJ Publication No. 170612). Washington, DC: U.S. Department of Justice.

Fein, R. A., & Vossekuil, B. (1999). Assassination in the United States: An operational study of recent assassins, attackers, and near-lethal approachers. *Journal of Forensic Sciences, 44,* 321–333.

Fuselier, G. D. (1981a). A practical overview of hostage negotiations, part 1. *FBI Law Enforcement Bulletin, 50,* 2–6.

Fuselier, G. D. (1981b). A practical overview of hostage negotiations, part 2. *FBI Law Enforcement Bulletin, 50,* 10–15.

Fuselier, G. D. (1988). Hostage negotiation consultant: Emerging role for the clinical psychologist. *Professional Psychology: Research and Practice, 10,* 175–179.

Fuselier, G. D., Lanceley, F. J., & Van Zandt, C. R. (1991). Hostage/barricaded incidents: High risk factors and the action criteria. *FBI Law Enforcement Bulletin, 60,* 6–12.

Galyean, K. D., Wherry, J.N., & Young, A.T. (2009). Valuation of services offered by mental health professionals in SWAT team members: A study of the Lubbock, Texas SWAT team. *Journal of Police and Criminal Psychology, 24,* 51-58.

Gelles, M. (2001). Negotiating with emotionally disturbed individuals: Recognition and guidelines. In M. J. McMains & W. C. Mullins (Eds.), *Crisis negotiations: Managing critical incidents and hostage situations in law enforcement and corrections* (2nd ed., pp. 229–288). Cincinnati, OH: Anderson.

Gelles, M. G., & Palarea, R. (2011). Ethics in crisis negotiation: A law enforcement and public safety perspective. In C. H. Kennedy & T. J. Williams (Eds.), *Ethical practice in operational psychology: Military and national intelligence applications* (pp. 107–123). Washington, DC: American Psychological Association.

Giebels, E., Noelanders, S., & Vervaeke, G. (2005). The hostage experience: Implications for negotiation strategies. *Clinical Psychology and Psychotherapy, 12,* 241–253.

Hatcher, C., Mohandie, K., Turner, J., & Gelles, M. (1998). The role of the psychologist in crisis/hostage negotiations. *Behavioral Sciences and the Law, 16,* 455–472.

Hickman, D. (2010). An assessment of hostage negotiators' attitudes toward mental health professionals' involvement in hostage negotiation. *Dissertation Abstracts International: Section A. Humanities and Social Sciences,* p. 3392.

Hughes, J. (2009). A pilot study of naturally occurring high-probability request sequences in hostage negotiation. *Journal of Applied Behavior Analysis, 42,* 491–496.

Kennedy, C. H. (2012). Institutional ethical conflicts with illustrations from police and military psychology. In S. Knapp & L. Vandecreek (Eds.). *APA handbook of ethics in psychology: Vol. 1. Moral foundations and common themes* (pp. 123–144). Washington, DC: American Psychological Association.

Kennedy, C. H., & Williams, T. J. (Eds.). (2011). *Ethical practice in operational psychology: Military and national intelligence applications.* Washington, DC: American Psychological Association..

McMains, M. J. (1988, October). *Current uses of hostage negotiators in major police departments.* Paper presented to the Society of Police and Criminal Psychology, San Antonio, TX.

McMains, M. J., & Mullins, W. C. (1996). *Crisis negotiations: Managing critical incidents and hostage situations in law enforcement and corrections.* Cincinnati, OH: Anderson.

McMains, M. J., & Mullins, W. (2001). *Crisis negotiations: Managing critical incidents and hostage situations in law enforcement and corrections* (2nd ed.). Cincinnati, OH: Anderson.

Meloy, J. R. (1992). *Violent attachments.* Northvale, NJ: Jason Aronson.

Metz, A. (2005, March 16). *She relied on instincts, faith.* Retrieved May 26, 2012, from *www.newsday.com/news/she-relied-on-instincts-faith-1.665117.*

Miron, M. S., & Goldstein, A. P. (1979). *Hostage.* New York: Pergamon Press.

Mohandie, K., Meloy, J. R., & Collins, P. I. (2009). Suicide by cop among officer-involved shooting cases. *Journal of Forensic Sciences, 54,* 456–462.

Monahan, J. (1992). Mental disorder and violent behavior: Perceptions and evidence. *American Psychologist, 47,* 511–521.

Ochberg, F. M. (1980). What is happening to the hostages in Tehran? *Psychiatric Annals, 10,* 186–189.

Schlossberg, H. (1979). Police response to hostage situations. In J. T. O'Brien & M. Marcus (Eds.), *Crime and justice in America* (pp. 209–220). New York: Pergamon Press.

Strentz, T. (1979). Law enforcement policy and ego defenses of the hostages. *FBI Law Enforcement Bulletin, 4,* 2–12.

Taylor, P. J. (2002). A cylindrical model of communication behavior in crisis negotiations. *Human Communication Research, 28,* 7–48.

Taylor, P. J., & Donald, I. (2004). The structure of communication behavior in simulated and actual crisis negotiations. *Human Communication Research, 30,* 443–478.

Taylor, P. J., & Thomas, S. (2008). Linguistic style matching and negotiation outcome. *Negotiation and Conflict Management Research, 1,* 263–281.

Turner, J. T., & Gelles, M. G. (2003). *Threat assessment: A risk management approach.* Binghamton, NY: Haworth.

Van Hasselt, V. B., Baker, M. T., Romano, S. J., Sellers, A. H., Noesner, G. W., & Smith, S. (2005). Development and validation of a role-play test for assessing crisis (hostage) negotiation skills. *Criminal Justice and Behavior, 32,* 345–361.

Van Hasselt, V. B., Flood, J. J., Romano, S. J., Vecchi, G. M., de Fabrique, N., & Dalfonzo, V. A. (2005). Hostage-taking in the context of domestic violence: Some case examples. *Journal of Family Violence, 20,* 21–27.

Vecchi, G. M., Van Hasselt, V. B., & Romano, S. J. (2005). Crisis (hostage) negotiation: Current strategies and issues in high-risk conflict resolution. *Aggression and Violent Behavior, 10,* 533–551.

Webster, M. (2003). Active listening and beyond: Compliance strategies in crisis negotiation. *Crisis negotiations: A compendium.* Quantico, VA: U.S. Department of Justice; Federal Bureau of Investigation, FBI Academy.

Wilson, M. A. (2000). Toward a model of terrorist behavior in hostage-taking incidents. *Journal of Conflict Resolution, 44,* 403–424.

Zakrzewski, D. R. (2003). *Crisis negotiation.* Jacksonville, AL: ZAK.

CHAPTER 12

Survival, Evasion, Resistance, and Escape (SERE) Training

Preparing Military Members for the Demands of Captivity

Anthony P. Doran
Gary B. Hoyt
Melissa D. Hiller Lauby
Charles A. Morgan III

This chapter is dedicated to former SERE instructor GYSGT Ronald Baum, who is remembered as a valued friend, a dedicated family man, a talented SERE instructor, a leader, and a warrior. GYSGT Baum was killed in Iraq in May 2004 after having served the United States Marine Corps for 18½ years.

Becoming a prisoner of war (POW) has historically meant that a service member may experience brutality, torture, coercion, loneliness, and isolation, among many other forms of deprivation and exploitation. Each of these experiences is designed to accentuate human dependence on captors and, through these deprivations, achieve maximum exploitation. The immediate and lifelong effect of these experiences cannot be overstated. Service personnel captured and detained as POWs have significantly higher rates of emotional and physical trauma than service members not so detained (Babic & Sinanovic, 2004; Solomon, Neria, Ohry, Waysman, & Ginzburg, 1994), exhibiting as a group the highest rates of posttraumatic stress disorder (PTSD) and other mental health conditions (Sutker & Allain, 1996).

During World War II (WWII) roughly half of the military members captured in Germany and Japan developed PTSD (Goldstein, van Kammen, Shelly, Miller, & van Kammen, 1987; Zeiss & Dickman, 1989), which remained symptomatic throughout their lifetimes (Port, Engdahl, & Frazier, 2001; Tennant, Fairley, Dent, Sulway, & Broe, 1997). Sutker and Allain (1996) suggest that between 88 and 96% of Korean War POWs experienced a mental health condition related to their captivity. It has also been reported that POWs from WWII had extremely high mortality rates (Cohen & Cooper, 1954) and cognitive difficulties, such as visuospatial and memory deficits, decreased planning abilities, and impulse control problems (Sutker, Allain, & Johnson, 1993). In later life, surviving POWs who developed dementia were found to have higher rates of paranoia (Verma et al., 2001). Some of these problems are presumed to be related to the severe malnutrition often experienced by POWs; those who lost 35% or more of their body weight during captivity have had the greatest degree of verbal and visual learning and memory deficits (Sutker, Allain, Johnson, & Butters, 1992; Sutker, Vasterling, Brailey, & Allain, 1995). Also, in comparison with non-POW veterans, POWs have more adjustment disorders (Hall & Malone, 1976; Ursano, Boydstun, & Wheatley, 1981), alcohol abuse (Rundell, Ursano, Holloway, & Siberman, 1989), depressive disorders (Page, Engdahl, & Eberly, 1991), anxiety disorders (Hunter, 1975; Query, Megran, & McDonald, 1986), binge eating (Polivy, Zeitlin, Herman, & Beal, 1994), relationship difficulties (Cook, Riggs, Thompson, Coyne, & Sheikh, 2004), gastrointenstinal and musculoskeletal disorders (Creasey et al., 1999), and premature aging (e.g., Russell, 1984). (For a comprehensive review of the experiences of POWs through the various wars as well as their outcomes, see Moore, 2010.)

HISTORY OF SURVIVAL SCHOOLS

The military has long recognized the need for training programs to help service members effectively deal with survival in harsh environments, evasion from an enemy, and capture by a hostile force. The earliest survival schools focused on the use of life rafts, taught stereotyped traits of the Japanese, and provided the admonition, if captured, to disclose only the "Big Four" (name, rank, service number, and date of birth). Following WWII, when the Air Force was created in 1947, basic survival schools were set up in Nome, Alaska; Thule, Greenland; and Goose Bay, Labrador. Since the primary Air Force mission at that time was defending Alaska and preventing attacks over the North Pole, these schools were subsequently created to prepare service members for cold weather environments and taught such skills as building makeshift airstrips for rescue (J. Rankin & M. Wilson, personal communication, February 2002).

It was the Korean conflict, however, that dramatically changed the focus of the survival schools. Although the Korean War has been referred to as the "forgotten war" (fought between WWII and the Vietnam War), this description marginalizes the physical and psychological injuries suffered by many of these POWs. Forty percent of the more than 7,000 POWs in Korea died in captivity. The only POW death rate that was higher was American POWs held by the Japanese during WWII. Following the Korean War, 21 service members agreed to stay in Korea, having signed false confessions. Many interrogation experts and consultants believe that these confessions were the result of physical and psychological torture. Following these events, former POWs and senior military leaders began to take a long and serious look at how to better prepare our service men and women in survival training (Carlson, 2002).

Survival, evasion, resistance, and escape (SERE) training schools in their current form were the brainchild of the surviving Korean POWs, developed by a working group established by President Eisenhower, and implemented by the Air Force in 1961. The Air Force survival school is presently located in Spokane, Washington. The Navy SERE schools came online in 1962 (desert survival in Coronado, California, and cold weather survival in Brunswick, Maine), followed by the Army in 1963 (Fort Bragg, North Carolina). The Marine Corps initially developed a SERE school at Cherry Point, North Carolina, but ultimately chose to use the Navy schools, which are both now staffed with a detachment of Marines. In 2006, the Marine Corp created a specialized SERE program for their special operations community, which became fully accredited in 2008.

The Air Force initially used the term "survival" training to encompass everything from preparing for evasion and capture through recovery periods. The Navy coined the term SERE in the 1970s, according to the manner in which instructors divided the tasks to be taught (survive, evade, resist, and escape). The Army later followed the Navy, and the Air Force survival school became standardized with the other services, incorporating SERE in the 1980s (J. Rankin & M. Wilson, personal communication, February 2002).

Prior to the Korean conflict, the training for those at high risk of capture was to give only the Big Four, as taught during WWII. Because of the formidable task of enduring years of interrogation without revealing something other than name, rank, service number, and date of birth, other strategies were devised to help POWs manage interrogation without betraying their country and/or antagonizing their interrogators (Ruhl, 1978). After the Vietnam POWs returned in 1972, a number of them aided their SERE schools by teaching students about their experiences with torture, lengthy interrogations, threats of execution, disease, physical injuries, communications with fellow POWs and, most important, the means to keep hope alive. The most significant recommendation from the Vietnam veterans was to standardize training across the services.

Over the years, several joint organizations were developed to meet this challenge until ultimately the Joint Personnel Recovery Agency (JPRA) was established in 1999 under U.S. Joint Forces Command. The strategic purpose of this agency is to provide operational support and products to meet personnel recovery challenges; to provide training and education to prepare for, prevent, and respond to isolating events; to provide guidance and oversight in the standardization of training; to analyze personnel recovery capabilities and processes; and to ensure that relevant personnel recovery technologies are compatible and interoperable with existing command and control architectures (JPRA, 2011).

In 2011 after the disestablishment of U.S. Joint Forces Command, the Joint Chiefs of Staff was assigned as the executive agent for the JPRA. Today the JPRA continues to provide the oversight for all SERE and Military Code of Conduct training. In addition to providing regular oversight inspections of each SERE schoolhouse, the JPRA hosts annual training forums for program directors, SERE psychologists, and personnel recovery specialists, and planners to adjust and provide standardized guidance to all of the SERE schools and personnel recovery personnel. Viewed as integral training by all military service departments, SERE schools continue to develop and evolve to meet current challenges and ensure all students are adequately trained to handle today's threats. The JPRA has recently published new guidance on joint standards for SERE training in support of the Code of Conduct and on joint standards for SERE training role-playing activities in an effort to ensure best practices and the safety of both students and staff in this high-risk training environment (JPRA, 2010a, 2010b) . The Air Force has developed a Level B SERE course, Evasion and Conduct After Capture, which provides academic survival, evasion, and recovery lessons along with the intensive captivity role play laboratory. The Marine Corps and Navy have both developed specialized SERE courses for their special operations forces to more thoroughly cover issues and situations more likely to be encountered by these specialized groups.

OVERVIEW OF CURRENT SERE TRAINING

SERE instructors provide survival training to those military personnel designated as high risk of isolation, capture, kidnapping, or governmental detention (e.g., aviation personnel, snipers, members of Special Forces, and intelligence gatherers). SERE training is built around stress inoculation training (Meichenbaum, (1985). The concept of stress inoculation (Meichenbaum, 1985) is very much akin to the concept of preventing illness through vaccination. Like a vaccine, stress inoculation occurs when training stress is high enough to activate the body's psychological and biological coping mechanisms but not so great as to overwhelm them. When stress inoculation occurs, an individual's performance is likely to improve when stressed again. To work within this model, students are presented with didactic information in the classroom as well as opportunities to further acquire the skills through classroom-based role plays. Training culminates in an *in vivo* laboratory exercise to further refine and use their skills in an environment that is as realistic as possible.

There are two key components in the training: field and resistance. The field component of training is designed to give students the skills to survive the elements, navigate unfamiliar territory, and evade capture. The resistance component encompasses skills to survive captivity, including how to use situational awareness, to resist and degrade exploitation and interrogation methods, to plan an escape if feasible, and to return with honor by following the Code of Conduct. To best prepare today's service men and women, all SERE schools prepare students for a variety of captivity contingencies, including peacetime/governmental detention, POW captivity, and various abduction and hostage scenarios. Given its sensitive nature and content, only an overview of the unclassified portion of the training may be provided here.

Students are provided academic lessons that review personal survival skills, navigation and evasion, as well as techniques to assist in successfully resisting interrogation and exploitation methods. Following academic lessons, students are provided with more in-depth and practical experiences in the field such as land navigation lessons covering skills to navigate through unknown territory and how to procure potable water, hunt and trap small animals, build small shelters, and differentiate edible from poisonous

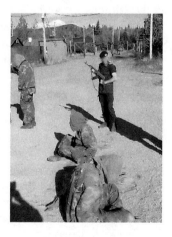

FIGURE 12.1. Students are exposed to some of the stressors of captivity.

plants. During this time, students are forced to deal with hunger, uncertainty, fatigue, and discouragement in an experiential manner rather than in an academic format. In the field component, students officially begin the live evasion portion of their training. Their primary task initially is to reach various navigation objectives (i.e., make contact with friendly forces) several miles away by successfully moving through hostile territory. During the captivity phase, students are captured by simulated hostile entities, where they are confronted with various captivity scenarios in which they must use their situational awareness, newly acquired resistance techniques, and the Code of Conduct to successfully survive captivity. This is indeed the most memorable, and ultimately the most physically and psychologically demanding, aspect of the training (see Figures 12.1 and 12.2).

THE SERE PSYCHOLOGIST

Little has been written about the varied roles of a SERE psychologist. In the past, SERE psychologists received their mandates from a variety of resources that included several U.S. Department of Defense Directives (DoDD) and Instructions (DoDI) that articulated some of the roles and training requirements: DoDD 1300.7 (DoD, 2000a), DoDD 2310.2 (DoD, 2000b), DoDI 2310.4 (DoD, 2000c), and DoDI 1300.21 (DoD, 2001). In response to the need for a better articulated instruction, the JPRA published the "Guidance on Qualification Criteria and Use of Department of Defense (DoD) Survival, Evasion, Resistance, and Escape (SERE) Psychologists in Support of the Code of Conduct" (2010c). This document clearly articulates the qualifications needed to work in the SERE community as well as the roles and responsibilities of psychologists in both the schoolhouse and personnel recovery environment.

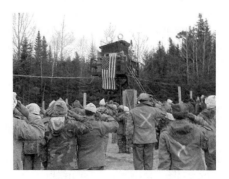

FIGURE 12.2. A SERE class completes the captivity phase.

The 2010 guidance delineates three levels of SERE qualifications for psychologists. A SERE-oriented psychologist is a DoD psychologist who has completed a JPRA-approved SERE oriented psychologist course. A SERE-oriented psychologist is able to assist JPRA and SERE-certified psychologists in the reintegration processes of repatriated service members and beneficiaries. A SERE-certified psychologist is a DoD psychologist who is certified by JPRA to assist JPRA, combatant commands, and services during the reintegration process and may serve as the psychologist on the reintegration team. Certification requirements include the orientation course as well as having an in-depth knowledge in the dynamics of captivity, isolation, and exploitation; how to promote resilience in returnees; and how to support reintegration. Additionally, the SERE-certified psychologist must participate regularly in reintegration exercises, complete continuing education in the field, and most importantly complete a Level C SERE course. By having the experience provided by the course, especially the emotional and physical strain of being taken prisoner and the pressures of countering interrogation efforts and exploitation, the psychologist is better able to achieve far greater empathy and understanding of what is necessary for survival in captivity, thus resulting in a greater ability to work in the various roles required as a SERE psychologist. Last, a third SERE psychology qualification is the RT qualified-SERE psychologist. An RT-qualified SERE psychologist is a DoD psychologist who is a certified-SERE psychologist who has been assigned to a DoD SERE school or a high-risk unit and has obtained the necessary training and experience to oversee Code of Conduct high-risk training.

PRIMARY ROLES OF THE SERE PSYCHOLOGIST

The roles and functions of the SERE psychologist will depend greatly upon assignment, although they fall into five general categories: evaluator, safety observer, educator, consultant/researcher, and repatriation. According to the JPRA 2010 guidelines, an RT-qualified SERE psychologist will be the commander's primary representative to ensure close supervision of training, including risk monitoring and assessment, training effectiveness and evaluation, assessment and selection, and ongoing evaluation of instructors. Additionally, the RT-qualified SERE psychologist will provide instructor training to reduce risk to students and increase training effectiveness, provide interventions to students and staff as needed, and provide a debrief to SERE students at the completion of their training. SERE-certified psychologists may also be called upon to assist in the reintegration of isolated personnel (JPRA, 2010c).

Evaluator

A key function of the SERE psychologist is the performance of screening assessments to evaluate a candidate's suitability as a SERE instructor. All SERE instructors, without exception, must undergo an intensive psychological evaluation prior to reporting. Given that one of the most important and potentially dangerous roles of the SERE instructor is role-playing the character of a captor, guard, or interrogator, this evaluative screening becomes paramount in importance. Many of the procedures at the SERE school for the selection and training of instructors are a direct result of the prison experiment conducted at Stanford University (Haney, Banks, & Zimbardo, 1973). This study examined the behavior of 24 individuals who had been carefully evaluated and selected for emotional stability. They were randomly assigned to either a "guard" or "prisoner" group. The experiment was initially designed to last 2 weeks, but it was discontinued after 6 days because of increasing and arbitrary antisocial behavior in the role-playing environment. The subjects who were pretending to be guards became overly "negative, hostile, affrontive, and dehumanizing" (p. 80) in effect, ceasing to perceive the prisoners as research participants. The subjects pretending to be prisoners became overly compliant, docile, and conforming, and five of them had to be released prior to the premature end of the experiment because they developed "extreme emotional depression, crying, rage, and acute anxiety" (p. 81).

A reevaluation of this decades-old experiment tells us that these lessons continue to have just as much merit today. Haney and Zimbardo (1998) suggest that prison environments must be carefully evaluated and regulated, and they warn that social contexts with significant power differentials left unchecked can interact to produce dehumanizing environments. They further suggest that psychological assessment for prison personnel must include situationally sensitive models that tap specific situations likely to occur in a prison environment. Essentially, an intrinsically problematic social context can significantly affect the behavior of normal individuals and contribute to their participation in behavioral drift (consciously or unwittingly). More recent events at Abu Ghraib continue to support the fact that when certain factors come into play (e.g., combat stressors, inadequate training, role immersion), ordinary people placed in the role of prison guards can perform unforeseen acts of cruelty (Bartone, 2010; Fiske, Harris, & Cuddy, 2004).

Since it is clear that individuals who are screened for emotional stability can still exhibit pathological behavior (Haney et al., 1973), selection as a SERE instructor necessarily entails an arduous and extensive process, with months of follow-up training that includes annual training on recognizing and preventing behavioral drift and self-care. A general profile of the

SERE instructor indicates that the average individual is over 30 years of age (approximately 10 years older than the college students used in the prison study), has more than 15 years of military service, is married, has numerous personal awards, was their previous command's top performer, and has no legal, substance abuse, or disciplinary history. For screening purposes, a comprehensive psychological evaluation is provided, consisting of an in-depth clinical interview, medical record review, reports from previous supervisors, and psychological testing (e.g., Minnesota Multiphasic Personality Inventory, second edition). Psychologically the SERE instructor has a high need for achievement, has a high frustration tolerance, enjoys being part of a group (Doran, 2002), and is able to tolerate the intense scrutiny of not only the evaluation process but, more important, the constant observation and oversight that occurs throughout a tour at the SERE school.

Safety Observer

Perhaps the most important lesson from the prison experiment in relation to SERE training is the necessity of maintaining the physical and psychological health of participants through consistent monitoring of individuals and systematic evaluation of the process itself. SERE training necessarily incorporates certain levels of emotional and physical distress to maintain the integrity and efficacy of the training experience, essentially integrating many of the lessons learned from prior POW experiences. For example, captors (e.g., Germans and Japanese in WWII and North Koreans and Vietnamese during these respective conflicts) have generally utilized four tactics with captured personnel: isolation, deprivation, abuse, and interrogation (Sherwood, 1986). Isolation consists of not only physical separation from other prisoners but also a more general isolation strategy of breaking ties with family, country, and, most significantly, a former identity of oneself. Deprivation consists of withholding food, water, adequate clothing and shelter, sleep, access to constructive physical and cognitive activity, medical care, and adequate means of maintaining personal hygiene. Psychological abuse, such as threatening to harm or kill prisoners, and coercive physical abuse have been commonly reported historically. Last, interrogations for the purpose of gathering military intelligence have been routinely performed, often utilizing combinations of the first three tactics.

Because these imprisonment strategies are brutal in and of themselves, and approximating them for learning purposes in training scenarios is an extremely sophisticated task, the existence of stringent guidelines and protocols is basic for effective functioning. The just-mentioned issues illuminate the need for in-depth training of staff in positions of power as well as in regimented safety procedures. The safety observer position was implemented to ensure that "captors and guards" do not cross the line and that "prisoners" do not become unduly traumatized by their experience. Consequently, the role of safety observer is one of the key responsibilities of the SERE psychologist.

During SERE training, there are at least three to five personnel whose sole responsibility is to be safety observers, ensuring the well-being of those participating in training. Although all SERE personnel at times act as safety observers, the psychologist's specific duty in this role is to monitor the instructors for cues that a "guard" or "captor" might be taking the role too seriously or too far. Other than the obvious scenario of a too-aggressive instructor, the psychologist looks for subtle changes in instructors' typical mode of operating, which may indicate that they are having some difficulties. Some instructors might become more outspoken when they are typically quiet, become too gentle during an interrogation, exhibit real affect during or after an exercise, or even subtly or unconsciously target a specific student. Some of the more general indicators of behavioral drift include observed diffusion of responsibility, dehumanizing tendencies, or reliance on anonymity for decreased accountability. A key concept in training for instructors is "performing" the role versus "becoming" the role. The instructor must maintain the mind-set that he or she is an instructor, not an interrogator or guard, and that the purpose of the exercise is for the student to demonstrate resistance techniques.

In addition to the monitoring in the training environment, instructors are also monitored outside of it. Accepting a job at SERE places a strain on even a healthy marital relationship, as much of the job cannot be discussed at home because of its classified nature. The combination of possibly bringing power roles home to spouses and children and being unable to discuss workday occurrences and stressors can be difficult on these military families. SERE personnel are taught how to monitor each other for warning signs, such as increases in irritability or alcohol consumption, decreased military bearing, or any new shifts in behavior that might affect their ability to perform. The SERE psychologist formally and informally encourages instructors to decompress from the training environment through the use of healthy stress management techniques (such as physical exercise, relaxation strategies, and humor). Also, the SERE psychologist is one of many personnel who help ensure that SERE instructors are rotated from position to position. This not only helps to promote cross-training but also helps to move SERE instructors out of power roles for extended periods of time.

Although a main thrust of the safety observer's role is to closely monitor the instructors, the observers are ultimately there to maintain the integrity and realism of the training experience for the benefit of the students. Not unexpectedly, some students have strong, maladaptive reactions to certain aspects of the training. Given the nature of the highly dedicated and trained SERE students (e.g., Special Forces members, aircrew and pilots, and intelligence operators), they are not always amenable to psychological intervention or performance direction. Although significant anxiety, irritability, and even hallucinations are considered normal, interventions may be initiated when they arise. Generally, this early intervention and assessment of psychological status is best done by a technician (e.g., corpsman, medic, psychological technician) or a psychologically minded senior instructor to reduce stigma, although still under the supervision of the psychologist. Having a psychologist immediately intervene may create the perception that the SERE student is incapable of completing training or that his or her reaction is not normal (True & Benaway, 1992).

Educator

The SERE psychologist provides multiple types of education for both staff and student trainees. All SERE personnel receive training in the dangers of role-playing situations in which individuals have power over others. The psychologist reviews in-depth information related to role immersion, the prison study findings, and the ethics involved in the mock imprisonment described earlier (Zimbardo, 1973). All personnel must exhibit a comprehensive understanding of the concepts raised by this research in order to work at SERE. In addition, the operational psychologist teaches the safety observers what signs to look for, in both the instructors and the students that would indicate a problem so that appropriate intervention can be initiated.

In addition to regular training, the SERE psychologist also educates the trainees. In this role as educator, the operational psychologist explains the normal reactions to severe uncontrollable stress—including fear, anger, negative self-statements, crying, illusions and hallucinations, dissociation, somatic complaints, and memory problems—and how long they are expected to last (Dobson & Marshall, 1997; Engle & Spencer, 1993; Mitchell, 1983; Sokol, 1989; Yerkes, 1993). This education has proven to be an integral part of the success of captured service members. A number of factors help individuals to be more resilient under stress (Morgan, Wang, Mason, et al., 2000); Morgan, Wang, Southwick, et al. (2000). From Korea and Vietnam POWs to the more recent EP-3 crew detained in China, service members reported that whereas their military training aided in the survival of a particular incident, it was the experiential nature of SERE training that facilitated their survival in captivity (Doran, 2001).

In addition to successfully completing SERE training, individuals who functioned well in captivity possessed several characteristics, including a strong faith in their country, in each other, and in God. Those who focused on factors under their internal control, such as thinking about future plans (e.g., designing their dream house, down to the smallest detail) or developing a personal exercise program in their cell, were also much more successful (Ursano & Rundell, 1996). Successful former POWs had a tremendous sense of humor (Henman, 2001), were older and had higher levels of education at the time of their imprisonment (Gold et al., 2000), and had an ability to reframe their situation even under the most dire circumstances. Research on former POWs from the Vietnam War has consistently demonstrated that this group is fairly resilient (Coffee, 1990), and that SERE training provided experiential anchors and cues to help them effectively cope with the demands of captivity. An example of the ability to reframe events comes from the comments of a commanding officer who kept a piece of shrapnel on his desk and would explain to the curious: "That is a piece of shrapnel that flew over my head during the Vietnam War when I was serving as a corpsman. When I am having a bad day, I realize things could be a lot worse" (CAPT A. Shimkus, personal communication, November 2003).

Consultant and Researcher

Acquainted with the results of stress research (Meichenbaum, 1985), the U.S. military designs training to be physically and psychologically demanding and lifelike in stress intensity. Challenging and realistic training develops trainees' ability to perform on the battlefield, and exposure to realistic levels of stress is intended to inoculate them from the negative effects of operational stress. In the roles of consultant and researcher, the SERE psychologist explores a wide variety of research topics related to the effects that severe stress has on humans. SERE offers a unique opportunity to validate training parameters, establish predictors of superior performance, and develop new tools and techniques for the war on terrorism. These topics have particular military relevance, and a brief synopsis of some of this research follows.

Validation of Training Parameters

Over the past decade, civilian and military research teams have assessed the impact of acute stress on psychological, neurohormonal and physiological parameters in students enrolled in U.S. and in non-U.S. military survival school training (Eid & Morgan, 2006; Demoulis et al, 2007; Morgan, Wang, Mason, et al., 2000; Taylor et al., 2000; Morgan et al., 2001, 2002, 2006, 2009; Morgan, Hazlett, et al., 2004; Taylor, Sausen, Mujica-Parodi, et al., 2007; Taylor, Sausen, Potterat, et al., 2007; Morgan, Southwick, et al., 2004; Morgan, Wang, Southwick, et al., 2008, 2009, 2011, 2012). This research has had the overarching goal of assessing the impact of realistic stress in healthy humans and to elucidate the factors that explain why and how people differ in their response to stress. It is hoped that by elucidating the factors that contribute to stress resilience, this research will lead to better treatment strategies for individuals who suffer from trauma-related mental health problems. Given this overarching goal, the initial purpose of studies conducted at SERE was to assess whether or not SERE represented a venue in which valid studies of acute stress in humans could be conducted. Specifically, it was important to learn whether the stress experienced by participants was comparable to real-world stress (Morgan, Wang, Mason, et al., 2000; Morgan, Wang, Southwick, et al., 2000; Morgan et al., 2001, 2002). Investigators examined the overall impact of each phase of SERE training (classroom, evasion, and detention) as well as several specific components. The results of these studies provide the following evidence:

1. SERE stress is within the range of real-world stress and of a magnitude necessary for stress inoculation (Morgan, Wang, Mason, et al., 2000; Morgan, Wang, Southick, et al., 2000; Morgan et al., 2001, 2002).
2. Students who undergo SERE training recover normally and do not show a negative effect from having experienced this type of military training (i.e., stress sensitization; Morgan et al., 2001, 2002, 2006; Morgan, Hazlett, et al., 2004; Morgan, Southwick, et al., 2004).
3. Students' physiology and biological measures indicate a normal recovery from the various physical interrogation aspects of SERE training (Morgan et al., 2001, 2002).

Establishment of Predictors of Superior Performance during Stress

The SERE research conducted to date has also provided clues as to why and how some students perform better under stress than others. More specifically, this team of investigators has examined why and how some students remain mentally clear and experience fewer stress-induced cognitive deficits when the stress increases. The researchers evaluated specific capacities such as resistance techniques, simple and complex problem-solving abilities during stress, and visual and verbal memory capacity (Morgan, Hazlett, et al., 2004; Morgan, Southick, et al., 2004; Morgan et al., 2006; Morgan, Aikins, et al., 2007; Morgan, Hazlett, et al., 2007). The results of this line of research indicate the following:

1. Specific psychological and biological differences at baseline predict objective performance during stress. (For a review of the neurobiological and neuroanatomical elements of acute stress, see McNeil & Morgan, 2010.) For example, students who exhibit high heart rate variability, low

levels of neuropeptide Y (NPY)—a 36-amino-acid peptide related to the release of norepinephrine and involved in the regulation of noradrenergic system functioning (Morgan, Wang, Southwick, et al., 2000; Morgan et al., 2002)—and baseline symptoms of dissociation do significantly worse under stress (Eid & Morgan, 2006; Morgan et al., 2001, 2002).

2. There are specific biological differences in circulating hormones during stress that explain why some students are more focused, more clear-headed during stress, and show more accuracy in cognitive and memory tests after stress. For example, students who do well when exposed to training stress release greater levels of dehydroepiandrosterone (a steroid hormone that can convert into estrogen and testosterone) and NPY during stress than those who do poorly. These individuals are more accurate in descriptions of what they encountered during stress. These studies can help us develop specific interventions to enhance operational abilities (Morgan, Southwick, et al., 2004; Morgan, Aikins, et al., 2007; Morgan, Hazlett, et al., 2007; Taylor et al., 2007, 2008, 2009, 2011, 2012).

New Tools and Techniques for Professions Engaged in the War on Terrorism

In response to issues raised by the September 11, 2001, terrorist attacks on the United States, the Director of National Intelligence issued a report on what is currently known about interrogations: "Educing Information: Interrogation: Science and Art, Foundations for the Future" (Fein, Lehner, & Vossekuil, 2006). As noted in the report, there is little empirical evidence for most of the methods and techniques employed by law enforcement or government officials who conduct interrogations. A significant barrier to conducting research that could help determine whether specific questioning techniques or technologies (such as the polygraph) are effective is that most research laboratories cannot ethically expose research subjects to realistic stress comparable to that of a person being questioned in real-life circumstances. However, as noted by stress studies described previously, SERE training is a venue in which one can ethically examine the issue of efficacy of some methods currently used by U.S. officials, such as the polygraph. Determining whether a traditional method (like the polygraph) loses efficacy when used on people who are experiencing significant stress would be extremely helpful. Clarifying whether or not techniques that purportedly detect deception actually work under stressful conditions may provide empirical data that would inform law enforcement agencies as well as government officials about whether spending taxpayer money on these techniques, or believing the information gained by using such techniques, is valid.

A team of investigators has recently completed a study with SERE students that was designed to test the accuracy (sensitivity and specificity) of the traditional polygraph in detecting concealed knowledge. Analysis of the data indicated that traditional measures of the polygraph did no better than chance in detecting the guilty subjects. These findings are important and provide powerful evidence that officials should *not* rely on such techniques to detect deception in people who are experiencing significant stress. This said, it is possible that new approaches, such as assessments of RSAnorm, can be used to accurately determine when a person is engaged in telling a deceptive story while under conditions of stress. While promising, these data need to be replicated in populations of SERE students who are not members of special operations units in order to assess whether the findings are likely to generalize to other members of the population.

One future direction of SERE stress research is to look at differences between men and women. Dimoulas et al. (2007) examined dissociation and somatic complaints in female SERE students and compared them with previous samples of male students that included Special Forces troops and general infantry soldiers. The research highlighted three points. First, both men and women who report previous trauma from which they thought they might die tend to experience greater levels of dissociation. Second, baseline measures of dissociation indicated that the female participants' dissociation measures were most similar to those of the Special Forces comparison group and, as a sample, were lower than those of the general infantry students. One possible explanation for this is that women who self-select careers that require SERE training are most likely a very stress-hardy group, having already completing physically and mentally challenging training (i.e., flight school, officer candidate school) in their career pathways. Last, women with higher levels of dissociation tend to report more somatic complaints ($r = .76, p < .0001$) compared with their male counterparts ($r = 0.54$, $p < .02$). Unfortunately, this study was limited in that it was not able to determine whether this finding is due to differences in pathophysiology or the homogeneity of this particular sample. Future research will determine whether women's stress response mechanism is similar to males or controlled by different brain and neurohormone mechanisms (Dimoulas et al., 2007). A study currently under way at Navy SERE West will specifically examine gender differences as it pertains to these very important questions. Ultimately, all of this research is geared toward enhancing our understanding of stress and improving the performance of our sailors, soldiers, aircrews, and Marines during combat.

Repatriation

A critical role for the SERE psychologist is the repatriation process. Verifying both the applicability and efficacy of SERE training to real-world situations can be a difficult task, given the significant hurdles or confounds of validation research of POW occurrences. However, one of the primary vehicles utilized by the DoD for assessment of individual performance and SERE training in general is the process of repatriation. DoDI 2310.4 (2000c), concerning personnel recovery, indicates that preserving the life and well-being of personnel who are placed in harm's way is one of the highest priorities. It states that "personnel recovery is a critical element in the DoD ability to fulfill its moral obligation to protect its personnel, prevent exploitation of U.S. personnel by adversaries, and reduce the potential of captured personnel being used as leverage against the United States" (p. 2).

In general, there are four basic types of personnel recovery. First and foremost, isolated individuals have an obligation to evade potential captors and, if captured or detained, to effect their own escape within the parameters of the Military Code of Conduct and Geneva Conventions (in essence, to facilitate their own recovery). The term *isolated* is used here to describe personnel who are supporting a military mission and are temporarily separated from their units in an environment requiring them to survive and evade capture or to resist and escape if captured. The second form of personnel recovery is characterized as conventional combat search and rescue (CSAR), wherein trained military forces on land or sea recover the isolated individual. An example would be the recovery of a downed pilot, in danger of being captured but not yet detained. The third form of recovery, typically a far more fluid and dangerous proposition, is described as an unconventional assisted recovery. In this situation, trained Special Forces might be inserted into the equation to contact, authenticate, and extract detained U.S. personnel. In essence, the CSAR mission becomes an armed recovery from enemy forces, with the goal of returning detainees to U.S. control. Certainly, this can be fraught with danger, for both the detainees and recovery forces, and will have important implications in the repatriation process debriefings. The fourth method of personnel recovery involves a negotiated release, typically with diplomatic initiatives between governments. Of course, these four methods are general descriptions and contain a number of variants and convergences as the situation dictates.

Once isolated or detained personnel are recovered and returned to U.S. control, the work of repatriation begins. Repatriation can be thought of as an established process that bridges two entirely different contexts: the readjustment from captivity back into life as a U.S. citizen and/or service member. The repatriation of recovered DoD personnel is an extraordinarily important process for the well-being of the individual and for U.S. government interests. Certainly, one of the primary aims is to restore the health of formerly isolated personnel through a process of psychological decompression. Other critical concerns include the lessons learned from recovery incidents or methods, the tactical and strategic intelligence that may have been gleaned from or transferred to enemy combatants, and the applicability or efficacy of the SERE training course. DoDI 2310.4 (2000c) explicitly states, "The well-being and legal rights of the individual returnee shall be the overriding factors when planning and executing repatriation operations. Except in extreme circumstances of military necessity, they must take priority over all political, military or other considerations" (p. 3). Subsequently, the operational aspects of each stage of the repatriation process will be carried out in accordance with thoughtful consideration of the hardships endured and the physiological, psychological, and spiritual needs of the returnee. Other inclusive aims involve the recovery of personal dignity and pride that may have been affected by captivity and the restoration of confidence in one's person and country.

Repatriation is accomplished in three phases. Phase I begins when recovered personnel are returned to U.S. control. If possible, they are met by an operational psychologist, a medical officer, a carefully selected key unit member, a chaplain, a public affairs officer (PAO), and a legal officer. At times, because of logistical complications, the presence of the entire repatriation team is not possible during Phase I and instead becomes available during Phase II. An essential component of the first phase is the immediacy of medical and psychological stabilization for the returnees. The initial medical and psychological triage of the individuals involved and the subsequent assessment of their health will significantly influence their handling and processing in each phase. Of course, these assessments will differentiate between actual detainment status and being isolated behind enemy lines, and they will also consider the duration and treatment in captivity, along with the type of recovery method utilized (conventional vs. unconventional).

Another key component in Phase I repatriation is transportation to a designated secure area nearby. This secure area can be in the same theater of operations and is intended to allow for safe and efficient repatriation. Also, in the event of a relatively short period of isolated experience or evasion, and if no medical, psychological, or operational contraindications exist, the individual might very well return to duty from this location. There is a greater degree of flexibility in assessing recovered personnel who have been isolated but not detained. The decision to return to duty from this secure area is consistent with the BICEPS concept of combat stress control: *Brevity* of treatment, *Immediacy* of the response, *Centrality* of the treatment area, *Expectancy* of recuperation, *Proximity* of treatment near the incident location, and *Simplicity* of the interventions. Since the returnees are considered not in need of psychological services, the focus can be directed at transitioning them back to duty unless their condition suggests otherwise. They would still complete critical operational and/or intelligence debriefings for immediate dissemination but then would be allowed to return to their primary duty.

If the returnees have experienced a prolonged period of evasion from or detention by hostile forces, then the Phase I secure area will probably be a short transition point en route to a Phase II location, typically a major regional medical center near that theater of operation. General duties of the operational psychologist during this phase may include (1) initial and ongoing psychological assessment to address the needs and psychological status of the returnees, which will subsequently direct future interventions and debriefing operations for them; (2) education of the returnees (and their chain of command) about what they may expect in the near future; and (3) the moderation of their activities and public or familial exposure to aid in decompression and transition. These factors will continue to be revisited and adjusted as needed while the SERE psychologist accompanies the returnee to the Phase II location.

In general, most returnees continue on to Phase II of the repatriation, where more thorough medical and psychological assessment takes place. Also, most of the formal debriefing occurs during this time. A variety of debriefings occur in Phase II and often carry over into Phase III. These might include operational or intelligence debriefs, SERE training debriefs, or psychological decompression debriefs. They are carried out separately to avoid convergence of details or facts and are generally moderated by an operational psychologist in accordance with the psychological condition of the returnees. The operational psychologist monitors for situations that detract from the returnees' readjustment and advocate for protocols that maximize the accuracy of recalled information. Each of these debriefs are part of a larger decompression effort formulated to allow returnees maximum reintegration success in their military and civilian lives. The minimum time frame to complete these processes is 3 days.

Operational and intelligence debriefs are oriented toward the returnee's mission. Military members in general are routinely asked to complete postmission debriefs with superiors, often focusing on successes and failures, lessons learned, intelligence gleaned from the enemy or given away (if contact was made), or changes in standard operating procedures (should the situation warrant it). These military debriefs are carried out in a professional manner, are behaviorally or factually focused, and are tactical or strategic in nature. Operational and/or intelligence debriefers in a repatriation context try to mirror routine, typical debriefs. There is an important decompressing element as well, since returnees are able to obtain relevant feedback from authorities who can answer nagging concerns or questions they may have about their own performance. In this manner, returnees are allowed conceptually to "complete the mission." The relevant information from these debriefs is immediately disseminated to the appropriate commanders for tactical purposes.

Psychological debriefing primarily provides decompression for the returnees through a guided process of "telling their story." This process can be particularly helpful when there is more than one returnee, as experiences are shared and each recipient receives a fuller understanding of the situation and experiences. Furthermore, since returnees are not necessarily considered psychologically impaired as a result of their experiences, much effort is expended to educate and normalize their psychological reactions to the situations they encountered. The returnees generally find significant comfort in understanding their past and/or current reactions as "normal human responses to abnormal events" and the knowledge that these reactions will improve over time. Some of the typical psychological reactions to release from captivity are sleep disruption (nightmares, insomnia, or hypersomnia), changes in concentration (memory deficits or disorientation), mood fluctuations (irritability, hostility, depression, guilt, anxiety, or euphoria), and reevaluation of life goals and convictions. The extent of these symptoms largely depends on the preexisting traits of the individual, the level of sleep and sensory deprivation or isolation experienced, the type of duress and coercive attempts endured, and possibly the duration of captivity. Much of the psychological decompression occurring in Phase II involves the operational psychologist's ability to (1) educate and normalize the returnees' reactions to the events they experienced and (2) clarify the context in which their actions occurred, with the goal of providing meaning and connectedness to their actions.

A reciprocal benefit of SERE debriefs is the ability to provide feedback to the SERE training institutions in a research and development continuum. In other words, clarifying difficulties encountered with personnel recovery, learning about the enemy's interrogation methods or aims of exploitation, or assessing the treatment of captives is directly applicable to the validation efforts of the current training methodologies and course of instruction. It is important in this educative process that returnees are able to ask direct questions and receive direct feedback about their own performance. Since military members are held to the standards of the Military Code of Conduct, it is often part of their psychological decompression to know that they have comported themselves well and "returned with honor."

In Phase II, reintegration with the returnee's family also begins. Generally, the initial contact with family is by telephone, as personal visitation in Phase II has been found to be problematic in the past. Although this principle would seem to be counterintuitive in some ways, experience has shown that the returnees' immediate integration with their families can be conflictive with their own long-term psychological decompression needs as well as with the general efforts of a repatriation operation. For instance, there may have been significant shifts in family roles during detention, or family issues may have already existed, making it difficult for the returnees to receive assistance in decompressing while engaged in familial needs. Accordingly, a PAO and legal officer are also assigned to the returnee to assist with any information or interview requests, as well as any relevant legal concerns caused by the detention. Again, with the returnee's needs foremost, the operational psychologist will generally work closely with the PAO to jointly decide on the appropriate level of media exposure. A "key unit member" also aids the decompression process by providing familiarity to predetention life, liaison assistance between the returnee and the unit, and assistance with any other administrative or logistical concerns.

Phase III occurs in the continental United States and is the opportunity for the returnees to be physically reunited with their families, unit members, and friends. Despite the probable desire to be immediately sheltered away by family, loved ones, or friends, it is equally important for returnees to maintain some form of contact with their military unit or captivity peers upon returning home, particularly for those who had been held in group captivity and were repatriated together. Generally, there may have been some unique experiences and psychological reactions that are best worked through with the same repatriated peers or with guides familiar with the psychology of captivity. Continued affiliation with groups that have experienced traumatic or difficult events together has proven helpful in the past. If significant changes occurred in the family structure because of the returnee's absence, a period of transition or adaptation may be indicated. Furthermore, if family members wish to address their own needs or concerns related to the returnee's absence, it can be provided by contact with the military unit or through JPRA and SERE psychologists.

For the returnee's aftercare, medical needs will continue to be attended to as necessary, along with follow-up by the affiliated SERE psychologist for any ongoing psychological needs. By protocol, the SERE psychologist will continue to be available and provide aftercare as indicated throughout the following year. Also, all detainees and repatriated POWs are eligible for annual screenings and continued medical and psychological services through the Robert Mitchell Center for Repatriated POW Studies Center in Pensacola, Florida (see Moore, 2010).

SUMMARY

SERE training aids and equips service members to cope with the unthinkable demands of captivity. Although SERE training may induce temporary psychological changes and demands while being held captive by a simulated enemy for several days, the psychological and physical effects of truly being held prisoner can result in permanent damage. One of the key functions of SERE training, and the experiential learning and preparation therein, is to give service members the tools and the confidence needed to mitigate problematic future effects of the demands of captivity.

The operational psychologist plays a vital role in this training environment as an evaluator, safety observer, educator, researcher, and consultant. When service members are recovered, the SERE psychologist functions as a consultant and clinician during the repatriation process. The SERE environment is a laboratory of realistic stress, and over time the research conducted can provide far greater understanding of how to enhance performance under severe stress.

REFERENCES

Babic, D., & Sinanovic, S. (2004). Psychic disorders in former prisoners of war. *Medical Archives, 58,* 179–182.

Bartone, P. T. (2010). Preventing prisoner abuse: Leadership lessons of Abu Ghraib. *Ethics and Behavior, 20,* 161–173.

Carlson, L. (2002). *Remembered prisoners of a forgotten war: An oral history of the Korean War POWs.* New York: St. Martin's.

Coffee, G. (1990). *Beyond survival: Building on the hard times.* New York: Putnam.

Cohen, B., & Cooper, M. (1954). A followup study of WWII POWs. *Veterans Administration Medical Monograph.* Washington, DC: U.S. Government Printing Office.

Cook, J. M., Riggs, D. S., Thompson, R., Coyne, J. C., & Sheikh, J. I. (2004). Posttraumatic stress disorder and current relationship functioning among World War II ex-prisoners of war. *Journal of Family Psychology, 18,* 36–45.

Creasey, H., Sulway, M. R., Dent, O., Broe, G. A., Jorm, A., & Tennant, C. (1999). Is experience as a prisoner of war a risk factor for accelerated age-related illness and disability? *Journal of the American Geriatric Society, 47,* 60–64.

Dimoulas, E., Steffian, L., Steffian, G., Doran, A. P., Rasmusson, A. M., & Morgan, C. A. (2007). Dissociation during intense military stress is related to subsequent somatic symptoms in women. *Psychiatry, 4,* 66–73.

Dobson, M., & Marshall, R. (1997). Surviving the war zone: Preventing psychiatric casualties. *Military Medicine, 162,* 283–287.

Doran, A. (2001). *Summary of repatriation of EP-3 crew.* Unpublished mission summary.

Doran, A. (2002). *Descriptive factors of SERE instructors at Brunswick, Maine, from 2000–2002.* Unpublished raw data.

Eid, J., & Morgan, C. A. (2006). Dissociation, hardiness and performance in military cadets participating in survival training. *Military Medicine, 171(5),* 436–442.

Engle, C., & Spencer, S. (1993). Revitalizing division mental health in garrison: A post Desert Storm perspective. *Military Medicine, 158,* 533–537.

Fein, R. A., Lehner, P., & Vossekuil, B. (2006). *Educing Information. Interrogation: Science and art. Foundations for the future.* National Defense Intelligence College. Retrieved October 16, 2011, from *www.fas.org/irp/dni/educing.pdf.*

Fiske, S. T., Harris, L. T., & Cuddy, A. J. (2004). Why ordinary people torture enemy prisoners. *Science, 306,* 1482–1483.

Gold, P. B., Engdahl, B. E., Eberly, R. E., Blake, R. J., Page, W. F., & Frueh, B. C. (2000). Trauma exposure, resilience, social support, and PTSD construct validity among former prisoners of war. *Social Psychiatry and Psychiatric Epidemiology, 35,* 36–42.

Goldstein, G., van Kammen, W., Shelly, C., Miller, D., & van Kammen, D. P. (1987). Survivors of imprisonment in the Pacific theater during World War II. *American Journal of Psychiatry, 144,* 1210–1213.

Hall, R., & Malone, P. (1976). Psychiatric effects of prolonged Asian captivity: A 2 year follow-up. *American Journal of Psychiatry, 133,* 786–790.

Haney, C., Banks, C., & Zimbardo, P. (1973). Interpersonal dynamics in a simulated prison. *International Journal of Criminology and Penology, 1,* 69–97.

Haney, C., & Zimbardo, P. (1998). The past and future of U.S. prison policy: Twenty-five years after the Stanford prison experiment. *American Psychologist, 53,* 709–727.

Henman, L. (2001). Humor as a coping mechanism: Lessons from POWs. *Humor, 8,* 141–149.

Hunter, E. (1975). *Isolation as a feature of the POW experience: A comparison of men with prolonged and limited solitary confinement.* San Diego, CA: Center for Prisoner of War Studies, Naval Health Research Center.

Joint Personnel Recovery Agency (JPRA). (2010a). *Guidance on Joint Standards for survival evasion, resistance, escape (SERE) training role play activities in support of the Code of Conduct,* Spokane, Washington.

Joint Personnel Recovery Agency (JPRA). (2010b). *Guidance of Joint Standards for survival, evasion, resistance escape (SERE) training in support of the Code of Conduct ,* Spokane, Washington.

Joint Personnel Recovery Agency (JPRA). (2010c). *Guidance on qualification criteria and use of Department of Defense (DOD) survival, evasion, resistance, and escape (SERE) psychologists in support of the Code of Conduct ,* Spokane, Washington.

Joint Personnel Recovery Agency (JPRA). (2011). *About the Joint Personnel Recovery Agency.* Retrieved from *www.jpra.mil/Military/about/goals.htm.*

McNeil, J. A., & Morgan, C. A. (2010). Cognition and decision making in extreme environments. In C. H. Kennedy & J. L. Moore (Eds.), *Military neuropsychology* (pp. 361–382). New York: Springer.

Meichenbaum, D. (1985). *Stress inoculation training.* New York: Pergamon Press.

Mitchell, J. (1983). When disaster strikes: The critical incident stress debriefing process. *Journal of Emergency Medical Services, 8,* 36–39.

Moore, J. L. (2010). The neuropsychological functioning of prisoners of war following repatriation. In C. H. Kennedy & J. L. Moore (Eds.), *Military neuropsychology* (pp. 267–295). New York: Springer.

Morgan, C. A., Aikins, D., Steffian, G., Coric, V., & Southwick, S. M. (2007).

Relation between cardiac vagal tone and performance in male military personnel exposed to high stress: Three prospective studies. *Psychophysiology*, *44*, 120–127.

Morgan, C. A., Doran, A., Steffian, G., Hazlett, G., & Southwick, S. M. (2006). Stress induced deficits in working memory and visuo-constructive abilities in special operations soldiers. *Biological Psychiatry, 60, 722–729.*

Morgan, C. A., Hazlett, G., Baranoski, M., Doran, A., Southwick, S. M., & Loftus, E. (2007). Accuracy of eyewitness identification is significantly associated with performance on a standardized test of recognition. *International Journal of Law and Psychiatry, 30,* 213–223.

Morgan, C. A., Hazlett, G., Doran, A., Garrett, S., Hoyt, G., Thomas, P., et al. (2004). Accuracy of eyewitness memory for persons encountered during exposure to highly intense stress. *International Journal of the Law and Psychiatry,* 27(3), 265–279.

Morgan, C. A., Hazlett, G. A., Southwick, S. M., Rasmusson, A., & Lieberman, H. (2009). . Effect of carbohydrate administration on recovery from stress induced deficits in cognitive function: A double blind, placebo controlled study of soldiers exposed to survival school stress. *Military Medicine, 174,* 132-138.

Morgan, C. A., Rasmusson, A., Wang, S., Hoyt, G., Hauger, R., & Hazlett, G. (2002). Neuropeptide-Y, cortisol, and subjective distress in humans exposed to acute stress: Replication and extension of previous report. *Biological Psychiatry, 52,* 136–142.

Morgan, C. A., Southwick, S., Hazlett, G., Rasmusson, A., Hoyt, G., Zimolo, Z., et al. (2004). Relationships among plasma dehydroepiandrosterone in humans exposed to acute stress. *Archives of General Psychiatry, 61,* 819–825.

Morgan, C. A., Wang, S., Mason, J., Southwick, S., Fox, P., Hazlett, G., et al. (2000). Hormone profiles of humans experiencing military survival training. *Biological Psychiatry, 47,* 891–901.

Morgan, C. A., Wang, S., Rasmusson, A., Hazlett, G., Anderson, G., & Charney, D. (2001). Relationship among plasma cortisol, catecholamines, neuropeptide-Y, and human performance during exposure to uncontrollable stress. *Psychosomatic Medicine, 63,* 412–422.

Morgan, C. A., Wang, S., Southwick, S. M., Rasmusson, A., Hazlett, G., Hauger, R. L., et al. (2000). Plasma neuropeptide-Y concentrations in humans exposed to military survival training. *Biological Psychiatry, 47,* 902–909.

Page, W., Engdahl, B., & Eberly, R. (1991). Prevalence and correlates of depressive symptoms among former prisoners of war. *Journal of Nervous and Mental Disorders, 179,* 670–677.

Polivy, J., Zeitlin, S. B., Herman, C. P., & Beal, A. L. (1994). Food restriction and binge eating: A study of former prisoners of war. *Journal of Abnormal Psychology, 103,* 409–411.

Port, C. L., Engdahl, B., & Frazier, P. (2001). A longitudinal and retrospective study of PTSD among older prisoners of war. *American Journal of Psychiatry, 158,* 1474–1479.

Query, W., Megran, J., & McDonald, G. (1986). Applying post-traumatic stress disorder MMPI sub-scale to WWII POW veterans. *Journal of Clinical Psychology, 42,* 315–317.

Ruhl, R. (1978, May). The Code of Conduct. *Airman,* 63–66. Available at *www. au.af.mil/au/awc/awcgate/au-24/ruhl.pdf.*

Rundell, J., Ursano, R., Holloway, H., & Siberman, E. (1989). Psychiatric responses to trauma. *Hospital and Community Psychiatry, 40,* 68–74.

Russell, J. F. (1984). The captivity experience and its psychological consequences. *Psychiatric Annals, 14,* 250–254.

Sherwood, E. (1986). The power relationship between captor and captive. *Psychiatric Annals, 16,* 653–655.

Sokol, R. (1989). Early mental health intervention in combat situations: The USS *Stark. Military Medicine, 154,* 407–409.

Solomon, Z., Neria, Y., Ohry, A., Waysman, M., & Ginzburg, K. (1994). PTSD among Israeli former prisoners of war and soldiers with combat stress reaction: A longitudinal study. *American Journal of Psychiatry, 151,* 554–559.

Sutker, P., & Allain, A. (1996). Assessment of PTSD and other mental disorders in WWII and Korean POWs and combat veterans. *Psychological Assessment, 8,* 18–25.

Sutker, P., Allain, A., & Johnson, J. (1993). Clinical assessment of long-term cognitive and emotional sequelae to World War II prisoners-of-war confinement: Comparison of pilot twins. *Psychological Assessment, 5,* 3–10.

Sutker, P., Allain, A. N., Johnson, J. L., & Butters, N. M. (1992). Memory and learning performances in POW survivors with history of malnutrition and combat veteran controls. *Archives of Clinical Neuropsychology, 7,* 431–444.

Sutker, P. B., Vasterling, J. J., Brailey, K., & Allain, A. N. (1995). Memory, attention, and executive deficits in POW survivors: Contributing biological and psychological factors. *Neuropsychology, 9,* 118–125.

Taylor, M. K., Markham, A. E., Reis, J. P., Padilla, G. A., Potterat, E. G., Drummond, S. P., et al. (2008). Physical fitness influences stress reactions to extreme military training. *Military Medicine, 173,* 738–742.

Taylor, M. K., Mujica-Parodi, L. R., Padilla, G. A., Markham, A. E., Potterat, E. G., Momen, N., et al. (2009). Behavioral predictors of acute stress symptoms during intense military stress. *Journal of Traumatic Stress, 22*(3), 212–217.

Taylor, M. K., Padilla, G. A., Stanfill, K. E., Markham, A. E., Khosravi, J. Y., Dial Ward, M. D., et al. (2012). Effects of dehydroepiandrosterone supplementation during stressful military training: A randomized, controlled, double-blind field study. *Stress, 15*(1), 85–96.

Taylor, M. K., Sausen, K. P., Mujica-Parodi, L. R., Potterat, E. G., Yanaqi, & Kim, H. (2007). Neurophysiologic methods to measure stress during survival, evasion, resistance, and escape training. *Aviation Space Environmental Medicine, 78,* 224–230.

Taylor, M. K., Sausen, K. P., Potterat, E. G., Mujica-Parodi, L. R., Reis, A. E., Markham, A. E., et al. (2007). Stressful military training: Endocrine reactivity, performance, and psychological impact. *Aviation Space Environmental Medicine, 78,* 1143–1149.

Taylor, M. K., Stanfill, K. E., Padilla, G. A., Markham, A. E., Ward, M. D.,

Koehler, M. M., et al. (2011). Effect of psychological skills training during military survival school: A randomized, controlled field study. *Military Medicine, 176*(12), 1362–1368.

Tennant, C., Fairley, M. J., Dent, O. F., Suway, M., & Broe, G. A. (1997). Declining prevalence of psychiatric disorder in older former prisoners of war. *Journal of Nervous and Mental Disease, 185*, 686–689.

True, B., & Benaway, M. (1992). Treatment of stress reaction prior to combat using the "BICEPS" model. *Military Medicine, 157*, 380–381.

U.S. Department of Defense. (2000a, December 8). *Training and education to support the code of conduct* (CoC) (DoD Directive 1300.7). Washington, DC: Author.

U.S. Department of Defense. (2000b, December 22). *Personnel recovery* (DoD Directive 2310.2). Washington, DC: Author.

U.S. Department of Defense. (2000c, November 21). *Repatriation of prisoners of war (POW), hostages, peacetime government detainees and other missing or isolated personnel.* (DoD Directive 2310.4). Washington, DC: Author.

U.S. Department of Defense. (2001, January 8). *Code of conduct training and education* (DoD Directive 1300.21). Washington, DC: Author.

Ursano, R., Boydstun, J., & Wheatley, R. (1981). Psychiatric illness in US Air Force Vietnam POWs: A five year follow-up. *American Journal of Psychiatry, 138*, 310–314.

Ursano, R. J., & Rundell, J. R. (1996). The prisoner of war. In R. J. Ursano & A. Norwood (Eds.), *Emotional aftermath of the Persian Gulf War: Veterans, families, communities, and nations* (pp. 443–476). Washington, DC: American Psychiatric Press.

Verma, S., Orengo, C. A., Maxwell, R., Kunik, M. E., Molinari, V. A., Vasterling, J. J., et al. (2001). Contribution of PTSD/POW history to behavioral disturbances in dementia. *International Journal of Geriatric Psychiatry, 16*, 356–360.

Yerkes, S. (1993). The "un-comfort-able" making sense of adaptation in a war zone. *Military Medicine, 58*, 421–423.

Zeiss, R. A., & Dickman, H. R. (1989). PTSD 40 years later: Incidence and person situation correlates in former POWs. *Journal of Clinical Psychology, 45*, 80–87.

Zimbardo, P. G. (1973). On the ethics of intervention in human psychological research: With special reference to the Stanford prison experiment. *Cognition, 2*, 243–256.

CHAPTER 13

The Psychology of Terrorists

Nazi Perpetrators, the Baader–Meinhof Gang, War Crimes in Bosnia, Suicide Bombers, the Taliban, and Al Qaeda

Eric A. Zillmer

> While nothing is easier than to denounce
> the evildoer, nothing is more difficult than
> to understand him.
> —FYODOR DOSTOYEVSKY

"They're all gone," announced Jim McKay, the ABC TV announcer covering the 1972 Munich Summer Olympics. The tragic killing of 11 Israeli athletes by Palestinian terrorists illustrated how little West German authorities and the media knew about the mind-set of the perpetrators they were dealing with. In the early morning of September 5, members of a unit of the terrorist group Black September climbed the fence of the Olympic village and forced their way into the Israeli Olympic team's quarters, shooting two athletes and taking nine hostage. As the next 16 hours unfolded before millions of television viewers and climaxed in a botched rescue attempt at a nearby military airport, it became clear that the police and armed forces units were completely unprepared for such an international crisis. At the end of the day, 11 Israeli athletes, one German policeman, and 10 terrorists were dead; three of the terrorists were captured. The Munich Olympics terrorist attack demonstrated how a small number of terrorists who demanded the release of Palestinian prisoners in Israel could touch the psyche and resilience of an international audience watching as extensive media coverage magnified the event's social and political impact. Since then, much has changed in terms of not only establishing specialized antiterrorism military and police units but also understanding the psychology and the culture of terrorists (for more on hostage incidents, see Chapter 11, this volume).

The 9/11 terrorist attacks by Al Qaeda on the United States have brought terrorism on a grand scale to local soil and have changed the collective psychology of our nation and our perception of the threat of terrorism (see Figure 13.1). This danger has led the military and law enforcement agencies to pose many questions for psychologists:

- How and under what circumstances do terrorists get recruited?
- What is the terrorists' decision-making process?
- Under what social context are terrorist acts most likely to occur?
- What are the specific personalities that may be involved in terrorist atrocities?

There has been a strong effort by the psychology community to conduct research and consultation in these arenas, which has provided opportunities for both scientific and clinical contributions. In the fight against the threat of terrorism, psychologists may find themselves progressively more involved as consultants to the military, security firms, federal and state

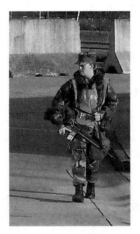

FIGURE 13.1. "There is no more dangerous time in the history of our nation than today . . . approximately 1,500 terrorist organizations in more than 200 countries are being tracked" (General Peter J. Schoomaker, former Chief of Staff, U.S. Army, personal communication, November 10, 2006). Photo courtesy of Eric A. Zillmer, by permission.

governments, intelligence agencies, and the police (see Kennedy & Williams, 2011). Given that terrorism on a large scale has become increasingly possible because of the availability of explosive materials, modern communication, global financial transactions, and the relative ease of travel, it has become essential to understand the terrorist's frame of mind. As a result, a primary strategy on the current Global War on Terror includes an understanding of the psychological prerequisites for terrorist acts.

As a result, the "how" and the "why" of terrorism have become an important emerging research and practice area for psychology (Zillmer, 2004). Working from psychological data, biographical information, and historical accounts, this chapter examines several assumptions concerning how and under what circumstances humans are most likely to be recruited for and engage in terrorism. The findings in this chapter are based on different theaters of terrorism and genocide and primarily suggest that the threshold for terrorist participation is much lower than is commonly expected. Terrorists often commit acts of terror based on a rational risk–reward paradigm for what they believe are justifiable and logical reasons.

HISTORY OF TERRORISM

Terrorism has a long history, but the psychological study of terrorists covers a relatively short time period. During the past two millennia, political violence has proliferated throughout the world (Reich, 1998). Naturally, explanations of terrorism have been a focus for many researchers, and there have been a number of findings, often contradictory, that typically focus on social as well as individual factors. For example, some believe that terrorism is simply a moral problem (Moghaddam, 2005), or it has been assumed that those who commit terrorist attacks must be financially disadvantaged or developmentally immature or have been raised in broken families. On the basis of their fanatic actions, terrorists cannot possibly be well educated, must have been brainwashed, and are most likely unskilled, unemployed, and ignorant. Terrorists must have weak minds, be religious zealots, or present a history of criminal behavior. It is often assumed that terrorists must suffer from mental illness; how else could one explain some of the most hideous terror attacks involving innocent children? Some have even suggested that the answer to terrorists lies within the study of the psychology of human evil (Bartlett, 2005). As we shall see, the modern notion of the psychology of terrorists is in stark contrast with almost all of these common conceptions, especially for organized terrorist groups: that terrorists perpetrate their actions with deliberation and a realistic knowledge of the consequences. A modern understanding of the psychology of terrorists views them as a formidable enemy.

DEFINITION OF TERRORISM

The label "terrorist" is a negative term that even so-called terrorists do not like to use. Most terrorists, in fact, do not regard themselves as terrorists at all but rather as soldiers, liberators, martyrs, legitimate freedom fighters, or revolutionaries for a noble social cause. As a result, the term *terrorist* and defining an act of terrorism are controversial concepts, and different groups often accuse each other of terrorist acts.

There are more than 100 competing definitions of terrorism. A broad, but useful, definition is proposed by Laqueur (1987, p. 144): "The unlawful use or threat of violence against persons or property to further political or social objectives. It is usually intended to intimidate or coerce a government, group, or individual to modify their behavior or politics." Acts of terrorism can include punishment, threats, violence, kidnapping, extortion, torture, hate crimes, rape, child abuse, stalking, domestic violence, and even bullying. This definition demonstrates that terrorist behaviors are widely engaged in by everyday individuals. Thus, without any systematic psychological study, it should be apparent that terrorism as defined by Laqueur might have a much lower threshold than most people believe.

There are at least four types of terrorist group activity (Bartlett, 2005): those between groups (e.g., organized crime), those between groups and states (e.g., Al Qaeda and the United States), those between states and groups (e.g., Nazi genocide), and those between states (i.e., war). Thus, it is useful to differentiate between terrorism from above, perpetrated by dictators and governments, and terrorism from below, involving rebels, revolutionaries, and protestors (Hacker, 1980).

RELEVANT PSYCHOLOGICAL STUDIES: ASCH, MILGRAM, AND ZIMBARDO

Several landmark studies have laid the groundwork for understanding the possible psychological operations involved in the capacity to harm. An initial question about those who engage in terrorism is whether they are unique individuals, that is, outside of the norm. If this were true, it would make it less likely for everyday individuals to become involved in terrorism, and it would make it more difficult for terrorist organizations to recruit for the simple reason that there would be smaller populations to recruit from. Three important psychological experiments have suggested that the threshold for individuals to conform, even in the face of obvious contradictory evidence and at times resulting in potential harm to others, is much lower than commonly expected. These classic comparative experimental studies include:

- Asch's (1952) experiments on social conformity.
- Milgram's (1974) studies of obedience to authority.
- Zimbardo's (1972) investigation of prison life.

Briefly, Solomon Asch (1952), a social psychologist, showed how powerful the tendency to conform to others could be. Faced with a simple, unambiguous task (matching the length of a line with one of three unequal lines), a large majority of the subjects ignored their own intuition and agreed with the obviously incorrect choice made by a group of strangers; actually confederates of the experimenter. The "Asch effect" showed how readily most people will go along with a decision that their own judgment tells them is wrong, even when no coercion or force is used. For example, millions of people in the Middle East felt ambivalent toward the 9/11 attacks. Or polls of Palestinians who supported suicide bombings in the second intifada show how a significant proportion still said that they disagreed with it in principle (Nichole Argo, personal communication, December 11, 2005). Many terrorists, however, do not join a terror cell just because they think they should go along with the group. More often, they actually believe that they are doing the right thing.

Guessing the length of a line is, of course, not comparable to participating in terrorist activities. However, Stanley Milgram (1974) showed that obedience to authority relieves many people of moral responsibility, thus making them more likely to behave with considerable cruelty. Milgram had originally designed his experiment in response to the Adolf Eichmann trial, in part to understand why ordinary people in Germany had participated in the murder of millions of innocent victims during World War II (WWII; Zillmer, Harrower, Ritzler, & Archer, 1995). The results he obtained at Yale University, however, made it clear that he did not have to leave the United States. Milgram recruited subjects through advertisements in a local newspaper for a "Study in Memory." In one of the experiments, almost one-third of the subjects were willing to hold a "learner's" hand against a metal plate to force him to receive an electric shock. Milgram's study clearly demonstrated that, under certain circumstances, the tendency to obey an authority figure is very strong, even when causing harm to an innocent person. This may explain why terrorists who sacrifice themselves through suicide bombs are vulnerable to the command of those perceived as authority figures.

In yet a different experiment, psychologist Philip Zimbardo (1972) asked a group of ordinary college students to spend time in a simulated prison. Some were randomly assigned as guards—given uniforms, billy clubs, and whistles—and were instructed to enforce certain rules. The remainder became prisoners and were locked in barren cells and asked to wear humiliating outfits. After a short time, the simulation became very real, as the guards devised cruel and degrading routines. The prisoners, one by one, broke down, rebelled, or became passively resigned. After only 6 days, Zimbardo had to terminate the study, demonstrating that, for many of us, what we do may be what we gradually become.

In summary, these psychological experiments can be applied to modern terrorist motivation and suggest the following:

- Those who follow a majority's viewpoint may disagree in principle with the means of terror (i.e., violence), but they may endorse the effects of the terror (e.g., political change).
- The masterminds of terror operations may have significant social authority and emotional influence over their followers, and often a simple request is all that is necessary for a terrorist act to be initiated.
- Once someone is assimilated into a terror cell, it may be surprisingly easy to take on the role of a terrorist.

If Asch, Milgram, and Zimbardo are correct, it may be that law-abiding men and women with conventional virtues are indeed capable of committing terrorist acts once the command is given and necessary social mechanisms are set in motion. These three experiments laid the foundation for an understanding of the social and group characteristics in which potentially dangerous behavior can occur. But what are the psychological prerequisites for individual terrorist acts? To help answer this question, it may be useful to first examine the psychological database on more than 200 war criminals of the Third Reich, who committed state-sponsored terrorism and genocide (Zillmer et al., 1995).

NAZI PERPETRATORS AND COLLABORATORS

The Third Reich revealed to the world the surprising and concerning comprehension that large groups of individuals, who were integrated into Western culture, could engage in state-sponsored terrorism against others as well as their own people. One surprising account of the Third Reich was the scale of terror; that is, between 150,000 and 200,000 perpetrators were actively responsible for committing war crimes. Of those, approximately 35,000 have been captured, brought to trial, and convicted. Many theories were developed in reaction to the Nazi crimes against humanity, the Holocaust, and the creation of concentration and death camps. One popular notion was to attempt the psychological profiling of Nazis. Subsequently, at the end of WWII, theories of the sadistic personality (Miale & Selzer, 1975) or the German authoritarian personality (Adorno, Frankel-Brunswick,

Levinson, & Sanford, 1950) were formulated. The basic notion of those researchers was to suggest that the behavior of the Nazi perpetrators must have been related to some type of uniform pathology (Dicks, 1972).

The problem, however, with the concept of a uniform Nazi personality theory was twofold. First, one could not think of a more heterogeneous group of individuals involved in the atrocities and state-sponsored terrorism during the Third Reich (Browning, 1993). People from all walks of life, including non-German collaborators, were involved. It is impossible to find simple psychological characteristics for such a diverse group of individuals and such a heterogeneous and complex collection of behaviors. Second, many of the characteristics proposed by the theorists of a uniform Nazi personality can be attributed to individuals who played no role in the creation of Nazi terror. For example, many offenders who committed crimes and were sent to jail had little or any connection to Nazi ideology.

The idea of a uniform pathological Nazi personality was later revised by Hannah Arendt (1958, 1963), who argued that Nazis were not sadists or even aggressive individuals intent on doing harm to others for depraved satisfaction, just ordinary, conscientious, moderately ambitious bureaucrats who were more interested in simply obeying orders. Arendt based her theory on the 1961 Adolf Eichmann trial in Jerusalem. Many observers, including Arendt, were surprised by Eichmann's personality, that is, the quality or lack of it. Arendt argued that the banality of Eichmann's personality kept him from having compunction or even second thoughts about his job, which was to keep trains running to concentration camps on schedule (see Figure 13.2). Arendt's controversial thesis simply implies that many of the Nazis were banal, morally indifferent, mundane, and without a feeling of hatred or any ideological malice toward their victims. In fact, she concluded that they were quite ordinary.

Arendt's concept of the banality of evil has merit because it implies that ordinary men in the right circumstances can perform evil deeds. But it also assumes the presence of a relatively homogeneous personality prototype that others have argued to be sinister and vicious, not ordinary. Each of these hypotheses, the "evil Nazi personality" and "the banality of evil," starts with a divergent bias concerning the behavior of Nazis. Both assume a relatively homogeneous personality type—one vicious, sadistic, and antisocial, the other obedient, indifferent, and mundane. Both have naturally stirred much debate and controversy. Arendt's theory, however, differs from those endorsing the "mad Nazi" hypothesis in a very important way, for she suggests that the potential for behaving like a Nazi exists in many.

The psychological data on more than 200 Nazi perpetrators and collaborators from the Copenhagen War Crime Trials and the Nuremberg International Tribunal did not indicate a uniform Nazi personality (Zillmer et al., 1995). However, there were important findings that have implications

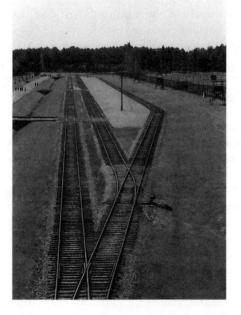

FIGURE 13.2. Auschwitz–Birkenau, which was established by the Nazis in 1940, has become a symbol of terror, genocide, and the Holocaust. Psychological analysis proved to be useful in separating the psychological characteristics of Nazi followers from those who were considered the Nazi leadership. Nazi rank and file, including guards, were found to be simple thinkers who were easily influenced by authority. Pictured here is the end of the train line at Birkenau concentration camp, where 2,000 to 3,000 Jews and other prisoners were brought via cattle cars on freight trains. After a "Selektion" by Nazi officials, many were immediately escorted to gas chambers. Photo courtesy of Eric A. Zillmer, by permission.

for contemporary terrorism among those accused of state-sponsored terrorism, genocide, and war crimes. For example, an analysis of the psychological data suggests that it is important to differentiate between those who created the Nazi regime from those who were rank-and-file members. The Nazi elite was involved in the creation of concentration camps, initiated aggressive warfare, and was considered to be in authority. The rank and file, in contrast, were made up of Nazi officials, guards, military personnel, and bureaucrats who were largely responsible for implementing state terrorism. In fact, it still seems appropriate to consider modern terrorists in these two categories with different psychological attributes: the terrorist mastermind who initiates the mission and provides the orders, and the followers who execute them.

The Nazi psychological data on the rank and file suggest that they engaged in a unique information-processing style, which can be described as oversimplified. That is, they were not creative thinkers, were easily influenced by authority, were vulnerable to acts of impulsiveness, and were attracted to the rigid and quasi-military Nazi hierarchy. They were not complex individuals but rather preferred to seek out external structure, guidance, and reassurance. They believed that they were simply following orders and that they had little to do with the concentration camps (see Figure 13.3). In fact, this was a frequent defense of those rank-and-file Nazis who were captured and put on trial. They felt that they were victims of circumstance and that their behaviors were not entirely under their control. It does not excuse their actions, but it explains why so many may have participated with little deliberation. As a group, they relied heavily on denial and were missing an internal moral compass. They were lacking in confidence and felt socially frustrated.

Socially and interpersonally, the rank and file may not have been as shallow and aloof as they have been portrayed in the media and film industry. They actually sought out social relationships and were eager about joining a fraternity (Kameradschaft), which gave them a sense of belonging and structure. Thus, as a group, rank-and-file terrorists may demonstrate a cognitive simplicity that is consistent with an oversimplified problem-solving style. Since the capacity for terrorist evil seems easily accessible to many, it is very possible that there are tens of thousands of disillusioned individuals who are highly vulnerable to recruitment by terrorist cells.

In contrast, the psychology of Nazi leadership was different. The Nazi elite was overconfident, entitled, arrogant, manipulative, and egocentric. They were well educated and bright, in fact having average to superior intelligence (Zillmer et al., 1995). A deficiency in their ability to empathize with others was characteristic, being similar to individuals who would be considered psychopaths. It is a mistake to underestimate terrorists' leaders' intelligence and psychological influence. The elusive nature of Osama bin Laden, Muammar Gaddafi, and Saddam Hussein indicates that there may be some validity to this hypothesis.

The final analysis of the Nazi data suggests that they could not plead insanity in the court of universal justice. No definitive, specific inclination was found toward violence, aggression, or sadism. Ordinary, well-educated, middle-class, family-type people became involved in atrocities and did not demonstrate any particular inclination toward violence. In fact, those with criminal records or with psychiatric histories were excluded from participating in the Nazi establishment. They were not deemed sufficiently reliable. Hitler's men were more different from each other in terms of their personality than they were alike.

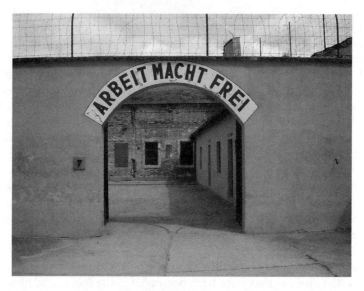

FIGURE 13.3. "Arbeit macht frei"—"Work sets you free." Nazi administrators placed the infamous slogan over the entrances of many concentration camps during the height of the Third Reich, including Dachau and Auschwitz. Pictured here is the entrance to Terezin in the Czech Republic

POLITICAL TERRORISM:
THE BAADER–MEINHOF GANG

The daily insecurity in the United States after the 9/11 attacks has been a familiar one for the West German population, who lived through almost a decade of unpredictable terror. The Baader–Meinhof terror group inflicted on West Germany its first internal social–political crisis. In fact, the years 1968 through 1977 represented the most tumultuous era in the Federal Republic of Germany's short history. The Baader-Meinhof Gruppe (*Gruppe* is German for "group"; however, the "group" is also commonly referred to as a *Bande*, or gang) grew out of the West German 1968 student movement in West Berlin, whose mission was to resist capitalism, U.S. "occupation," and state-sponsored authority. The Baader–Meinhof gang was named after their leader, Andreas Baader, and one of its founding members, Ulrike Meinhof. Baader, the leader of the violent leftist group, along with his girlfriend, Gudrun Ensslin, were convicted of the 1968 arson bombing of a Frankfurt department store. He escaped from police custody in May 1970 with the help of the journalist Meinhof, giving birth to the so-called Baader–Meinhof gang. National issues related to the Cold War, German national unity, the Vietnam War, the proliferation of nuclear weapons, and the large presence of U.S. military and North Atlantic Treaty Organization troops in West Germany resulted in large-scale student protests. Many leftist students wanted a revolution and naïvely sought to kick-start the cause through terrorism in prosperous West Germany. What followed was a series of bombings, kidnappings, bank robberies, and murders, which left Germany in a wake of terror unlike any seen in an industrialized country (Rasch, 1979).

One surprising phenomenon that emerged from this terrorist activity, and which is now thought to be an essential ingredient in the effectiveness of the Baader–Meinhof gang, was its surprising popularity among average West Germans. In fact, German polls showed that an extraordinarily high number, approximately 10 to 20%, of Germans supported its cause in one way or another. This was a remarkable finding because it suggested that millions of ordinary Germans sympathized with Baader–Meinhof's terror initiatives. In addition, popular and well-known intellectuals sympathized with the cause, which added to its authenticity, including Günter Grass, Heinrich Böll, Jean-Paul Sartre, Rainer Werner Fassbinder, and Rudi Dutschke. The word *sympathizer* literally means to show pity or compassion and to share ideas with someone else. Sympathizers may have been reluctant to agree with Baader–Meinhof's radical methods of terror and violence, but somehow their anti-American cause struck a chord with the German public. As a result, the term *sympathizers* of terrorist groups was coined and became a focus in the study of terrorism.

In fact, sympathizers are now considered an essential prerequisite in any large-scale terror movement. If there were no sympathizers, there would most likely not be a financial, intellectual, or ideological basis for a terror movement. This appears relevant historically in the case of anti-Semitism and the Holocaust (Goldhagen, 1996) as well as with terror groups, such as the Islamic Resistance Movement (Hamas), the Irish Republican Army (IRA), the Basques of northern Spain, Hezbollah, Taliban, and Al Qaeda. Even though the Baader–Meinhof gang engaged in illegal criminal behavior, many German citizens, including well-known, popular, and established authors and lawyers, said publicly that some of their actions were ideologically justified. Like many of their generation, "they had opposed the old form of Fascism and what they thought was its new face" (Aust, 2008, p. 419). In the end, the Baader–Meinhof gang's support fizzled when they began to rely solely on violence, merely robbing banks and committing murders. The "German Autumn" comprised years of underground terror in the Federal Republic of Germany and left a balance sheet of 47 dead.

Most of the leaders of the Baader–Meinhof gang were captured in 1972. Their followers would kidnap and kill close to a dozen people over the next 5 years in an effort to secure their leaders' release from prison. However, the West German government had no intention of releasing them.

On October 17, 1977, the leaders committed suicide while in jail, perhaps related to a failed attempt to secure their release through an airplane hijacking by Palestinian comrades. The Baader–Meinhof era was officially over.

Another important development related to the Baader–Meinhof group was the government's response. The West German government organized antiterrorism efforts with a specific police task force, which underwent specialized training and was centrally organized. This marks one of the first responses of a specialized, federal antiterror strike force in any country. Once the terrorists were captured, the German Ministry of the Interior set out to understand how this terror movement evolved and was sustained. A five-volume set, published in the German language in the early 1980s, includes an analysis of more than 220 members of the Baader–Meinhof gang. One volume was dedicated entirely to the psychological understanding of the group (Jager, Schmidtchen, & Sullwold, 1981). This study of the psychosocial causes of the Baader–Meinhof group indicates that all of the terrorists shared a common political ideology (Weltanschauung), which made them feel entitled to commit acts of violence. For example, Baader would admit publicly to being "politically" responsible for the violence but not "personally" responsible. In their own minds, their actions were justified and reasonable in the pursuit of their cause. At his trial, Baader accused the German legal system of "state terrorism," and members of the gang declared their collaborator's suicide in jail resulting from his hunger strike as murder by the state.

A psychological investigation of those imprisoned shows no conclusive evidence for the assumption that a significant number of the terrorists were disturbed or abnormal. In fact, most of the supporters were well educated, from middle-class families, favored BMWs for transportation, and were part of an intellectual elite of university students. The members of the Baader–Meinhof gang did share a common conception of disillusionment (Urmisstrauen) or disappointment caused by a frustrated ideal. This appears to be a common ingredient of terrorist cells, that is, a feeling of frustration, which then leads to action. Personality investigations suggest that, similar to the Nazi rank and file, members of the terror group exhibited significantly poor self-esteem (Minderwertigkeitsgefühle). An important mechanism of their terror affiliation centered on the fact that many of them were friends who felt solidarity (Solidarität) with each other and frequented the same social circles. This desire for a social network (soziale Rollenfindung) was similar to a Gemeinschaftsgefühl among the Nazi groups and, in fact, appears to play an important role in any terror cell. This terrorist group phenomenon was later described as "within-group love" compared with "outside-group hate" (Sageman, 2004).

In general, however, the psychosocial studies of participants of the Baader–Meinhof gang do not reveal a uniform terrorist personality but do indicate a number of prerequisites for such a terror movement. These characteristics centered on the fact that many members of the gang felt frustrated and disillusioned and many of them were or became friends who ultimately committed suicide in prison together.

The study of the political and psychological aspects of group terrorist membership, such as the Baader–Meinhof gang, brought to the forefront the advent of sympathizers and supporters, without which a terror movement would not be possible. Today, the white supremacy movements in the United States generally lack any support by the general population and are essentially ineffective. In contrast, the Lebanese terror organization Hezbollah enjoys widespread support from their constituents and is able to mobilize demonstrations of hundreds of thousands, and many members of the group hold high and relevant administrative positions in their communities. Hamas, a political party that the United States considers a terrorist group, won a majority of seats in the Palestinian Parliament in the January 2006 elections. On an individual level, the former pop singer Cat Stevens, famous for his coffeehouse style ballads that celebrated peace and understanding, was found to have supported the militant terror group Hamas financially and consequently was denied entry into the United States and Israel.

Thus, the Baader–Meinhof phenomenon demonstrated that political terrorism does not occur in a psychological vacuum, but is supported by the mainstream, possibly even by individuals with moderate views but who embrace part of the message of the terrorist group. With sympathizers on board, terrorist groups represent a daunting threat. Thus, addressing sympathizers who potentially support terrorist groups—doing so through education and propaganda—is now considered an important step in fighting terrorism.

WAR CRIMES IN BOSNIA

The former Yugoslavia was a multiethnic republic for more than four decades under communist ruler Marshal Tito. After the death of the republic's leader, Yugoslavia fragmented along ethnic lines. In early 1992, and related to bitter tension between the ethnic groups that had been simmering for generations, Slovenia, Croatia, Macedonia, and Bosnia and Herzegovina were recognized as independent states. However, in April 1992, the remaining republics of Serbia and Montenegro declared a new Federal Republic of Yugoslavia. Under President Slobodan Milosevic, nationalist Serbian paramilitary units led numerous interventions to unite ethnic Serbs located in neighboring republics into a "Greater Serbia."

As a result, Bosnia, which is roughly the size of Maine, was burdened by a civil war that pitted three different ethnic groups against each other (see Figure 13.4). There were reports of mass executions and graves, and under a program of "ethnic cleansing," paramilitary groups "created conditions of comprehensive oppression; systematically raped, tortured, and murdered civilians; appropriated and pillaged civilian property" (Waller, 2002, p. 259). Brčko, on the border with Croatia, was the scene of some of the worst atrocities during the war. Here, more than 20,000 Muslims—constituting a majority population—were forced into exile, and at least 7,000 Croat and Muslim civilians were killed, buried in mass graves. In addition, it was reported that more than 1,000 Muslims were executed in a factory near Svebrenica after they were separated from their families.

Since the end of the war in 1995, 2 million people have been displaced and more than 1 million land mines remain unaccounted for. The country's physical infrastructure remains in shambles. The civic institutions that many take for granted, including banks, police, garbage disposal, a judicial system, and public utilities, either barely exist or are corrupted. After the war there was no economy to speak of, and a simulated, nontradable currency, the Bosnian Convertible Mark, had to be introduced. There has been, however, significant progress in restoring peace and stability, credited mostly to a 12-nation peacekeeping force organized by the United Nations

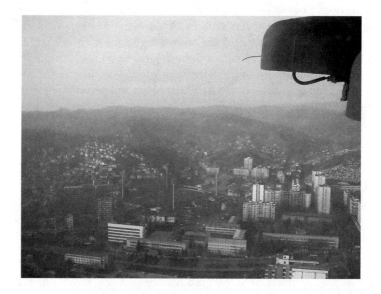

FIGURE 13.4. "It is complete chaos," a U.S. soldier offered. "The only thing left for them to do is to kill each other—Christians, Muslims, and Islam, they all hate each other. It has been going on for generations and generations." Pictured in an aerial view of Tuzla, one of the many "hot spots" in Bosnia. Photo courtesy of Eric A. Zillmer, by permission.

(UN). Through special programs, such as Operation Harvest, the peace-keeping forces assisted in the disarming of Bosnian civilians and provided for a safe, stable, and secure Bosnia. The success of the multinational peace-keeping force stems not only from the cooperation of the dozen countries participating, each with its own assigned territory, but also the fact that Bosnians, by and large, welcomed the international delegation. As a result, supervised elections have been held, the railroad system has recently been restored, and a program of taxation has begun.

Bosnia is a modern-day reminder of the fragility of any social structure, how an entire nation can self-destruct, and how easily an organized outbreak of hostilities can be realized. This terror occurred in a country that had been integrated into Europe, which had catered to millions of tourists over the years, staged the 1984 Winter Olympics in Sarajevo, and is located only several hundred miles from many European cultural centers. In response to the terror, the UN formed an International Criminal Tribunal in The Hague, Netherlands, to address war crimes and crimes against humanity. The 2001 arrest of Slobodan Milosevic, who still enjoyed strong popularity among his supporters, allowed for his subsequent transfer to the tribunal to be tried for crimes against humanity. The Hague tribunal is modeled after the Nuremberg International Tribunal, which was formed after WWII and pioneered many of the international laws that are now in place. The geographical areas of Albania, Kosovo, and Bosnia remain a political hot spot, and the lessons learned from this most recent terror include how quickly a genocidal warfare engulfed a country as neighbor literally turned against neighbor, with the world standing by (Neuffer, 2001).

Bartlett (2005) suggests that the terrorist shares many of the same emotional characteristics that are found in those who commit genocide. The pursuit of an ethnically homogeneous state resulted in a thinly disguised terror/genocide campaign and included deportation and murder of ethnic communities that had previously cohabitated in shared territories. The recent human rights violation in Rwanda or Uganda deserves mention here as well and serves as an additional reminder of the cruelties so easily engaged in by individuals who have seemingly lived together in peace for decades. Ordinary people, who did not demonstrate any particular inclination toward violence and who lived peacefully together for decades, committed crimes against humanity once certain political, economic, and social catalysts were set in motion.

SUICIDE BOMBERS

Nothing is more disturbing than reports of human bombers infiltrating a public gathering such as a discotheque (Israel), a wedding (Jordan), or a subway station (London) and setting off explosives. More recently, in Iraq almost weekly suicide bombings at checkpoints or at local gatherings disrupted the coalition's peacekeeping efforts. It seems inconceivable to most individuals that anyone would go to this extreme in order to engage in political violence. Are suicide bombers more evil than others? Surely, those who commit these acts of terror, in which they sacrifice their own lives, must be depraved individuals with nothing else to lose. Profiling suicide bombers' psychological characteristics is tempting because it may allow for a screening or early detection of potential threats.

Suicide bombings have been on the rise: "Suicide terrorists sought to compel American and French military forces to abandon Lebanon in 1983, Israeli forces to leave Lebanon in 1985, Israeli forces to quit the Gaza Strip and the West Bank in 1994 and 1995, the Sri Lankan government to create an independent Tamil state from 1990 on, and the Turkish government to grant autonomy to the Kurds in the late 1990s" (Pape, 2003, p. 343). Several researchers have examined the cause of suicide terrorism. Kobrin (2010) used a psychoanalytic framework to understand Islamic suicide bombing. She suggests that a "suicide murderer's personality does not arise de novo; rather, it is shaped very early by his or her first relationship in life, that with the mother" (p. 36). Kobrin suggested that Islamic infants are at risk to have their "deck of cards" stacked against them and are at risk of growing into suicide bombers who have impaired thinking. Contextual factors, of course, are not sufficient to explain why some individuals become suicide bombers and others do not, even though they may have been exposed to the same situation. Most agree, however, that there is not one psychological profile of suicide bombers (Merari, 2004) and that they are a heterogeneous group of men and women. Merari (2010) suggested that suicide terrorism is a complex phenomenon affected by many factors, including political grievances, strategic goals, cultural traits, and the individual psychology of the suicide bomber. He points out that, while there may be many sympathizers of suicide bombing among different Islamic populations ranging in the millions, only very few (perhaps an estimated 2,000) have been willing to cease their own life for the purpose of a greater cause. The number of suicide terrorists is a very small fraction when compared with terrorists in general. Thus, within the psychological framework of the individual suicide bomber, most assume that there must be something psychologically abnormal or that there must be some psychological characteristics among healthy individuals who commit suicide for a political cause.

The first studies of suicide bombers reported on the Japanese kamikaze pilots in WWII. During the Battle of Okinawa in April 1945, for example, several thousand Japanese planes crashed their fully fueled fighters into hundreds of U.S. Navy ships, killing more than 5,000 sailors.

A psychological analysis of those selected for suicide missions, however, found them to be relatively average citizens, actually reserve soldiers who engaged in terrorist actions for the Japanese cause (Morris, 1975; Taylor, 1988). The modern suicide bomb is a stealthier but equally deadly weapon as the Kamikaze pilots. The Palestinian suicide bombers, who have been studied in most detail, do not seem to share the same psychological characteristics as almost all individuals who commit traditional suicide, such as an affective disorder, depressed mood, or experience of loss or grief. Thus, it has been suggested that the appropriate term for those terror perpetrators should be "human bombs," not suicide bombers or homicidal bombers (Argo, 2006). Since one can commit acts of violence without suicide, some researchers argue that the additional act of suicide may be significant in terms of the psychological makeup of the perpetrator. For example, Lester, Yang, and Lindsay (2004) suggest that suicide bombers may be characterized by risk factors that increase the probability of suicide. They posit that the authoritarian personality might provide a good fit for the personality and psychodynamics of terrorists and suicide bombers. The authoritarian personality has been implicated before in the psychological makeup of terrorists, for example, in the discussion of Nazis, with little support.

Researchers studying Palestinian suicide bombers in Israeli prisons found them to be a hetergeneous group, similar to the findings for Nazis, the Baader–Meinhof gang, and the ideologies of those who committed war crimes in Bosnia. For example, Nichole Argo (2003) interviewed 15 preempted Palestinian bombers and three would-be bombers in Israeli prisons—all males between the ages of 16 and 37. Of the 18, 5 were born to refugee families; 14 were single, two were married, and two were engaged. These were not just brainwashed young individuals but also middle-aged, employed, and married adults.

A psychological analysis of the interviews reveals a general absence of psychopathology; the would-be suicide bombers were not lunatics, extremists, maniacs, or depressed persons. They had compassion and showed empathy for their potential victims, but they also felt completely justified for their acts and showed no remorse. There was little evidence of despair and poverty. Thus, judging on these interviews, their prebombing quality of life was relatively good and they sacrificed everything for their cause. In fact, almost all interviewees in this study exhibited a sense of loyalty to an intimate cohort of peers, which would speak against the common conception that suicide bombers are loners. Similar to the common thread of friendship in other terror groups, they were prepared to die for one another. Also similar to other studies reported in this chapter, the preempted suicide bombers shared a common religion and a nationalist ideology. This appears to transcend all aspects of Palestinian bomber motivation, although there was much variance in level of religiosity among the bombers. Although all were Muslim, some were far more observant than others and some even called themselves secular.

Pape (2005) examined the database of suicide bombers between 1980 and 2003, for a total of 315 cases worldwide. He found that suicide attackers did not have a criminal background and were not illiterate or poor. Rather, they came mostly from secular, educated, middle-class families. For example, the 2005 London subway bombings were committed by suicide bombers who were friends, some older, married, and employed. Consequently, suicide bombers have much to lose. The notion of sacrifice is an important concept in the psychological operations of suicide attackers. Suicide terrorists through their actions make a symbolic offering for what they believe is the larger good of their people. Atran (2003) reports that in summer 2002, for example, 70 to 80% of Palestinians endorsed or sympathized with martyr operations. Without the sacrifice, the act of terror may not be as meaningful to the terrorist and thus may be an important prerequisite. Thus, the prevailing view is that suicide bombers lack psychopathology (Merari, 2010): "Contrary to what seems to be the public impression, the currently prevailing opinion among scholars is that suicide terrorists are psychologically normal" (p. 248). That does not mean that there are not individuals who act alone and act from a framework of mental illness. For example, individuals who have committed terrorist acts and who are most likely mentally unstable typically act alone and not within a political or social framework include shoe bomber Richard Reid, Olympic bomber Eric Rudolph, and Unabomber Theodore Kaczynski. A more recent example of an individual committing a terrorist act is the case of Major Nidal Malik Hasan, who on November 5, 2009, went on a shooting spree at Fort Hood, Texas, and killed 13 U.S. Department of Defense employees and wounded 32. The Fort Hood shooting represented the worst terrorist attack on U.S. soil since September 11, 2001. Major Hasan, a U.S. Army officer and psychiatrist, was arrested and is standing trial for murder and other charges in military court-martial proceedings. Hasan's case is interesting because, like the prior examples, he acted alone; however, he also engaged in e-mail correspondence with a radical Islamic leader and was known to have extreme religious beliefs, many of which were counter to his role as a U.S. military officer. These should have raised a red flag to superiors and opened up discussions regarding his potential to act as a terrorist. Even within the military and perhaps because of his status as a psychiatrist, those around him either did not take him seriously or were unaware of his transformation to Islamist extremism. In the final analysis by the FBI, Hasan was deemed a ticking time bomb, which necessitates better capability to counter the threat of homegrown terrorism (Lieberman & Collins, 2011). More recently, an American soldier allegedly opened fire and killed 17 innocent Afghan civilians in cold blood, which came on the heels of a spate of events, including the desecration of Taliban corpses by four Marines. This points to the toll that the war is taking on U.S. troops and the need to include a better understanding of the cross-cultural challenges that are likely to be encountered when men and women in the armed forces are deployed into foreign combat zones like Afghanistan (Zillmer, 2012).

Within organized group terrorism, compared with terrorists acting alone, a great majority of suicide bombings and missions are almost always planned in detail, executed according to specific timed criteria, and perpetrated by nonpathological individuals who do not seem to suffer from a psychological disorder (Atran, 2003).

THE TALIBAN

The Taliban is an Islamist militant and political group that rules large parts of Afghanistan, which is slightly smaller than Texas and has a population of approximately 28 million. The Taliban's roots are the Mujahedeen (Afghan fighters) who have a long history of participating in civil unrest and are perceived as being an experienced and battle-tested enemy. The Taliban climbed to political control in the mid-1990s after the withdrawal of Soviet forces and the resultant anarchy and warlordism that arose. They have proven to be a difficult adversary for the United States, elusive and strategic with a loyal following. They are financed by the opium trade and Taliban-friendly governments. The "new" Taliban have specialized in asymmetrical warfare (see Figure 13.5), which has become a staple of terrorist groups, including sniper attacks using spotters, thousands of improvised explosive devices, and the use of indirect fire (i.e., rocket and mortar attacks). The Taliban not only have improved tactically in the field, but are also educated in managing public relations among their constituents and well organized in terms of their directives and focus on Afghanistan.

The Taliban movement has been criticized by the West for their strict interpretation of Muslim doctrine and their harsh treatment of women. As a terrorist group, the Taliban operate mostly in Afghanistan and northwest Pakistan and engage in the attack and control of civilian populations to further their political and ideological goals. Before the attempted Soviet occupation of Afghanistan and the Global War on Terror, Afghanistan had a history of sheltering terrorist groups and providing training grounds for them (e.g., the Baader–Meinhof gang, Al Qaeda).

The Taliban are important to understand from a psychological perspective because their terror focuses equally on winning the war of ideas and on geopolitical warfare. For the West, the Taliban are difficult to comprehend. They rule a great majority of Afghanistan through threat, war,

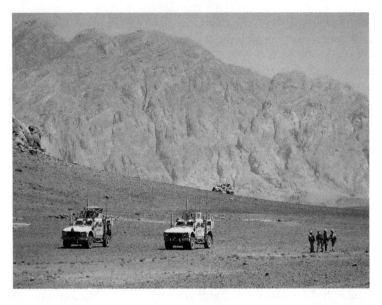

FIGURE 13.5. The difficult terrain of Afghanistan has enabled the Taliban's brand of asymmetrical warfare, including sniper attacks and improvised explosive devices. Photo courtesy of Gunnery Sergeant Brendan McInerney, USMC.

and corruption. But they do provide a form of security and political structure that is not easily obtained otherwise. The Taliban and their followers are united in part by a deep mistrust of foreigners invading Afghanistan. Centuries of war have hardened their resolve. A major fear by the West is that if Afghanistan does not have open relations with the international community, it could once again become a safe haven for Al Qaeda and other terrorist groups.

Of interest to the intelligence and psychological community is how the Taliban is structured sociologically. Similar to the Hezbollah and Hamas, the Taliban leadership plays multiple roles, from community to military leaders. The Taliban uses many tactics to gain political and economic control, including corruption, threats, extortion, and the opium trade. In this sense, the Taliban reflects more a group of warlords than international terrorists, more criminals than political terrorists. Little if any psychological analysis has been attempted on the Taliban, because the West is still trying to understand the characteristics of this reclusive group. Much information has come from TV and print media journalists who have made contact with the Taliban (e.g., Taliban: *The Unknown Enemy* by Fergusson, 2010). More academic approaches to the Taliban (Giustozzi, 2009) have focused on regional differences and clashes of the Taliban rather than on their organizational infrastructure or psychological biographies of their leaders. Thus, there is scant published information about them individually and collectively.

It is understood that the Taliban have a deep resentment for foreigners and that they do not operate in an open society or cooperate with international directives by the UN or the United States. Estimated literacy rates in Afghanistan are 43% for men and 12% for women. Afghanistan has made some advances in increasing basic education, however. More than 10,000 schools are providing educational services to over 7 million children, representing a sixfold increase in enrollment since 2001. Under the Taliban regime, no girls are registered in schools (U.S. Department of State, 2011). Unemployment is approximately 35%. While the U.S. forces stationed in Afghanistan attempt to interact as much as possible with local communities, the fact remains that they are outsiders who mostly are stationed on temporary bases, located away from population centers, and operate mostly on mission-based initiatives. Language barriers, cultural differences, and a deep resentment of the U.S. presence have made it difficult to deal and negotiate directly with the Taliban. Largely uneducated and illiterate, much of the general population is held in terror by the Taliban, who operate through threats, corruption, extortion, blackmail, and intimidation.

There are some insights that one can learn from those who have served in Afghanistan and those who have researched the Taliban's culture and rise to power. First, the Taliban is a loosely organized group that more closely resembles the organizational structure of a clan or a tribe. Similar to other terrorist movements, membership is vague and more often is locally or regionally regulated (e.g., the Taliban in Zabul or the Taliban in the northern exposure). As such, the Taliban do not resemble other social governing systems in terms of supervising their initiatives through on-field site visits or a centralized organizational structure, with deputies regularly traveling to the provinces (Giustozzi, 2009). As a result, the Taliban leadership is at a disadvantage in gaining reliable information on the ground. This may seem like a significant weakness in the face of the better equipped and funded U.S. force. However, this is not the case, because, similar to other terrorist movements, the Taliban's decentralization allows them to absorb as much damage as possible without compromising the overall operational capability of the group.

The social structure of the Taliban also fits that of other terrorist groups, in that they seemingly represent a heterogeneous collection of individuals from their communities. In this respect, the Taliban resembles other modern terrorist groups that can be divided into two categories, with each having different psychological attributes. The regional Taliban leader enjoys significant authority over others and initiates missions and provides orders. Several journalists have made contact with Taliban leaders and have described them as intelligent, creative, and manipulative. They rule through fear and crime. In that sense, they are organizationally more like the Mafia or warlords in Somalia or Yemen. As criminal terrorists, they engage in acts of terror based on a rational risk–reward paradigm for what they believe are justifiable and logical reasons, including threats, corruption, extortion, or the opium trade. As such, the Taliban operate with deliberation and have significant social authority and emotional influence over their followers.

The Taliban are at their most formidable in imposing an asymmetrical warfare unto their opponents. It is as if they are defined by these conflicts, which provides an ideological and psychological context for them. Once in power, they are actually not very efficient at enforcing their style of government. Financially supported through the opium trade and possibly by other Taliban-friendly foreign governments, they represent a very resistant and challenging terrorist enemy.

AL QAEDA

Al Qaeda is an international terrorist group ideologically fueled by the jihad, which followers of Al Qaeda interpret as a religious war with those who are nonbelievers. The term *Al Qaeda* is used when known associates of Al Qaeda plan or execute terrorist attacks, if the perpetrators declare themselves to be members of Al Qaeda or if the political goal of the attack is consistent with Al Qaeda ideology. Al Qaeda terrorist attacks include, among many other incidents, the 1999 bombing of Los Angeles International Airport, the 2000 USS *Cole* bombing, the 9/11 attacks, the 2003 Istanbul bombings, and the 2004 Madrid train bombings. In some cases, there is clear evidence of a directive for the attack from Al Qaeda leadership (e.g., 9/11; National Commission on Terrorist Attacks upon the United States, 2004); in other attacks, only indirect connections can be established (e.g., Istanbul). Al Qaeda terrorist activity has developed both in isolation (aka homegrown) without any traceable evidence of communication with Al Qaeda leaders and in the form of highly organized terrorist activity across international borders involving complicated banking transactions and elaborative planning and deception. Al Qaeda is a loosely organized, decentralized terrorist network that is bound together by a common anti-Western ideology and is difficult to track and engage because of their elusive networking structure and lack of a linear organizational hierarchy. Al Qaeda's terrorist tactics differ from those of prior terrorist groups because of their willingness to attack soft targets, including unprotected civilians. In contrast, the Baader–Meinhof gang concentrated on political targets, state-owned banks, U.S. military installations, and right-wing politicians.

An important connection in understanding the psychology of Al Qaeda is to examine what kind of individual joins the jihad and under what circumstances. While millions may support the jihad ideologically, only a very small number of those "sign up" for Al Qaeda to fight for the cause. Little is known about Al Qaeda, but by studying the biographies of known Al Qaeda members it is thought that a great majority of Al Qaeda followers decide to join the social terrorist network based on preexisting friendships formed either in childhood or through a social circle at cultural or religious centers. Anonymous recruitment, the influence of a secular education, or kinship or marriage is thought to play a smaller part in Al Qaeda recruitment. For example, the four London bombers first met each other as friends at a local cultural center and later killed 52 people in the London Underground and on a double-decker bus in 2005. The Fort Dix Six were friends who in 2007, inspired by Al Qaeda and bin Laden, plotted to stage an attack against U.S. military personnel stationed at Fort Dix in New Jersey before FBI agents arrested them. Women play an important role in the practice of Al Qaeda. They provide the glue for their invisible social infrastructure, encourage relatives and friends to join the jihad, and solidify their commitment by marrying the brothers of other members, further deepening the loyalty and bond to the Al Qaeda movement (Sageman, 2004).

Another aspect of Al Qaeda recruitment is the location, which is overwhelmingly on foreign soil. For example, all 18 of the 9/11 hijackers were recruited into Al Qaeda outside of their country of origin. Thus, it appears that those who see value in joining Al Qaeda are more likely to do so if they feel alienated from society and removed from culture and family and friends of origin (Sageman, 2004). This disillusionment in potential Al Qaeda terrorists living abroad, their need for social bonding, and their search for external structure should be considered a main component for how and why potential terrorists are recruited—not because of fear or even ideology but because of a need for affiliation. Many followers of Al Qaeda are not creative thinkers, are easily influenced by authority, and are attracted to the quasi-military hierarchy and structure of terrorist cells. They are vulnerable to being manipulated by the terrorist leader, who is most likely intelligent, narcissistic, and charismatic. Al Qaeda followers are being asked to make a sacrifice in the name of the cause, their community, their family, and their leader. Without the sacrifice, the act of terror may not be as meaningful to the terrorist and is an important prerequisite in his or her motivation to complete the terrorist act. Conversely, disobeying a command would be associated with shame. Thus, psychological concepts of loyalty, attachment, sacrifice, indoctrination, and disillusionment appear to play a common and important role in the recruitment of terrorists.

A further important step in understanding Al Qaeda is the examination of them as individuals. Sageman (2004) investigated more than 400 biographies of Al Qaeda and found that less than 1% had a criminal background or psychiatric history. A majority were married and many had children or were employed. Thus, one of the lessons of the psychology of Al Qaeda—and indeed almost all terrorist groups—is that those least likely to do harm individually are most able to do so collectively. Thus, the psychology of the Al Qaeda phenomenon is based on group dynamics rather than on individual pathology. Those who join Al Qaeda do not have evidence of a pathological past.

Once individuals are known to be associated with Al Qaeda, international intelligence organizations track them as well as other terrorist associates who may be collaborating with them. Al Qaeda is best thought of as an international network of terrorist cells with operational groups as large as 20 or as small as one. A majority of the interaction is among the cell members and little communication exists outside of the terrorist cell. Therefore, intelligence gathering from suspects who are known Al Qaeda terrorists is essential in learning more about the group's network.

In support of the war on Al Qaeda, psychologists may be called on to interact with terrorists or more likely to educate military leadership and personnel about the psychology of these individuals (Sageman, 2004). Thus, an understanding of their psychological makeup is important. For example, the threshold for joining Al Qaeda is much lower than previously thought. Once an individual becomes a member of Al Qaeda, there is a motivation to participate in its missions based on group dynamics and social bonding. In fact, this social bond is thought to be difficult for a terrorist to abandon, without betraying his closest friends and family. Consider, for example, the Baader–Meinhof gang, which comprised mostly friends. Once incarcerated, they all committed suicide together as an act of loyalty. Al Qaeda's motivation to harm the United States is based on this same intense loyalty and a modus operandi that is based on an actuarial assessment of the terrorist's plan for failure or success.

To date, the Global War on Terror has been successful in disrupting Al Qaeda's ability to function financially and operationally. Certainly, the elimination of Al Qaeda's leader Osama bin Laden in 2011 represents an important victory. Nevertheless, Al Qaeda remains a challenging political and terrorist threat because of its size, its global influence, and its vast number of sympathizers, including millions of moderate Arabs as well as numerous Al Qaeda-friendly state governments. Among the sympathizers of Al Qaeda, the terrorists' actions and anti-West sentiment are tolerated, appreciated, and condoned by a much larger group. In fighting Al Qaeda it is important to engage behavioral scientists and psychologists alike to optimize psychological science for use in counterterrorism endeavors (see Figure 13.6). Advancing psychological science directly and indirectly in these areas will benefit the security of our nation as well as the discipline of psychology.

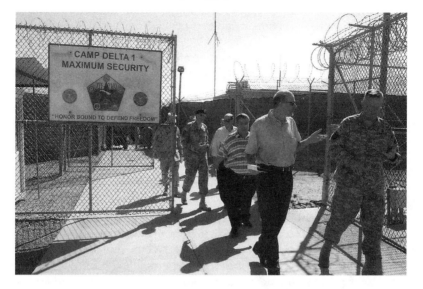

FIGURE 13.6. In the Global War on Terrorism, knowledge is an essential military tool. Interrogations of terrorists have become one of the controversial ingredients of the current war on Al Qaeda (see Chapter 14, this volume). U.S. Navy photo by MC3 Remus Borisov; UNCLASSIFIED//Cleared for Public Release; CDR Robert T. Durand, JTF-GTMO PAO.

SUMMARY

Over the last decade, the nature of military engagement has changed significantly. This is related to the geopolitical transformation after the Cold War, the Persian Gulf War, and the wars in Iraq and Afganistan. In addition, recent terrorist attacks have brought a new psychological complexity to how terrorist groups are conceptualized. As a result, there has been a demand for the development of an increasingly mobile and modern military and a renewed interest in understanding terrorist motivation, that is, to get inside the "enemy's head." This chapter reviewed historical and current theaters of terrorism in order to understand the psychology of terrorists. Major findings include:

- The threshold for terrorist participation is much lower than is commonly expected.
- Terrorists do not show any striking psychopathology or predisposition toward terrorism.
- The most common characteristic of terrorists is their normality (e.g., slip through airport security, live in foreign countries undetected).

- Most terrorists are not crazed fanatics and have no history of criminal behavior.
- Terrorist acts appear to the perpetrator to be reasonable and a necessary part of a rational strategy, with calculable costs and benefits.

Research on WWII Nazi perpetrators (Zillmer et al., 1995), modern German terrorists (Rasch, 1979), Japanese kamikaze pilots (Taylor, 1988), IRA terrorists (Bartlett, 2005), Palestinian terrorists (Laqueur, 1987), and Italian Red Brigade terrorists (Reich, 1998) found no consistent patterns of psychopathology. In fact, most terrorists consider themselves soldiers, and perhaps it is best to think of them psychologically as such. Even though it has become common to think of terrorists as flawed, even deranged individuals, those who committed atrocities as part of an organized group and in a variety of different venues ranging from genocide to suicide missions showed a surprising absence of any psychopathology, uniform abnormality, psychiatric history, or criminal history. Thus, psychological data indicate that ordinary people who did not demonstrate any prior inclination toward violence became involved in atrocities.

In addition, terrorists are difficult to profile psychologically and appear to represent a heterogeneous population. Thus, there is very little evidence of a terrorist-specific personality profile. The most common characteristic of terrorists, in fact, is their heterogeneity and their normality, which allows them, for example, to slip through airport security or blend into society to avoid detection. This explains why former Nazi concentration guards as well as modern terrorists, including Al Qaeda, can live in the United States or other countries for prolonged periods of time and remain undetected (i.e., a sleeper cell).

The great majority of terrorists are not crazed fanatics and have no history of criminal behavior. Those who are mentally ill are unlikely to possess the discipline and fortitude required of effective terrorists and expected by their leaders. Fanatics are generally not recruited by terrorist cells because of their possible mental instability. In fact, terrorist groups often expel from their midst emotionally disturbed individuals, since they are a security risk and unreliable.

In order to influence their followers, terrorist leaders are most likely to be educated, intelligent, manipulative, and charismatic. The current evidence on the psychology of terrorists suggests that it may be rooted far more in nationalist defiance or utilitarian strategy as a means of the preservation of their community rather than in religious extremism. An important finding is that, in almost all of the terror groups studied here, individuals entered the network as part of a social process through friends, family, or a need for interpersonal closeness and attachment, not necessarily prior ideological beliefs or radicalization (Argo, 2006; Sageman, 2004; Zillmer et al., 1995).

Argo (2006) summarized it as follows: "Emotion and social ties precede the acquisition of an ideology" (p. B15). Terrorists have a common worldview, which provides a cognitive and emotional cohesiveness to their group.

Political terrorists share an interpretation of the world—political, religious, or otherwise—whose construction is often immune to argument and resistant to contrary facts. In a sense, terrorists are educated. Thus, for the individual terrorist, the act of self-renunciation is meaningful and rational. The giving of one's life in an act of self-sacrifice is done in the name of the cause. Terrorists are engaging in terrorist acts for what they think are logical reasons. They are not forced to commit atrocities; rather, there is an overwhelming sense of loyalty and even affection for those who give the orders. This shared ideology and need for attachment and sacrifice includes the following realities:

- Emotion and social ties precede the acquisition of an ideology.
- Once in the terrorist movement, it is difficult to abandon it without betraying close friends and family.
- Terrorists share an interpretation of the world, an ideology (political, religious or otherwise), whose construction is resistant to argument.
- For the individual terrorist, the act off self-renunciation is meaningful and rational.
- Terrorists think they are not doing wrong, but that they are doing good. In their own minds they think they are idealists.

Terrorists are more formidable than we previously thought because they are a rational enemy. In the war on terror, a first line of defense should focus on the prevention of recruitment (Atran, 2003). Fighting terrorism by eliminating poverty and providing education appears to be naïve. One must reduce the member of sympathizers, since they are thought to be an essential ingredient for a terrorist movement. Most people have moderate views, and thus one has to counter psychological warfare with ideas and public relations in order to marginalize the terrorists. Finally, fighting terror networks through technology is a most recent and important approach because terrorist cells depend on cellular and electronic communication and financing through modern banking institutions.

REFERENCES

Adorno, T. W., Frankel-Brunswick, E., Levinson, D. J., & Sanford, R. N. (1950). *The authoritarian personality.* New York: Harper & Brothers.

Arendt, H. (1958). *The origins of totalitarianism.* New York: Meridian Books.

Arendt, H. (1963). *Eichmann in Jerusalem: A report on the banality of evil*. New York: Viking Press.

Argo, N. (2003). *The banality of evil, understanding today's human bombs* (Policy paper, Preventive Defense Project). Stanford, CA: Stanford University.

Argo, N. (2006, February 3). The role of social context in terrorist acts. *Chronicle of Higher Education*, pp. B15–B16.

Asch, S. E. (1952). *Social psychology*. New York: Prentice Hall.

Atran, S. (2003). Genesis of suicide terrorism. *Science, 7*, 1534–1539.

Aust, S. (2008). *Baader–Meinhof: The inside story of the R.A.F.* New York: Oxford University Press.

Bartlett, S. J. (2005). *The pathology of man: A study of human evil*. Springfield, IL: Charles C Thomas.

Browning, C. R. (1993). *Ordinary men: Reserve Police Battalion 101 and the final solution in Poland*. New York: Harper.

Dicks, H. V. (1972). *Licensed mass murder: A socio-psychological study of some SS killers*. New York: Basic Books.

Fergusson, J. (2010). *Taliban: The unknown enemy*. Philadelphia: Da Capo.

Giustozzi, A. (2009). *Decoding the new Taliban: Insights from the Afghan field*. New York: Columbia.

Goldhagen, D. J. (1996). *Hitler's willing executioners: Ordinary Germans and the Holocaust*. New York: Knopf.

Hacker, F. (1980). Terror and terrorism: Modern growth industry and mass entertainment. *Terrorism, 4*, 143–159.

Jager, H., Schmidtchen, G., & Sullwold, L. (1981). *Analysen zum terrorismus 2: Lebenlaufanalysen* [Analysis of terrorism: Life-course analysis]. Darmstadt: Seutscher Verlag.

Kennedy, C. H., & Williams, T. J. (2011). *Ethical practice in operational psychology: Military and national intelligence operations*. Washington, DC: American Psychological Association.

Kobrin, N. H. (2010). *The banality of suicide terrorism: The naked truth about the psychology of Islamic suicide bombing*. Washington, DC: Potomac.

Laqueur, W. (1987). *The age of terrorism*. Boston: Little, Brown.

Lester, D., Yang, B., & Lindsay, M. (2004). Suicide bombers: Are psychological profiles possible? *Studies in Conflict and Terrorism, 27*, 283–295.

Lieberman, J. I., & Collins, S. M. (2011, February). *A ticking time bomb: Counterterrorism lessons from the U.S. government's failure to prevent the Fort Hood attack*. A special report by Joseph I. Lieberman, Chairman and Susan M. Collins, Ranking Member, U.S. Senate Committee on Homeland Security and Governmental Affairs, Washington, DC. Retrieved from *www.scribd.com/doc/48113252*.

Merari, A. (2004). Suicide terrorism. In R. Yufit & D. Lester (Eds.), *Assessment, treatment and prevention of suicide*. New York: Wiley.

Merari, A. (2010). *Driven to death: Psychological and social aspects of suicide terrorism*. New York: Wiley.

Miale, F. R., & Selzer, M. (1975). *The Nuremberg mind: The psychology of the Nazi leaders*. New York: New York Times Book.

Milgram, S. (1974). *Obedience to authority*. New York: Harper & Row.

Moghaddam, F. M. (2005). The staircase to terrorism: A psychological exploration. *American Psychologist, 60*(2), 161–169.

Morris, I. (1975). *The nobility of failure: Tragic heroes in the history of Japan.* London: Secker & Warburg.

National Commission on Terrorist Attacks upon the United States. (2004). *The 9/11 Commission Report.* New York: Norton.

Neuffer, E. (2001). *The key to my neighbor's house: Seeking justice in Bosnia and Rwanda.* New York: Picador.

Pape, R. (2003). The strategic logic of suicide terrorism. *American Political Science Review, 97,* 343–361.

Pape, R. (2005). *Dying to win: The strategic logic of suicide terrorism.* New York: Random House.

Rasch, W. (1979). Psychological dimensions of political terrorism in the Federal Republic of Germany. *International Journal of Law and Psychiatry, 2,* 79–85.

Reich, W. (1998). *Origins of terrorism: Psychologies, theologies, and states of mind.* Washington, DC: Woodrow Wilson Center Press.

Sageman, M. (2004). *Understanding terror networks.* Philadelphia: University of Pennsylvania Press.

Taylor, M. (1988). *The terrorist.* London: Brassey's.

U.S. Department of State. (2011). *Background note: Afghanistan.* Retrieved from *www.state.gov/r/pa/ei/bgn/5380.htm.*

Waller, J. (2002). *Becoming evil: How ordinary people commit genocide and mass killing.* New York: Oxford University Press.

Zillmer, E. (2012). *The psychological toll of war: CNN Opinion.* Retrieved from *www.cnn.com/2012/03/13/opinion/zillmer-afghanistan-killing.*

Zillmer, E. A. (2004). National Academy of Neuropsychology: President's address—The future of neuropsychology. *Archives of Clinical Neuropsychology, 19,* 713–724.

Zillmer, E. A., Harrower, M., Ritzler, B., & Archer, R. P. (1995). *The quest for the Nazi personality: A psychological investigation of Nazi war criminals.* Hillsdale, NJ: Erlbaum.

Zimbardo, P. G. (1972). Pathology of imprisonment. *Society, 6,* 4, 6, 8.

CHAPTER 14

Ethical Dilemmas in Clinical, Operational, Expeditionary, and Combat Environments

Carrie H. Kennedy

Military psychology ethics has received significant visibility in recent years, with unprecedented use of psychologists in the current war. Psychologists have been asked to use psychometric expertise in assessing blast concussion in the combat zone, have been involved in intelligence-gathering activities, and continue to expand other evolving skill sets (e.g., prescription privileges, telehealth, embedded psychology, counterespionage, counterterrorism, assessment and treatment of combat stress disorders). In an organization in which consultation activities and clinical decisions can have dire consequences, military psychologists address a number of difficult ethical issues. While every area of psychological practice contends with potentially conflicting loyalties, guidance, and regulations, military psychology faces a high degree of ethical dilemmas, with the added dynamics and potentially conflicting interactions of the American Psychological Association's (APA) *Ethical Principles of Psychologists and Code of Conduct* (2010; hereinafter referred to as the Ethics Code), APA policy, military instructions, and military laws (i.e., Uniformed Code of Military Justice; see also Johnson, Grasso, & Maslowski, 2010). Given the complexity of some of these interactions, the sometimes ambiguous wording of ethics codes in general, and the impossibility of ethics codes to cover every potential situation, simply following the Ethics Code is insufficient for ethical decision making (Kitchener & Kitchener, 2012), especially for the military psychologist.

This chapter focuses on the four environments in which military psychologists practice—traditional military treatment facilities, operational environments, noncombat expeditionary environments, and the combat zone—and highlights the most prominent ethical dilemmas experienced in each locale. Finally, recommendations for prevention and mitigation of conflicts are presented.

TRADITIONAL MILITARY TREATMENT FACILITIES

Traditional military treatment facilities (MTFs) include both military and veteran's hospitals and clinics and encompass all aspects of mental healthcare, from outpatient evaluation and psychotherapy to inpatient treatment. Included in this conceptualization are facilities in which military psychologists provide clinical services to wartime detainees. Military providers in MTFs enjoy routine access to resources most clinical psychologists take for granted: electronic medical records, sound-proofed offices, support staff, consistently functioning office equipment, and generally predictable schedules and patient caseloads, to name a few. Ethical conflicts tend to be those normally associated with traditional mental health care with the added dynamics of military practice.

The practice of clinical psychology in military treatment facilities dates back to World War II (WWII), when many psychologists transitioned from primarily research and psychometric assessment to the provision of mental healthcare. This occurred largely because of the overwhelming mental health needs of WWII veterans and insufficient numbers of psychiatrists (see Chapter 1, this volume; see also Kennedy, Boake, & Moore, 2010). Consequently, a robust analysis of ethical dilemmas in the military comes from practice in traditional military treatment environments given the seven decades that military psychologists have been able to identify and examine these challenges. These primary ethical dilemmas include multiple/dual roles and subsequent multiple relationships (Johnson, 2008; McCauley, Hughes, & Liebling-Kalifani, 2008), competence (Johnson, 2008), informed consent, cultural/multicultural competency (Kennedy, Jones, & Arita, 2007; Reger, Etherage, Reger, & Gahm, 2008), confidentiality (Johnson, 2008; McCauley et al., 2008), and mixed/dual agency, particularly as it pertains to fitness for duty decisions (Stone, 2008; Kennedy & Johnson, 2009). A new treatment and ethical challenge presented by the current war is that of the mental health care of wartime detainees in military detention facilities (Kennedy, Malone, & Franks, 2009; Kennedy, 2011).

Multiple/Dual Relationships and Roles

In the day-to-day role of any active-duty military psychologist, dual roles and relationships are unavoidable. The psychologist is a military officer with inherent regulations and expectations given his or her rank, in addition to the fact that the psychologist is a member of the command and community with collateral duties, community involvement, friendships, and so on. In a large MTF, these relationships are fairly easy to mitigate given significant options for referral (e.g., other military providers within the MTF and civilian referrals outside of the MTF). However, multiple relationships are particularly common in solo and remote billets, and these can be harder to manage. It is not uncommon for a psychologist to have to enter into a clinical relationship with a subordinate, a senior officer, a roommate, or even a friend (Johnson, 2011; Staal & King, 2000). Standard 3.05, Multiple Relationships, states:

> (a) A multiple relationship occurs when a psychologist is in a professional role with a person and (1) at the same time is in another role with the same person, (2) at the same time is in a relationship with a person closely associated with or related to the person with whom the psychologist has the professional relationship, or (3) promises to enter into another relationship in the future with the person or a person closely associated with or related to the person.
>
> A psychologist refrains from entering into a multiple relationship if the multiple relationship could reasonably be expected to impair the psychologist's objectivity, competence, or effectiveness in performing his or her functions as a psychologist, or otherwise risks exploitation or harm to the person with whom the professional relationship exists.
>
> Multiple relationships that would not reasonably be expected to cause impairment or risk exploitation or harm are not unethical.
>
> (b) If a psychologist finds that, due to unforeseen factors, a potentially harmful multiple relationship has arisen, the psychologist takes reasonable steps to resolve it with due regard for the best interests of the affected person and maximal compliance with the Ethics Code.

Not all multiple relationships are contraindicated. It is important for the military psychologist to be able to objectively determine whether a dual role/multiple relationship could be potentially harmful prior to entering into the relationship (Sommers-Flanagan, 2012). Treating a member of the command who does not work in your department, for example, and then serving on the military ball committee with that same person is not likely to qualify as potentially harmful. It is important, however, that thorough informed consent be done with every military patient, since these dual relationships arise frequently and unexpectedly and are not always so benign. Take, for example, a military psychologist who had to do an emergency assessment of an individual in the chain of command and after interviewing the individual's wife learned that she was planning a murder–suicide subsequent to some of his recent illegal actions. This type of multiple relationship should be avoided whenever possible and when not possible should be mitigated by informed consent and other creative strategies.

Competence

Competence is a particularly complicated issue in the military because there are a wide variety of jobs that psychologists may be assigned (e.g., embedded in primary care, inpatient treatment, aviation command, operational billet, aircraft carrier). Although competence is clearly a matter for junior psychologists, this concern is not solely the domain of the new military psychologist. It is not uncommon for active-duty psychologists to hold disparately different jobs throughout their career, requiring new training for each position. As an example, one midcareer officer in the Navy has been assigned to an HIV clinic, an alcohol and drug rehab, an aviation command, a detainee mental health clinic, a combat zone hospital, and in a counterintelligence position. This wide variety of experiences is not unusual for a military psychologist; however, "the range of professional competence within psychology is sufficiently broad that expertise in one area does not necessarily readily translate into another" (Nagy, 2012, p. 170). Consequently, military psychology competence is a constantly moving target. Standard 2.01, Boundaries of Competence, states:

> (a) Psychologists provide services, teach, and conduct research with populations and in areas only within the boundaries of their competence, based on their education, training, supervised experience, consultation, study, or professional experience.
>
> (c) Psychologists planning to provide services, teach, or conduct research involving populations, areas, techniques, or technologies new to them undertake relevant education, training, supervised experience, consultation, or study.
>
> (d) When psychologists are asked to provide services to individuals for whom appropriate mental health services are not available and for which psychologists have not obtained the competence necessary, psychologists with closely related prior training or experience may provide such services in order to ensure that services are not denied if they make a reasonable effort to obtain the competence required by using relevant research, training, consultation, or study.

In addition to the routine reassignment of active-duty clinical psychologists, new demands have provided increasing challenges to competency, as is demonstrated in this War on Terror in many ways (see also Combat Zone section later). Within traditional MTFs, two of these ways are the increased utilization of telehealth and the inception of new and experimental treatments for posttraumatic sress disorder (PTSD), to include virtual reality exposure treatments. Note that these are simply two examples of evolving strategies in traditional military mental healthcare. Psychologists working with military members and in the clinical psychology field in general face advances and changes to treatment provision on a regular basis.

With sweeping budget cuts, military manning decreases, and the increased need for military mental healthcare, in addition to coincident advances in technology, telehealth is becoming an increasingly considered option for both active-duty and veteran service members. In addition, some propose that one of the ways to assist generalist providers in the war zone with specific problems, such as blast concussion (see also Combat Zone section later), is to utilize telehealth for such roles as patient interviewing and cognitive test interpretation. Studies of the efficacy and implementation of telehealth as a mainstream option for treatment in the nonmilitary population are beginning to grow. Military research into telehealth is currently limited, though is also increasing (see, e.g., Gros, Yoder, Tuerk, Lozano, & Acierno, 2011; Tuerk, Yoder, Ruggiero, Gros, & Arcieno, 2010). Although telehealth may prove to be a promising option for service members, providing greater access to treatment, ethical dilemmas ultimately arise. Specific concerns related to the various modalities of telehealth are risks to confidentiality, technological competence required by the provider, assessment of client appropriateness for telehealth, and availability and accessibility of emergency resources when needed (Ragusea, 2012).

A second area of increasing utilization is that of virtual reality treatments, particularly for PTSD (Rizzo et al., 2011). Virtual reality is based on the premise and efficacy of exposure therapy but with the ability to create a virtual combat zone with realistic pertinent variables (e.g., other service members, war zone landscape, explosions, incoming rockets; see Reger & Holloway, 2011). Although virtual reality exposure therapy treatment is promising, empirical support for use with combat trauma disorders is only just emerging. Should it gain widespread use in the military, military psychologists will require formal training and supervision in order to gain competency.

While maintaining competency in a wide array of jobs with a diverse population (see Cultural/Multicultural Competency section later) is a challenging task, the military provides the opportunity for a wide range of competency development. This is achieved through formal internships, fellowships and other training programs, mentorship programs, continuing education, supervision, and the encouragement of individual professional development, such as board certification by providing monetary bonuses to diplomates.

With regard to fellowship, between the three services, formal training is provided in prescribing medication (see Laskow & Grill, 2003, for an overview of the U.S. Department of Defense [DoD] Psychopharmacology Demonstration Project), neuropsychology, child psychology, forensic psychology, operational psychology, and health psychology. Fellowship training is approached differently between the three services, with some fellows training in military sites (e.g., Army neuropsychology postdoctoral fellows) and others in civilian sites (e.g., Navy child psychology postdoctoral fellows). Shorter formal training programs are offered in aerospace psychology, repatriation of prisoners of war and other detained individuals, and behavioral science consulting, to name a few, and mentoring programs are available for military psychologists.

Informed Consent

Informed consent is an integral part of all mental health evaluation and care, and it is essential for service members and other individuals whom the military psychologist will evaluate or treat. In addition to more traditional information included in informed consent, the military provider must also discuss military-specific privacy and confidentiality issues (see later discussion of confidentiality) related to military service or status of the individual in question (e.g., service member prisoner, enemy combatant) as well as all of the potential outcomes inherent with contact with military mental health providers (e.g., fitness-for-duty issues, potential loss of flight status). Standard 3.10, Informed Consent, states:

> (a) When psychologists conduct research or provide assessment, therapy, counseling, or consulting services in person or via electronic transmission or other forms of communication, they obtain the informed consent of the individual or individuals using language that is reasonably understandable to that person or persons except when conducting such activities without consent is mandated by law or governmental regulation or as otherwise provided in this Ethics Code.
>
> (b) For persons who are legally incapable of giving informed consent, psychologists nevertheless (1) provide an appropriate explanation, (2) seek the individual's assent, (3) consider such persons' preferences and best interests, and (4) obtain appropriate permission from a legally authorized person, if such substitute consent is permitted or required by law. When consent by a legally authorized person is not permitted or required by law, psychologists take reasonable steps to protect the individual's rights and welfare.
>
> (c) When psychological services are court ordered or otherwise mandated, psychologists inform the individual of the nature of the anticipated services, including whether the services are court ordered or mandated and any limits of confidentiality, before proceeding.

(d) Psychologists appropriately document written or oral consent, permission, and assent.

Informed consent should be thoroughly discussed in any first session with a military patient prior to any disclosures by that individual. Only in the case of a command-directed evaluation, which is governed by law, may a service member undergo involuntary mental health evaluation (see Chapter 2, this volume, for a discussion of command-directed and emergent evaluations), so it is important that the service member understand the potential career repercussions of any disclosure and have the option of not revealing information. Informed consent, particularly as it relates to confidentiality, the provision of information to the service member's command, and fitness for duty should be revisited in each session.

Cultural/Multicultural Competency

Although professional competence is paramount for military psychologists, cultural and multicultural competence must be equally considered. In the military, cultural competence generally refers to the ability to evaluate, treat, and make informed decisions for both service member patients and the organization in the context of rank, military occupational specialty (MOS)/rate, officer/enlisted, branch of service, military language, mission, military instruction, and military law. Multicultural competence, on the other hand, refers to the ability to evaluate, treat, and make informed decisions regarding a diverse array of individuals with differing backgrounds. Age, gender, race/ethnicity, religion, disability, socioeconomic status, and sexual orientation all play key roles in the psychological assessment and treatment of military members. One needs not only to establish competency to work within the military with different groups but also to address any issues of individual bias and prejudice toward these same groups (Nagy, 2012).

Some multicultural issues have little bearing on military practice given the military context (e.g., disability), while some of these factors interact significantly with cultural competence. For example, in 2008 women made up approximately 14% of enlisted ranks and 16% of officer ranks across the military (Office of the Under Secretary of Defense, Personnel and Readiness, n.d). However, rules pertaining to women in military service continue to be differentiated from the service of male counterparts. Despite some recent changes to policies regarding women and military service, women are excluded from some military jobs (DoD, 2012) and consequently continue to have conditions placed on their military service. (For an in-depth discussion of the integration of women into the military, see Kennedy & Malone, 2009.)

To explore the notion of cultural competence in military psychology, it is necessary to examine the various ways in which both civilians and active-duty psychologists come to be in the military or working in a military setting. Civilian military psychologists may have years of military experience (i.e., veterans) but in many cases may have none. In recent years, given increased demands for mental health care for veterans, an unprecedented number of civilian psychologists have been hired by MTFs and commissioned into the military as direct accessions. Individuals without some type of prior military experience (e.g., prior active duty, Reserve or National Guard) are especially at risk of decision-making mistakes because of a general lack of familiarity and understanding of the military culture (Johnson & Kennedy, 2010). Some of these errors can impact rapport (e.g., failing to use the individual's correct rank), and some can be dire, such as not understanding an individual's MOS/rate and returning him or her to duty when this is contraindicated.

With regard to multicultural competency, in 2008, the racial composition of the U.S. Navy was 62.8% white, 21.3% black, 5.2% American Indian, 6.3% Asian, 1% Pacific Islander, and 3.4% of people who identified themselves as belonging to two racial groups. Of the total group, 16% endorsed Hispanic ethnicity (Office of the Under Secretary of Defense, Personnel and Readiness, n.d.). In addition, approximately 8% of the U.S. military is foreign born, with 12.6% of these individuals serving in the U.S. military as non-U.S. citizens (Stock, 2009).

Standard 2.01, Boundaries of Competence, states:

> (b) Where scientific or professional knowledge in the discipline of psychology establishes that an understanding of factors associated with age, gender, gender identity, race, ethnicity, culture, national origin, religion, sexual orientation, disability, language, or socioeconomic status is essential for effective implementation of their services or research, psychologists have or obtain the training, experience, consultation, or supervision necessary to ensure the competence of their services, or they make appropriate referrals, except as provided in Standard 2.02, Providing Services in Emergencies.

Multicultural competence is of principle importance for the military psychologist. Not only does one work with the various ethnic, racial, and religious groups from within the United States, one works with U.S. service members from foreign countries (a person does not need to be a U.S. citizen to serve in the U.S. military; see prior discussion), with foreign nationals, and with wartime detainees. Perhaps one of the more salient examples illustrating the need for multicultural competency is the provision of mental healthcare to the detainees in wartime detention facilities. Since the beginning of Operation Iraqi Freedom, military mental health providers have provided mental health assessment and care to wartime detainees both in and out of the war zone (Toye & Smith, 2011; Kennedy, Malone & Franks, 2009; see Figure 14.1). These detainees are from a variety of countries, are predominantly Muslim, have widely disparate levels of education, and speak many different languages. Topping the list of challenging ethical dilemmas identified by mental health providers are informed consent, multicultural competence, and mixed agency (Kennedy et al., 2009; Kennedy & Johnson, 2009; Kennedy, 2011).

Confidentiality

Confidentiality is a continuous challenge for the military psychologist. Given the dual-role challenge (see prior discussion) and the mixed-agency challenge (see the following section), knowing when something needs to be reported and to whom while maintaining the best interests of service members is significantly complicated. Standard 4.01, Maintaining Confidentiality, states:

> Psychologists have a primary obligation and take reasonable precautions to protect confidential information obtained through or stored in any medium, recognizing that the extent and limits of confidentiality may be regulated by law or established by institutional rules or professional or scientific relationship.

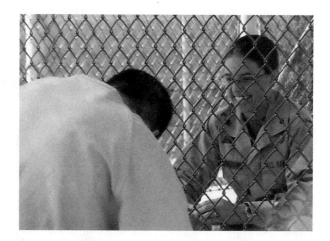

FIGURE 14.1. A detainee tells a joke during a therapy session in Guantanamo Bay. U.S. Navy photo by MC3 Remus Borisov; UNCLASSIFIED/Cleared for Public Release; CDR Robert T. Durand, JTF-GTMO PAO.

Service members understand that when they see military medical providers some of their information is not private. Their attendance at annual physical health assessments, whether or not they are up to date on immunizations, and the state of their dental readiness, for example, are all tracked by the command to ensure a state of continuous mission readiness. However, mental health evaluation and treatment is differentiated from this kind of routine medical maintenance. In August 2011, in an effort to decrease stigma and increase service members' willingness to get help, the military implemented an unprecedented instruction regarding confidentiality and mental healthcare. DoDI 6490.08 states "the DoD shall foster a culture of support in the provision of mental health care and voluntarily sought substance abuse education to military personnel in order to dispel the stigma" (DoD, 2011, p. 2). The instruction further states that "healthcare providers shall follow a presumption that they are not to notify a Service member's commander when the Service member obtains mental health care or substance abuse education services" (p. 2). This is negated when one of the following notification standards is met: harm to self, harm to others, harm to mission, special personnel, inpatient care, acute medical conditions interfering with duty, substance abuse treatment program, and command-directed evaluation. In these cases, however, the mental health provider is directed to "provide the minimum amount of information to the commander concerned as required to satisfy the purpose of the disclosure" (p. 2). This means that most service members who are considered fit for full duty may seek help from a military mental health provider in full confidence for a wide variety of problems (e.g., postdeployment adjustment, relationship problems, non-duty-limiting mental health concerns).

Finally, similar to rural communities, it is important for military psychologists to address with their military patients what their expectation is when seeing them in public. It is common knowledge among military psychologists that once they have been at the same duty station for about 12 months, they inevitably run into both active-duty and dependent patients almost every time they go to the commissary, exchange, gas station, and so on. Some military patients do not want to acknowledge their care provider so as to preserve confidentiality, while others want to say hello. It is recommended that this be addressed in the first session. Psychologists can instruct that they will wait for the patient's cue if they encounter each other in public.

Mixed Agency

Mixed agency is present in every professional interaction that a military psychologist has with a client. This is true in both active-duty and Veteran's Administration settings, given that many active-duty and Reserve personnel deploy multiple times (Stone, 2008). With every clinical decision made, the psychologist has a simultaneous responsibility to the service member patient, the military/organization, and to society at large. During wartime, the most common clinical psychological mixed-agency dilemma occurs in the context of returning a service member to duty. For example, when making a decision regarding the aeromedical qualifications of a military aviator, one must consider the aviator-patient, the branch of service (e.g., can the aviator currently meet mission requirements?), and society (e.g., is the aviator a hazard in the air and consequently a threat to others?). There are a variety of ethical standards pertaining to mixed agency, the three most pertinent of which are as follows:

- 1.02, Conflicts Between Ethics and Law, Regulations, or Other Governing Legal Authority, which states:

  > If psychologists' ethical responsibilities conflict with law, regulations, or other governing legal authority, psychologists clarify the nature of the conflict, make known their commitment to the Ethics Code, and take reasonable steps to resolve the conflict consistent with the General Principles and Ethical Standards of the Ethics Code. Under no circumstances may this standard be used to justify or defend violating human rights.

- 1.03, Conflicts Between Ethics and Organizational Demands, which states:

  > If the demands of an organization with which psychologists are affiliated or for whom they are working are in conflict with this Ethics Code, psychologists clarify the nature of the conflict, make known their commitment to the Ethics Code, and take reasonable steps to resolve the conflict consistent with the General Principles and Ethical Standards of the Ethics Code. Under no circumstances may this standard be used to justify or defend violating human rights.

- 3.11, Psychological Services Delivered to or through Organizations, which states:

  > (a) Psychologists delivering services to or through organizations provide information beforehand to clients and when appropriate those directly affected by the services about (1) the nature and objectives of the services, (2) the intended recipients, (3) which of the individuals are clients, (4) the relationship the

psychologist will have with each person and the organization, (5) the probable uses of services provided and information obtained, (6) who will have access to the information, and (7) limits of confidentiality. As soon as feasible, they provide information about the results and conclusions of such services to appropriate persons.

(b) If psychologists will be precluded by law or by organizational roles from providing such information to particular individuals or groups, they so inform those individuals or groups at the outset of the service.

Johnson and Wilson (1993) and Johnson (1995) reviewed three strategies military psychologists have used in the past to attempt to manage the mixed-agency dilemma: the military manual approach, the stealth approach, and the best-interest approach. To review, the military manual approach attempts to manage ethical conflicts by using literal applications of military rules. This approach is considered potentially harmful, tending to prevent the identification of ethical conflicts. The stealth approach is the other extreme, covering up issues that may impact the military and other military members by attempting to work solely in the context of the individual. While psychologists using this approach may believe they are working ethically in the best interests of the individual, this approach also has the potential to cause significant problems for the service member (e.g., occupational difficulty, life-threatening mistakes on the job). The best-interest approach, on the other hand, takes both the individual's and the military's needs into consideration and applies both the Ethics Code and military regulations. This approach involves the most creative problem solving and knowledge of pertinent ethical standards, military regulations, and laws but tends to demonstrate the best outcomes (see Kennedy & Johnson, 2009). This approach is advocated throughout this chapter as the only ethical approach of the three noted to manage the mixed-agency conflict.

While fitness for duty is the most frequently encountered mixed-agency dilemma for the clinical military psychologist, a second mixed-agency dilemma unique to the current war is that of mental healthcare for detainees. This war has marked the first time that detained enemy combatants have been provided mental healthcare during their incarceration. Some have criticized that this care is provided by military mental health providers as opposed to providers from an independent agency (Aggarwal, 2009). In 2008 members of APA voted to make it a violation of APA policy for military psychologists to work in wartime detention facilities except to treat service members (APA, 2008). Consequently, any military psychologist providing mental healthcare or forensic evaluation to detainees in wartime detention facilities or who are working as Behavioral Science Consultation Team (BSCT) members (see Operational Environment section) are in violation of APA policy. However, APA policy does not affect the APA Ethics Code, so psychologists may be in violation of policy while not committing an ethical violation (see Kennedy, 2012). This confusing situation, and consequent decision, is then left to individual psychologists as to whether or not to deploy to a wartime detention facility whether as a clinician, forensic expert, or a part of a BSCT.

Within this environment, military psychologists continue to provide care to wartime detainees. The mixed-agency triad consists of the detainee patient, the military/other government organizations involved, and society (e.g., innocent people who may be wounded/killed by terrorist activity). Military psychologists manage these conflicts using informed consent, peer consultation with prior detainee providers, and contact with senior military psychologists for mentorship when ethical dilemmas arise (see Kennedy, 2012).

OPERATIONAL ENVIRONMENTS

Operational psychology is "the application of the science and profession of psychology to the operational activities of law enforcement, national intelligence organizations, and national defense activities" (Kennedy & Williams, 2011b, p. 4). Operational psychological activities do not typically involve clinical responsibilities and include such activities as assessment and selection of personnel for high-risk jobs (e.g., special operations forces, embassy security guards, aviation personnel; Picano, Williams, Roland, & Long, 2011; see also Chapter 3, this volume), security clearance evaluations (Young, Harvey, & Staal, 2011), support for repatriated U.S. prisoners of war (see Chapter 12, this volume), counterintelligence and counterterrorism activities (Kennedy, Borum, & Fein, 2011), consultation to interrogation (Dunivin, Banks, Staal, & Stephenson, 2011), and crisis negotiation (Gelles & Palarea, 2011; Greene & Banks, 2009; Kennedy & Williams, 2011a; Kennedy & Zillmer, 2006; Shumate & Borum, 2006; see also Chapter 11, this volume).

Operational psychological activities are not as well established and studied as military psychology's clinical activities. Some of these less traditional applications of psychology have come under significant scrutiny, particularly as they pertain to the role of consultation to interrogation (see Figures 14.2 and 14.3). This singular issue has resulted in strong emotions and great debate (see Abeles, 2010; Galvin, 2008). Some psychologists believe that members of their profession should not perform this role, that psychologists who participated were involved in the engineering of torture,

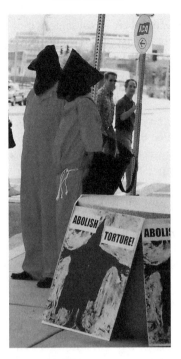

FIGURE 14.2. Protestors at the American Psychological Association convention in 2008. Photo courtesy of Cyndi Lenz.

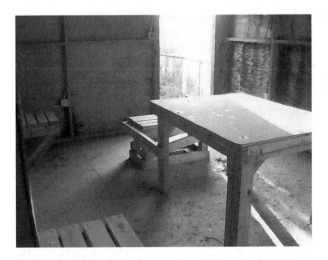

FIGURE 14.3. An abandoned interrogation room at Camp X-ray in Guantanamo Bay, Cuba. Photo courtesy of Carrie H. Kennedy.

and that the APA was complicit in these activities (e.g., see Soldz, 2008). Others believe that military psychologists are in a good position to influence policy, research, and practice (e.g., see Fein, Lehner, & Vossekuil, 2006) by focusing on issues such as memory distortion, effective questioning strategies, and the detection of deception (Loftus, 2011), thereby making a positive impact on current war efforts, increasing ethical and effective intelligence gathering, and preventing atrocities such as those that occurred at Abu Ghraib (Greene & Banks, 2009; Staal & Stephenson, 2006).

This singular disagreement within the field of psychology/APA has brought the ethics of operational psychology as a whole under significant examination. Kennedy and Williams (2011b) identify four primary ethical dilemmas in these environments, namely mixed agency, competence, multiple relationships, and informed consent. Note that there is considerable overlap of ethical dilemmas within each of the four practice environments. The reader is directed to the Traditional Military Treatment Facilities section for applicable ethical standards when indicated.

Mixed Agency

Mixed agency (also called dual agency, divided loyalty, and dual loyalty; see prior discussion for the pertinent ethical standards) occurs when a psychologist has a responsibility to two or more simultaneous entities. Within traditional clinical venues, this dilemma usually involves a service member, the military, and society at large. In operational psychological environments, this typically comes in the form of a responsibility to an individual, a government or military agency, and to society at large (Kennedy, 2012). Using crisis negotiations as an example (see also Chapter 11, this volume), the psychologist has a simultaneous responsibility to the law enforcement/military/government agency (i.e., the primary client), society at large (e.g., hostages, bystanders), and the individual in question (i.e., barricaded individual or hostage taker). It is notable that the psychologist in crisis negotiations will not have any face-to-face interactions with the hostage taker and the hostage taker will not know that there is a psychologist consulting, yet the purpose of the consultant psychologist is to optimize the chances of a peaceful surrender and minimize/prevent loss of life. Gelles and Palarea (2011) recommend that in order to ethically manage the mixed-agency and other dilemmas inherent in crisis negotiation consultation, the psychologist must identify the client, remain in the role of expert consultant (see also Mullins & McMains, 2011), remain autonomous in consultation and free from external influence, identify boundaries and delineate the boundaries between operational consultant and healthcare provider, appreciate the uniqueness of each crisis situation, and establish and maintain professional competence.

Competence

Operational psychology has grown into a subdiscipline of psychology; however, it is only in its infancy as it pertains to the development of a training curriculum and professional standards for competency. Standard 2.01, Boundaries of Competence, states (for other pertinent standards related to competency, see the prior MTF discussion above):

> (e) In those emerging areas in which generally recognized standards for preparatory training do not yet exist, psychologists nevertheless take reasonable steps to ensure the competence of their work and to protect clients/patients, students, supervisees, research participants, organizational clients, and others from harm.

Like the prior advances made by military psychologists during various conflicts, the evolution of the practice of operational psychology is growing on a grand scale. Fostered and predated by the work of psychologists in law enforcement, operational psychology has become a force for the war on terror. As with the development of clinical internships following WWII as a result of the relative newness of the field of clinical psychology (see Chapter 1, this volume), the expansion of operational roles for psychologists requires the same considerations for formal education and training. Staal and Stephenson (2006) recommend a formalized process that includes collaboration between all of the branches of service and involves a specialized postdoctoral fellowship in operational psychology as well as a formalized assessment and selection program geared toward identifying the most appropriate psychologists for this work. Beyond initial fellowship training, various training and conferences specific to operational psychologists (e.g., Special Applications in Psychology conference and survival, evasion, resistance, and escape [SERE] psychology conference) are available, as are mentorship programs and on-the-job training and supervision. Military psychologists may also be able to take advantage of board certification in the newest specialty recognized by the American Board of Professional Psychology—Police and Public Safety—as many of their functions mirror those in more traditional law enforcement. This provides for the highest formal standard of professional competency awarded to psychologists in any subspecialty.

Multiple Relationships

Multiple relationships occur in operational psychology environs as they do in traditional MTFs, although the circumstances differ significantly. A singular difference between operational psychologists and those military psychologists treating service members within MTFs is that operational psychologists typically do not perform clinical duties primarily. However, in any small, embedded, and/or deployed command, the military psychologist is at risk of having to manage the emergent mental health situation of a coworker or of being approached by a coworker for services. In an operational position, this may be a guard, police officer, or Special Forces personnel. This is the typical and most frequently occurring multiple relationship dilemma in the operational psychology environment. It should be mitigated whenever possible through referrals; however, when this is not possible because of an emergency or lack of referral source, thorough informed consent (see prior Traditional Military Treatment Facilities section and Informed Consent section next) is the primary way in which to mitigate the conflict until a more appropriate referral source can be obtained.

Informed Consent

Much of the work of operational psychologists differs dramatically from the work of traditional military clinical psychologists with regard to the individual in question. When working with a service member-patient, informed consent is a standard process that includes the individual (see prior discussion for pertinent standards). In some cases, informed consent is standard for operational psychologists as well, such as in cases of security clearance evaluations or assessment and selection procedures. In these instances, the individual is readily identifiable and involved in the process of obtaining/reviewing appropriateness for a security clearance or undergoing evaluation to obtain/maintain a special duty. However, in many cases, the psychologist will have no direct contact with the individual in question when performing operational psychological responsibilities (e.g., hostage negotiation consultation, interrogation consultation, counterterrorism consultation), and informed consent will be unable to be obtained for a variety of reasons. Take the case of a BSCT psychologist consulting to an interrogation as an example. BSCTs "are . . . not assigned to clinical practice functions, but to provide consultative services to support authorized law enforcement or intelligence activities, including detention and related intelligence, interrogation, and detainee debriefing operations" (U.S. Department of the Army, 2010, p. 4). Yet the BSCT psychologist is also "obligated, as are all service members, to report any actual, suspected, or possible violations of applicable laws, regulations, and policies, to include allegations of abuse or inhumane treatment" (p. 6). In addition, a BSCT psychologist who may be concerned about a detainee's mental health reports their concerns to a third party in order to generate a referral to a clinician, although they receive no feedback regarding any follow-up evaluation or treatment (Kennedy et al., 2009). Consequently, the psychologist maintains a duty to identifiable individuals even in cases where informed consent cannot reasonably be obtained and the individual does not know of the presence of the consulting psychologist (Koocher, 2009).

NON-COMBAT-ZONE EXPEDITIONARY ENVIRONMENTS

Expeditionary environments are those in which the psychologist is embedded within a military unit and provides the gamut of mental healthcare (i.e., prevention, early intervention, outpatient care, and at times inpatient treatment) to the members of that unit as well as consultation to its leadership. Common examples are Operational Stress Control & Readiness (OSCAR) providers who give clinical assessment, care, and consultation for U.S. Marine ground units (Hoyt, 2006), and Navy shipboard psychologists who are responsible for the crew of an aircraft carrier and the accompanying battle group (Wood, Koffman, & Arita, 2003). Expeditionary environments and embedded practice may or may not include duty within a combat zone. This section focuses on those noncombat roles and locations.

Embedded, or integrated, providers become well known to the leadership of a specific unit and to the service members within that unit. Routine interactions and a "one of us" conceptualization serve to establish a comfort level with the provider, who is seen as an approachable and credible resource. This credibility and acceptance, in turn, serve to significantly reduce stigma and increase receptiveness on the part of both individual service members and leadership to interventions and recommendations (Hoyt, 2006). In addition, the embedded provider provides continuity of care. This can be a significant problem for service members receiving care at a traditional MTF who require a course of psychotherapy. Not only do service member-patients deploy frequently but so do their MTF providers. Consequently, a traditional mental healthcare model can result in significant inconsistency and disruption of care (Ralph & Sammons, 2006). Embedded mental health is able to provide continuity of care since the providers are always with the unit wherever it might be. This embedded or expeditionary care is believed to be a powerful means to prevent problems, provide informed early interventions, facilitate better care when serious problems develop, and preserve the military's resources. For example, the billeting of a psychologist on each aircraft carrier has reduced the number of medical evacuations from Navy ships (Wood et al., 2003). However, with these significant advantages come increased ethical challenges. Johnson, Ralph, and Johnson (2005) describe dual agency and multiple roles as the most significant ethical challenges in these embedded environments.

Dual Agency and Multiple Roles

Dual or mixed agency and multiple roles are significant conflicts in all areas of military practice (see prior discussion on MTF and operational environments for the pertinent ethical standards and additional information). Although dual agency has already been described in depth and is highly similar to the dual agency found in traditional MTFs, multiple roles in expeditionary environments are the most magnified of any area of military psychology practice. This is because the psychologist is always a member of the same command hierarchy, is dedicated to provide care to the members of his or her same unit, and often does so in austere locations where there may be no referral sources of any kind.

As the sole mental healthcare provider, especially when deployed, the psychologist will find him- or herself in a position of multiple roles on a regular basis. Most of the time these roles are benign or manageable; however, at times they can be significantly problematic. Johnson et al. (2010), for example, describe a case of a carrier psychologist who has to perform a security clearance evaluation for a known patient, which resulted in the patient not receiving a clearance and consequently a better job. This secondary role placed the therapeutic alliance with that patient in serious jeopardy and compromised the service member's sole source of mental healthcare.

Johnson et al. (2005) provide considerable analysis of multiple relationships in expeditionary environments. These authors note several ways in which psychology practice is unique for the expeditionary psychologist.

1. The psychologist has multiple roles with every service member-patient, given that the psychologist is always an officer.
2. The psychologist has no choice as to whether or not to engage in a clinical relationship with someone. Because there are no other choices available, the psychologist cannot choose to begin a therapeutic relationship, transfer care, or even terminate treatment at times.
3. The psychologist will find him- or herself in a position of having to shift psychology roles with the same individual in order to make fitness-for-duty decisions, perform a forensic evaluation, or determine appropriateness for a security clearance (see prior example).
4. The psychologist represents a decision maker with absolute authority in some matters. "Embedded military psychologists frequently influence the client's life thoroughly, and salient go/no-go decisions by the psychologist commonly impact whether a client will achieve promotions or even remain on active duty" (p. 75).
5. The psychologist will have ongoing personal contact with patients. Within an embedded unit, encountering patients, for example, in

their work space, in the gym, or at command functions is a normal matter of course.

6. The psychologist will inevitably end up providing services to friends, coworkers, and even superiors.

Although it is believed that expeditionary/embedded psychology significantly reduces adverse outcomes and the need for medical evacuation, and increases service member's willingness and probability of seeking care, these are significant challenges that must be carefully and thoughtfully managed by the psychologist.

COMBAT ZONE

Duty in a combat zone brings all of the ethical hazards of expeditionary psychological practice (for embedded providers) as well as traditional practice in an MTF (for providers assigned to combat stress units), but in a physically more dangerous and emotionally charged environment where resources may be extremely limited. Psychologists in a combat zone may lack those things that are often taken for granted, such as routine access to electronic medical records, soundproofed offices (and in some cases even offices), office equipment, and predictable schedules and patient caseloads. Without basic resources, the other challenges become magnified.

Challenges develop beyond dual agency and multiple roles, as military psychologists are at increased risk of being asked to do something they are not trained to do as well as policy and nonmedical decision makers effecting clinical care. The dilemma of potential unlawful orders, professional competency, multicultural competency, and personal problems are also significant issues in the combat zone.

Dual Agency and Multiple Roles

Dual agency and multiple roles take on a new dimension in the combat zone, because without the dual roles psychologists can have a very difficult time treating service members and managing ethical dilemmas. In other words, psychologists must not only be skilled clinicians but also competent military officers. An understanding of the military hierarchy, the weapons, vehicles and other equipment used in the current conflict, military strategy, and military objectives in pertinent areas is not normally equated with skills needed by psychologists. However, understanding exactly what one's patients are being expected to do, where they may be returning to, and what operations are ongoing as well as the ability to interface effectively with the command are keys to clinical decision making and effective implementation of mental health interventions in a war zone. A competent military officer will make informed decisions regarding return to duty and will be able to effectively negotiate plans with the command, which are in the best interest of both the service member and the unit. Simply being an excellent clinician in the combat zone is insufficient to provide care for service members (see prior discussions of MTF and cultural competence).

Unlawful Orders

Occasionally, a psychologist in a combat zone may be ordered to do something either unlawful or inherently unethical. When this occurs, it is typically in the context of a superior officer (usually not an officer in the medical field) not understanding what he or she has asked the psychologist to do. Brief education on psychology/medical ethics and brainstorming to effectively troubleshoot the problem usually resolve any problems related to unlawful orders. In rare cases, however, this may become an issue. Kennedy (2009) presents a case of a junior psychologist, without prescriptive authority, being ordered by a senior medical officer to prescribe medication in the combat zone in the absence of a psychiatrist. The danger is that the junior psychologist will obey the order, even though it is not lawful. Recommendations for mitigation of unlawful orders if education and alternate problem solving are ineffective are to consult with senior members of the military psychology community and the local military lawyer.

Competence

Just because someone is an excellent clinician in garrison does not mean that he or she is going to enjoy the same efficacy in the combat zone. Treating combat trauma in a war zone requires competencies very infrequently used in a traditional mental health clinic. Everything changes in the combat zone to include diagnoses (e.g., acute combat stress vs. acute stress disorder, PTSD from a prior engagement now acutely exacerbated), risk mitigation, and treatment options. Each war also brings with it unique competency challenges for military psychologists. A modern example of an ethical dilemma is the situation involving blast concussion. Psychologists have been assigned the task of using neurocognitive assessment measures in theater, yet few have received formal training in neuropsychology, neurocognitive testing, or concussive/neurological injuries. Further complicating the issue are the facts that there is little published on acute blast concussion and little empirically validated basis for the use of these instruments in theater (Bush & Cuesta, 2010), so even trained neuropsychologists may be at a loss in some situations. Standard 9.07, Assessment by Unqualified Persons, states:

Psychologists do not promote the use of psychological assessment techniques by unqualified persons, except when such use is conducted for training purposes with appropriate supervision.

(For additional ethical standards relevant to competence, see prior Traditional Military Treatment Facilities section.) Issues regarding the Automated Neuropsychological Assessment Metrics and the requirement for neuropsychological evaluation in theater for those with multiple concussions (DoD, 2010) have provided significant pressure to generalists to practice neuropsychology without appropriate training.

Multicultural Competency

Another issue that arises in the combat zone is that of providing mental health services to the local population (see Tobin, 2005). In the current conflict, it is typically a member of the Afghan National Army (ANA) or Afghan National Police who has been brought to the emergency department following a suicide attempt or gesture. For example, a member of the ANA was brought to a combat hospital after jumping from a guard tower after receiving some bad news. He was physically unharmed but had voiced suicidal intent prior to jumping. The military psychologist was the only mental health provider available. To make matters more complicated, the combat hospital is only for acute admissions; there are no ANA mental health resources in that region; and there are no civilian mental health resources in that region. Having only minimal cultural competency to evaluate the individual and lacking any referral source at all, the military psychologist was presented with a complicated situation.

Personal Problems

In addition to the ethical challenges and logistical hurdles of managing patients outside of a traditional clinic or hospital, military psychologists are at risk of developing significant personal problems secondary to their own deployment stress and potentially traumatic incidents (Johnson et al., 2011). While there are no empirical studies addressing the psychological health of military mental health providers, the reality is that no one is truly impervious to the stressors of the combat zone, and the frequency and at times unpredictability of deployments is taking a toll on military psychologists (Johnson, 2008). Routine combat zone stressors for medical personnel can include fairly continuous exposure to the seriously wounded, dying, and dead; environmental stressors (e.g., sleep deprivation, extreme temperatures, wearing of heavy and restrictive personal protective equipment); taking indirect fire (i.e., rockets and mortars) or being fired at directly;

and "nearly constant vicarious exposure to trauma through the stories of traumatized clients" (Johnson & Kennedy, 2010, p. 299). This is in addition to any of the "normal" challenges encountered in trying to manage any unexpected problems on the homefront from a war zone. Maintaining one's own mental health is a significant challenge. Standard 2.06, Personal Problems and Conflicts, states:

> (a) Psychologists refrain from initiating an activity when they know or should know that there is a substantial likelihood that their personal problems will prevent them from performing their work-related activities in a competent manner.
> (b) When psychologists become aware of personal problems that may interfere with their performing work-related duties adequately, they take appropriate measures, such as obtaining professional consultation or assistance, and determine whether they should limit, suspend, or terminate their work-related duties.

While there are multiple conceptualizations of the stressors associated with secondary trauma, compassion fatigue, and burnout (for a review, see Maltzman, 2011; Seeley, 2008), there has been no empirical study of the experience of military mental health providers in the combat zone as it relates to potentially traumatic experiences, no follow-up beyond the routine postdeployment health assessments, and no exit assessments as to whether or not this is a factor in some military psychologists' decisions to leave the military. There also is little in the way of guidance in recognizing a detriment in professional competence and then acting upon it. Johnson et al. (2011) recommend the development of a "comprehensive program for both supporting and monitoring the health and competence of deployed military psychologists, both in theater and following their return to this country. Because many psychologists struggle with the transition from wartime triage to relatively mundane outpatient clinic work, reintegration programs should be established" (p. 97).

PREVENTING, MITIGATING, AND MINIMIZING RISK

While there are a multitude of ethical dilemmas that may arise in any work setting, there are also many strategies available to individual military psychologists, both active duty and civilian, that can assist significantly.

• *Know the Ethics Code, relevant state, federal and military laws, and relevant military instructions.* The practice of psychology (and even the issue of who can call themselves a psychologist) is governed by law, and complying with the Ethics Code is often a requirement of state licensure.

Understanding the requirements of the law as it relates to the field and general practice of psychology is a minimum prerequisite for psychologists (Behnke & Jones, 2012). Beyond the basic understanding of the regulation of psychology and in order to practice military psychology in an informed manner, one must be able to also apply relevant military laws and instructions (Johnson et al., 2010) and understand how these organizational regulations interact with the Ethics Code and APA policy (Kennedy, 2012).

• *Build a network of mentors, peers, and other pertinent professionals.* Military psychologists are expected to perform a wide variety of jobs, and requests for them to engage in unique duties or consultative roles occur daily. In order to manage these requests, it is essential that military psychologists have an existing network of professionals to consult (Johnson et al., 2005; Schank, Helbok, Haldeman, & Gallardo, 2010). At a minimum, it is recommended that each military psychologist have one to two senior mentors, have several peer consulting relationships, be in contact with an individual who had their job in the past, and have a good working relationship with a military lawyer (i.e., judge advocate general).

• *Take advantage of every training opportunity.* The military provides a vast amount of training, and the military psychologist should take advantage of any opportunities, even if they do not seem particularly relevant to current duties. Formal trainings such as rifle/pistol qualification; SERE training; Field Medical Service Officer school, and aeromedical officer training increase cultural competency and provide essential skills for future use.

• *Adopt a personal ethical decision-making model.* There are a number of ethical decision-making models (e.g., Barnett & Johnson, 2008), some of which are military specific (e.g., Staal & King, 2000). Psychologists are urged to evaluate and adopt a decision-making model in order to systematically and objectively evaluate ethical dilemmas as they arise (Johnson et al., 2010; McCutcheon, 2011).

• *Always work toward a best interest solution.* Considering the needs of both the individual and the military can be challenging, but there is usually a course of action that will benefit both parties (Johnson & Wilson, 1993; Johnson, 1995; Johnson et al., 2010). Cultural competence is key in being able to do this well.

• *Obtain appropriate informed consent.* In situations where informed consent can be obtained, military psychologists should discuss the realities of military instructions and laws on confidentiality, where and how records are kept, what the psychologist can reasonably do for the service member-patient, other treatment options, and how the various types of treatment/intervention may impact a current military career and/or future military career goals (Johnson, 1995; Johnson et al., 2005; Schank et al., 2010).

• *Become culturally savvy.* When just beginning to work in the military environment, one must make a concerted effort to understand the cultural differences between the services, military rank structure, military jargon and acronyms, and military law. Military psychologists should coordinate visits to the various commands that they serve, learn their mission, and understand the environments in which their patients operate.

• *Become multiculturally savvy.* The military psychologist should seek out both multicultural-specific continuing education and a diverse array of social events; travel to different areas and experience other cultures; explore and be open to one's own beliefs and personal biases (see Kennedy et al., 2007).

• *Within embedded and remote billets, the military psychologist should assume that everyone is a future patient.* Experienced military psychologists have reported how they can end up in a professional relationship with just about anyone in the command. Psychologists can prepare for this by remaining as neutral as possible on controversial issues, avoiding significant self-disclosure, and building a strong support system that is not a part of the command (see Johnson et al., 2005).

• *In remote and solo environments, have a backup plan should you have to provide an evaluation to someone that creates a potentially harmful situation for that person.* If this occurs, it will most likely be someone in your direct chain of command. These plans often include an agreement to send the military member elsewhere for evaluation (possibly to another service's base or to another country altogether) or, if the situation warrants it, to request an additional psychologist to travel to the command to perform the evaluation.

• *Within embedded and operational billets, educate the military chain of command.* With some of the newer roles for psychologists, not all commands and commanders understand both the breadth of services as well as the limitations of services that embedded/expeditionary and operational psychologists can provide. An upfront educational session for the chain of command and other pertinent members of the command can gain the psychologist significant support to keep the psychologist working within appropriate boundaries and avoiding ethical dilemmas.

• *Be prepared to say no.* In the very rare case where you may be asked to do something unlawful or something that you are not competent to do, be prepared to refuse the request and propose alternative options if appropriate. Preparation includes not only understanding the Ethics Code, your professional responsibilities, and being able to articulate the specific problem with the request, but also knowing who in your chain of command or the military psychology community you can consult and depend on for top cover.

• *Be active in your profession.* Join pertinent organizations in order to network and remain current on practice issues and advances.

• *Take care of yourself.* Our own mental health definitely impacts our abilities to provide care for others and make good decisions on the job. Military psychologists need to understand how a variety of life and job circumstances affect them (e.g., stressors, mood, medical issues, medication side effects, exposure to combat trauma, and secondary traumatization) and take action to make routine healthy lifestyle choices (Nagy, 2012) and create a network of support through other military psychologists and mentors (Johnson et al., 2011).

CONCLUSIONS

The current war has marked some unprecedented stressors for military mental health providers. In 2009 a U.S. Army soldier opened fire in a combat stress clinic in Iraq, killing an Army psychiatrist, a Navy social worker, and three service member-patients (Kaplan, 2009). Later that same year, a U.S. Army psychiatrist opened fire at Fort Hood, killing 13 people, many of whom were part of a combat stress team who were preparing to deploy, including a psychiatric nurse, a psychiatrist, and a psychologist. Military psychologists are deploying at unprecedented rates, are being directly exposed to wartime trauma, and then are actively assisting the warfighters in managing their own trauma.

As with past wars, the Global War on Terrorism has created a new group of challenges and opportunities for military psychologists. Telehealth and automated cognitive testing in the combat zone (e.g., for blast concussion) are creating the need for new competencies and bring into play a new set of ethical dilemmas (see Bersoff, DeMatteo, & Foster, 2012, for a review of ethical dilemmas in assessment and testing). Operational psychology continues to expand and has resulted in many new nontraditional jobs for psychologists. Embedded psychologists are on the ground with infantry units, instead of serving behind the frontlines. Once again, military psychology is poised to have a major impact on the practice of psychology.

REFERENCES

Abeles, N. (2010). Ethics and the interrogation of prisoners: An update. *Ethics and Behavior, 20,* 243–249.

Aggarwal, N. K. (2009). Allowing independent forensic evaluations for Guantanamo detainees. *Journal of the American Academy of Psychiatry and the Law, 37,* 533–537.

American Psychological Association. (2008). *Report of the APA Presidential*

Advisory Group on the implementation of the petition resolution. Retrieved March 6, 2011, from *www.apa.org/ethics/advisory-group-final.pdf.*

American Psychological Association. (2010). *Ethical principles of psychologists and code of conduct, 2010 amendments.* Retrieved February 5, 2011, from *www.apa.org/ethics/code/index.aspx#.*

Barnett, J. E., & Johnson, W. B. (2008). *Ethics desk reference for psychologists.* Washington, DC: American Psychological Association.

Behnke, S. H., & Jones, S. E. (2012). Ethics and ethics codes for psychologists. In S. J. Knapp, M. C. Gottlieb, M. M. Handelsman, & L. D. VandeCreek (Eds.), *APA handbook of ethics in psychology: Vol. 2. Practice, teaching, and research* (pp. 43–74). Washington, DC: American Psychological Association.

Bersoff, D. N., DeMatteo, D., & Foster, E. E. (2012). Assessment and testing. In S. J. Knapp, M. C. Gottlieb, M. M. Handelsman, & L. D. VandeCreek (Eds.), *APA handbook of ethics in psychology: Vol. 2. Practice, teaching, and research* (pp. 45–74). Washington, DC: American Psychological Association.

Bush, S. S., & Cuesta, G. M. (2010). Ethical issues in military neuropsychology. In C. H. Kennedy & J. L. Moore (Eds.), *Military neuropsychology* (pp. 29–55). New York: Springer.

Dunivin, D., Banks, L. M., Staal, M. A., & Stephenson, J. A. (2011). Behavioral science consultation to interrogation and debriefing operations: Ethical considerations. In C. H. Kennedy & T. J. Williams (Eds.), *Ethical practice in operational psychology: Military and national intelligence applications* (pp. 51–68). Washington, DC: American Psychological Association.

Fein, R. A., Lehner, P., & Vossekuil, B. (2006). *Educing information, interrogation: Science and art, foundations for the future.* Washington, DC: National Defense Intelligence College.

Galvin, M. (Producer/Director). (2008). *Interrogate this: Psychologists take on terror* [Motion picture]. (Available from MG Productions, 1112 Boylston St., #163, Boston, MA 02215)

Gelles, M. G., & Palarea, R. (2011). Ethics in crisis negotiation: A law enforcement and public safety perspective. In C. H. Kennedy & T. J. Williams (Eds.), *Ethical practice in operational psychology: Military and national intelligence applications* (pp. 107–123). Washington, DC: American Psychological Association.

Greene, C. H., & Banks, L. M. (2009). Ethical guideline evolution in psychological support to interrogation operations. *Consulting Psychology Journal: Practice and Research, 61,* 25–32.

Gros, D. F., Yoder, M., Tuerk, P. W., Lozano, B. E., & Acierno, R. (2011). Exposure therapy for PTSD delivered to veterans via telehealth: Predictors of treatment completion and outcome and comparison to treatment delivered in person. *Behavior Therapy, 42,* 276–283.

Hoyt, G. B. (2006). Integrated mental health within operational units: Opportunities and challenges. *Military Psychology, 18,* 309–320.

Johnson, W. B. (1995). Perennial ethical quandaries in military psychology: Toward American Psychological Association–Department of Defense collaboration. *Professional Psychology: Research and Practice, 26,* 281–287.

Johnson, W. B. (2008). Top ethical challenges for military clinical psychologists. *Military Psychology, 20,* 49–62.

Johnson, W. B. (2011). "I've got this friend": Multiple roles, informed consent, and friendship in the military. In W. B. Johnson & G. P. Koocher (Eds.), *Ethical conundrums, quandaries, and predicaments in mental health care practice* (pp. 175–182). New York: Oxford University Press.

Johnson, W. B., Grasso, I., & Maslowski, K. (2010). Conflicts between ethics and law for military mental health providers. *Military Medicine, 175,* 548–553.

Johnson, W. B., Johnson, S. J., Sullivan, G. R., Bongar, B., Miller, L., & Sammons, M. T. (2011). Psychology *in extremis*: Preventing problems of professional competence in dangerous practice settings. *Professional Psychology: Research and Practice, 42,* 94–104.

Johnson, W. B., & Kennedy, C. H. (2010). Preparing psychologists for high-risk jobs: Key ethical considerations for military clinical supervisors. *Professional Psychology: Research and Practice, 41,* 298–304.

Johnson, W. B., Ralph, J., & Johnson, S. J. (2005). Managing multiple roles in embedded environments: The case of aircraft carrier psychology. *Professional Psychology: Research and Practice, 36,* 73–81.

Johnson, W. B., & Wilson, K. (1993). The military internship: A retrospective analysis. *Professional Psychology: Research and Practice, 24,* 312–318.

Kaplan, A. (2009, July 6). Death of psychiatrist and other soldiers triggers inquiry into military's mental health care. *Psychiatric Times,* p. 26. Retrieved February 5, 2011, from *www.psychiatrictimes.com/display/article/10168/1426100.*

Kennedy, C. H. (2009). You want me to do what?: The case of the unlawful order. *Navy Psychologist, 2,* 9–10.

Kennedy, C. H. (2011). Establishing rapport with an "enemy combatant": Cultural competence in Guantanamo Bay. In W. B. Johnson & G. P. Koocher (Eds.), *Ethical conundrums, quandaries, and predicaments in mental health practice: A casebook from the files of experts* (pp. 183–188). New York: Oxford University Press.

Kennedy, C. H. (2012). Institutional ethical conflicts with illustrations from police and military psychology. In S. Knapp & L. VandeCreek (Eds.), *APA handbook of ethics in psychology: Vol. 1. Moral foundations and common themes* (pp. 123–144). Washington, DC: American Psychological Association.

Kennedy, C. H., Boake, C., & Moore, J. L. (2010). A history and introduction to military neuropsychology. In C. H. Kennedy & J. L. Moore (Eds.), *Military neuropsychology* (pp. 1–28). New York: Springer.

Kennedy, C. H., & Johnson, W. B. (2009). Mixed agency in military psychology: Applying the American Psychological Association's ethics code. *Psychological Services, 6,* 22–31.

Kennedy, C. H., Jones, D. E., & Arita, A. A. (2007). Multicultural experiences of U.S. military psychologists: Current trends and training target areas. *Psychological Services, 4,* 158–167.

Kennedy, C. H., & Malone, R. C. (2009). Integration of women into the modern military. In S. M. Freeman, B. A. Moore, & A. Freeman (Eds.), *Living and surviving in harm's way: A psychological treatment handbook for pre- and post-deployment of military personnel* (pp. 67–81). New York: Routledge.

Kennedy, C. H., Malone, R. C., & Franks, M. J. (2009). Provision of mental health services at the detention hospital in Guantanamo Bay. *Psychological Services*, 6, 1–10.

Kennedy, C. H., & Williams, T. J. (2011a). *Ethical practice in operational psychology: Military and national intelligence applications*. Washington, DC: American Psychological Association.

Kennedy, C. H., & Williams, T. J. (2011b). Operational psychology ethics: Addressing evolving dilemmas. In C. H. Kennedy & T. J. Williams (Eds.), *Ethical practice in operational psychology: Military and national intelligence applications* (pp. 3–27). Washington, DC: American Psychological Association.

Kennedy, C. H., & Zillmer, E. A. (2006). *Military psychology: Clinical and operational applications*. New York: Guilford Press.

Kennedy, K., Borum, R., & Fein, R. (2011). Ethical considerations in psychological consultation to counterintelligence and counterterrorism activities. In C. H. Kennedy & T. J. Williams (Eds.), *Ethical practice in operational psychology: Military and national intelligence applications* (pp. 69–83). Washington, DC: American Psychological Association.

Kitchener, R. F., & Kitchener, K. S. (2012). Ethical foundations of psychology. In S. J. Knapp, M. C. Gottlieb, M. M. Handelsman, & L. D. VandeCreek (Eds.), *APA handbook of ethics in psychology: Vol. 1. Moral foundations and common themes* (pp. 3–42). Washington, DC: American Psychological Association.

Koocher, G. P. (2009). Ethics and the invisible psychologist. *Psychological Services*, 6, 97–107.

Laskow, G. B., & Grill, D. J. (2003). The Department of Defense experiment: The psychopharmacology demonstration project. In M. T. Sammons, R. F. Levant, & R. U. Page (Eds.), *Prescriptive authority for psychologists: A history and guide* (pp. 77–101). Washington, DC: American Psychological Association.

Loftus, E. F. (2011). Intelligence gathering post-9/11. *American Psychologist*, 66, 532–541.

Maltzman, S. (2011). An organizational self-care model: Practical suggestions for development and implementation. *The Counseling Psychologist*, 39, 303–319.

McCauley, M., Hughes, J. H., & Liebling-Kalifani, H. (2008). Ethical considerations for military clinical psychologists: A review of selected literature. *Military Psychology*, 20, 7–20.

McCutcheon, J. L. (2011). Ethical issues in policy psychology: Challenges and decision-making models to resolve ethical dilemmas. In J. Kitaeff (Ed.), *Handbook of police psychology* (pp. 89–108). New York: Routledge.

Mullins, W. C., & McMains, M. J. (2011). The role of psychologist as a member of a crisis negotiation team. In J. Kitaeff (Ed.), *Handbook of police psychology* (pp. 345–361). New York: Routledge.

Nagy, T. F. (2012). Competence. In S. J. Knapp, M. C. Gottlieb, M. M. Handelsman, & L. D. VandeCreek (Eds.) *APA Handbook of ethics in psychology: Vol. 1. Moral foundations and common themes* (pp. 147–174). Washington, DC: American Psychological Association.

Office of the Under Secretary of Defense, Personnel and Readiness. (n.d.). *Population representation in the military services: Fiscal year 2008 report.* Retrieved November 13, 2011, from *ngycp.cna.org/PopRep/2008/summary/poprep-summary2008.pdf.*

Picano, J., Williams, T. J., Roland, R., & Long, C. (2011). Operational psychologists in support of assessment and selection: Ethical considerations. In C. H. Kennedy & T. J. Williams (Eds.), *Ethical practice in operational psychology* (pp. 29–49). Washington, DC: American Psychological Association.

Ragusea, A. S. (2012). The more things change, the more they stay the same: Ethical issues in the provision of telehealth. In S. J. Knapp, M. C. Gottlieb, M. M. Handelsmann, & L. D. VandeCreek (Eds.), *APA handbook of ethics in psychology: Vol. 2. Practice, teaching, and research* (pp. 183–198). Washington, DC: American Psychological Association.

Ralph, J. A., & Sammons, M. T. (2006). Future directions of military psychology. In C. H. Kennedy & E. A. Zillmer (Eds.), *Military psychology: Clinical and operational applications* (pp. 371–386). New York: Guilford Press.

Reger, G. M., & Holloway, K. M. (2011). Virtual reality exposure therapy. In B. A. Moore & W. E. Penk (Eds.), *Treating PTSD in military personnel: A clinical handbook* (pp. 90–106). New York: Guilford Press.

Reger, M. A., Etherage, J. R., Reger, G. M., & Gahm, G. A. (2008). Civilian psychologists in an Army culture: The ethical challenge of cultural competence. *Military Psychology, 20,* 21–35.

Rizzo, A., Parsons, T. D., Lange, B., Kenny, P., Buckwalter, J. G., Rothbaum, B., et al. (2011). Virtual reality goes to war: A brief review of the future of military behavioral healthcare. *Journal of Clinical Psychology in Medical Settings, 18,* 176–187.

Schank, J. A., Helbok, C. M., Haldeman, D. C., & Gallardo, M. E. (2010). Challenges and benefits of ethical small-community practice. *Professional Psychology: Research and Practice, 41,* 502–510.

Seeley, K. M. (2008). *Therapy after terror: 9/11, psychotherapists, and mental health.* New York: Cambridge University Press.

Shumate, S., & Borum, R. (2006). Psychological support to defense counterintelligence operations. *Military Psychology, 18,* 283–296.

Soldz, S. (2008). Healers or interrogators: Psychology and the United States torture regime. *Psychoanalytic Dialogues, 18,* 592–613.

Sommers-Flanagan, R. (2012). Boundaries, multiple roles, and the professional relationship. In S. J. Knapp, M. C. Gottlieb, M. M. Handelsmann, & L. D. VandeCreek (Eds.), *APA handbook of ethics in psychology: Vol. 1, Moral foundations and common themes* (pp. 241–277). Washington, DC: American Psychological Association.

Staal, M. A., & King, R. E. (2000). Managing a multiple relationship environment: The ethics of military psychology. *Professional Psychology, Research and Practice, 31,* 698–705.

Staal, M. A., & Stephenson, J. A. (2006). Operational psychology: An emerging subdiscipline. *Military Psychology, 18,* 269–282.

Stock, M. D. (2009). *Essential to the fight: Immigrants in the military eight years after*

9/11. Immigration Policy Center. Retrieved November 13, 2011, from *immigrationpolicy.org/sites/default/files/docs/Immigrants_in_the_Military_-_Stock_110909_0.pdf*.

Stone, A. M. (2008). Dual agency for VA clinicians: Defining an evolving ethical question. *Military Psychology, 20*, 37–48.

Tobin, J. (2005). The challenges and ethical dilemmas of a military medical officer serving with a peacekeeping operation in regard to the medical care of the local population. *Journal of Medical Ethics, 31*, 571–574.

Toye, R., & Smith, M. (2011). Behavioral health issues and detained individuals. In M. K. Lenhart (Ed.), *Combat and operational behavioral health* (pp. 645–656). Fort Detrick, MD: Borden Institute.

Tuerk, P. W., Yoder, M., Ruggiero, K. J., Gros, D. R., & Acierno, R. (2010). A pilot study of prolonged exposure therapy for posttraumatic stress disorder delivered via telehealth technology. *Journal of Traumatic Stress, 23*, 116–123.

U.S. Department of the Army. (2010, January). *OTSG/MEDCOM policy memo 09-053, behavioral science consultation policy*. Washington, DC: Author.

U.S. Department of Defense. (2010, June). *Directive type memorandum 09-033 policy guidance for management of concussion/mild traumatic brain injury in the deployed setting*. Washington, DC: Author.

U.S. Department of Defense. (2011, August). *Command notification requirements to dispel stigma in providing mental health care to service members* (Department of Defense Instruction 6490.08). Washington, DC: Author.

U.S. Department of Defense. (2012, February). *Report to Congress on the review of land policies and regulations restricting the service of female members of the U.S. armed forces*. Washington, DC: Author.

Wood, D. W., Koffman, R. L., & Arita, A. A. (2003). Psychiatric medevacs during a 6–month aircraft carrier battle group deployment to the Persian Gulf: A Navy force health protection preliminary report. *Military Medicine, 168*, 43–47.

Young, J., Harvey, S., & Staal, M. A. (2011). Ethical considerations in the conduct of security clearance evaluations. In C. H. Kennedy & T. J. Williams (Eds.), *Ethical practice in operational psychology: Military and national intelligence applications* (pp. 51–68). Washington, DC: American Psychological Association.

Index

Note: Page numbers in *italics* indicate figures and tables.